The Colon Cancer "Miracle"

How 17 Ordinary People Cured Themselves of Colon Cancer Naturally

By Ewan M. Cameron

Published by
Inspired Publishing Ltd
27 Old Gloucester Street
London
WC1N 3AX

ISBN- 978-1-78555-069-0

DISCLAIMER

The writer of this material believes that a natural and holistic approach to health and maintaining a balance within the human body are of extreme importance in experiencing energy, vitality, and vibrant health throughout life.

The author recognizes that within the scientific and medical fields there are widely divergent viewpoints and opinions. This material is written for the express purpose of sharing educational information and scientific research gathered from the studies and experiences of the author, healthcare professionals, scientists, nutritionists and informed health advocates.

None of the information contained in this book is intended to diagnose, prevent, treat, or cure any disease, nor is it intended to prescribe any of the techniques, materials or concepts presented as a form of treatment for any illness or medical condition.

Before beginning any practice relating to health, diet or exercise, it is highly recommended that you first obtain the consent and advice of a licensed health care professional.

The author assumes no responsibility for the choices you make after your review of the information contained herein and your consultation with a licensed healthcare professional.

None of the statements in this book have been evaluated by the Food & Drug Administration (FDA) or the American Medical Association (AMA).

ACKNOWLEDGEMENTS

I would like to thank tireless health advocates Dr. Robert O. Young, Anthony Robbins, Richard Moat, Ty Bollinger, Mike Adams, Dr. George Georgiou, Raj Bhachu, Dr. John Bergman, and Dr. Joseph Mercola for their inspirational and life-changing message. Your work has had a profound impact on my life and the life of my loved ones.

CONTENT

PART ONE:

Everything You Know About Health Is WRONG

PART TWO:

Everything You Know About Colon Cancer is WRONG

PART THREE:

The New Biology

PART FOUR:

17 Things In Your House That May Be Killing You

PART FIVE:

How To Experience Vibrant Health, Superhuman Energy, and Live Longer

FOREWORD

The information that you are about to read will probably shock you. The time has come for people to wake up and take back control of their health. You cannot delegate this responsibility to your doctor, your government, nor your country's medical establishment. You must empower yourself in this regard, for your sake and the sake of future generations. The process of healing from Colon Cancer naturally begins by educating yourself on the true causes of disease and *how to achieve vibrant health*, and no longer ignoring the daily chemical assaults on our health.

Preventable Diseases Are Reaching EPIDEMIC Proportions

Despite "advances" in medicine the human race has never been so diseased...

- ❑ 8 million people die from Cancer every year (14 million are diagnosed).

- ❑ 100 years ago, only 1 out of every 80 Americans were diagnosed with cancer (1.2%). Today, 26 times more will be diagnosed with cancer in their lifetime.

- ❑ One of every four deaths in the US is from cancer.

- ❑ 610,000 Americans a year die of Heart Disease.

- ❑ 6 million people die every year from smoking.

- ❑ 125 million people suffer from Eczema and Psoriasis.

- ❑ Multiple Sclerosis affects 2.3 million people worldwide.

- ❑ 44 million people are living with Alzheimer's (by 2050 this could exceed 135m)

- ❑ 350 million people worldwide suffer from Depression (source: WHO).

- ❑ An estimated 382 million people worldwide suffer from Diabetes (the IDF expects that number to rise to 592 million by 2035).

- ❑ 350 million people suffer from Arthritis.

- ❑ 500 million people worldwide are obese, including 64% of the US population.

95% of Americans will die of either Heart Disease, Cancer, or Diabetes (preventable, lifestyle-related and diet-related diseases). If you are an American that leads the same lifestyle as the average person, statistically-speaking this is your most probable outcome. We have the genetic potential to live to 140 years or more, and yet the average person in developed countries keels over at age 75.

In the US – an 18 trillion-dollar economy – the cost of treating patients has reached an astronomical $3.8 trillion as of 2014 (21% of the economy), and it is the *fastest* growing sector of the economy.

Despite billions of dollars being spent on discovering drugs for Cancer, Cancer has gone from being the #8 cause of death in the US in 1970 to the #2 cause currently, behind 'heart disease'. A child under the age of three in America currently has a 1 in 2 chance of developing Cancer in its lifetime.

This situation is quite simply horrific and unsustainable. A silent genocide is taking place. Since the 70's, the US has spent more on fighting cancer than on anything else except landing a man on the moon. And yet **not a single person has been cured by conventional means**, and now Cancer is an epidemic. Despite spending more on health care, per capita, than any other country in the world, the United States is only 37th in the world in *"overall health system performance"* by the World Health Organization. Clearly something is not quite right with the Western-style health system.

The U.S. spends more on healthcare than *all other countries in the world*, and yet they are:

- ❑ 92nd in healthfulness
- ❑ 60th in Longevity
- ❑ 41st in Live Births and First Months Survivability of Babies.

While a lot of the statistics mentioned so far are US-centric, the same problems are found in Europe and other 'Western', 'developed' economies. What is really going on? And what is the solution?

Unplugging From "The Matrix"

In 2003 I was working in a boring humdrum job in Montreal, barely eking out enough to make ends meet. I was extremely unhappy with my life, and this was compounded by my lack of energy, difficulty sleeping, chronic acne, and occasional mouth ulcers. When I attended a health seminar that year, the speaker revealed an alternative approach to health, one that flew in the face of conventional medicine. His approach was actually producing *results*. He showed us dozens of case studies of his patients overcoming arthritis, Multiple Sclerosis, obesity, diabetes, fibromyalgia, even cancer! And yet, instead of being embraced and spoken about openly, the medical establishment and the mainstream media sought to silence him and suppress his discoveries.

I began to realize that the medical system and the pharmaceutical companies had very little interest or incentive in keeping people healthy. On the contrary. Billions of dollars a year were at stake on maintaining us weak, sickly, and diseased, treating us with drugs that keep us just alive enough to continue feeding their profits, but never actually curing anything. Our health industry is really a "sickness industry". That is why it is *our job* to study the topic of 'Health', so that we can make smarter, more informed choices.

I also discovered how mass media monopolies depend heavily on advertising by Big Pharma, and that the major owners of pharmaceutical companies *also own the shares of the major television and press conglomerates*. That is why you will never hear the truth about the dangers of pharmaceutical drugs from your nightly news, television channels, newspapers, or magazines. It is down to the free alternative media and courageous health crusaders like *you and I* to spread the word about what is going on. Because truth be told, we are at war.

So far, they are winning the war for your *mind*. Their propaganda war over the past 100 years has achieved their aim of brainwashing the public into trusting them, at a cost of hundreds of billions of dollars. Today, we need to "de-program" you and *"unplug you from the Matrix,"* **so that you may finally see the truth about what is going on** and why you are experiencing your current symptoms.

Ultimately, it does not matter whether you believe a word I say in this book; their propaganda (lies and disinformation) may be engrained so deeply into your subconscious mind as to make the truth irrelevant. The truth about the Medical Establishment will mean nothing to you, for you will still believe and trust your doctors, your pill-pushers, and the "authorities". But keep in mind… in the final analysis… **all that matters is RESULTS**. Are they getting results? Are they *curing people?* Or are the alternative medicine practitioners trouncing them in that regard?

After attending that seminar in 2003, I could see where I had been going wrong. I embarked on a 30-day process of detoxification. I threw out all the processed food, junk food, chemicalized meats and dairy products from my fridge and cupboards, and *cleansed my system from the inside* out. The transformation was remarkable. Within a few days I started feeling better. My energy and vitality returned. My skin cleared up. I only needed 6 hours of sleep, instead of 9 or more. I enjoyed clear thinking for the first time in years. No more rashes or ulcers. *"This is working!"* I thought to myself.

I began seeking out the best alternative medicine practitioners – the ones that were getting *results*. I spoke with their patients. I spoke to dozens of people who had cured themselves naturally through detoxifying their bodies and using natural supplements and superfoods. Their stories were astonishing, and yet very few people knew had ever heard about them. That precious information was drowned out by a sea of disinformation and corporate propaganda intent on selling drugs.

Type in any disease into a search engine, and immediately thousands of websites will greet you with the same line: *"We don't know what causes this disease. We don't know how to cure it. But here are the* **drugs** *you need to take to 'treat' this disease."* The pharmaceutical companies spend millions of dollars a year to make sure that people find *these* websites, and *never find* the alternative medicine blogs and sites that reveal an altogether different story: "We DO know what causes this, we *know* how to reverse this condition, and whatever you do, DON'T use drugs that wreak havoc with the delicate chemical balances in your body, create more harm than good, and NEVER cure anything!"

I began sharing my discoveries almost immediately. I knew that if I didn't do something to actively get the word out, people would suffer immeasurably and even die. Even if I only reached 1000 people, it would have been a worthwhile exercise. It motivated me to persevere.

Within two years, 32,000 people had bought my books and 140,000 people had downloaded my free reports. Before long, my readers started writing in, sharing their stories of personal transformation. Industry insiders leaked information to me, urging me to publish this explosive content, but it was too controversial. The public wasn't ready. This book represents the next chapter in this saga.

Take Responsibility for Your Health

The majority of people do not choose to educate themselves about Health. Instead, they choose to leave it in the hands of others. Doctors, the government, drug companies... They avoid taking responsibility for the number one force they have to carry them through life – *their own body.*

Chances are the information I will be sharing with you over the next few pages is unlike anything else you will have heard before. Immensely powerful financial interests are fighting tooth and nail to keep this information suppressed. This information is a radical departure from what the current medical establishment preaches. You will have to decide who you are going to believe; the medical establishment and drug companies, or alternative medicine practitioners? You will have to ask yourself: *"What makes sense to me? Who should I _trust_? What actually produces RESULTS?"*

And you will start asking yourself, *"Why do our healthcare and educational systems fail to educate the public on how to prevent and cure diseases with nutrition?"*

You Take This Miracle For Granted

Your health is the single most important thing you need to take care of. And yet we often neglect what we know is most important – only to regret our decisions when our lifestyle catches up with our health.

Stop and think for a second about how magnificent the workings of your body truly are. Without you even having to think about it, and despite all the demands you make of it, your body produces millions of new cells every second, allows your senses to hear, feel, see, smell, taste… regulates your temperature… operates this incredibly powerful super-computer called your brain… a beautifully created, perfectly and delicately balanced self-healing organism that puts any man-made technology to shame. **And yet most of us take this miracle completely for GRANTED!** Worst, still… we abuse it!

Honour your body. Respect it. Your body is your vessel of life. To not take care of your body is to reject life. And know this: you always end up paying the price – or reaping the rewards – for your life choices. Every moment of your life you have a *choice*. What you put in your mouth, whether to exercise or not, whether to smoke, take drugs, drink alcohol… or not. Vibrant Health or *'Pain & Disease'* you will discover, is a choice. The time has come for you to choose Health.

The 2-Billion-Year-Old Car Metaphor

Imagine that you are driving a 2-billion-year-old car. An all-natural, all-organic, living, breathing car. For 2 billion years, this car has been using fuel such as water, seeds, nuts, grasses, herbs, roots, fruits, vegetables, cereals, and *most* of these were eaten raw (not processed until all their natural goodness is totally and utterly destroyed…). *That's* the fuel this vehicle is used to.

Then, suddenly, after two billion years, that car switches over – *for the last 100 years* – to a new, modern mixture of: sugar, sweets, biscuits, crisps, 'fruit juices', chocolate, ice cream, coffee, tea, Coca-Cola, fats & oils, cigarettes, alcohol, pharmaceutical drugs, mercury-laden vaccinations, brain-deadening fluoride *water*, chemicals, pesticides, and preservatives, Genetically Modified Organisms (GMO), hormone and antibiotic-laden meats and milk (with any remaining natural 'goodness' destroyed by heat, a.k.a. 'pasteurization'), refined carbohydrates with ZERO nutritional value (white rice, white flour, white sugar, pasta, bread…), etc.

What do you think would happen to this 'vehicle'? That's right – *it would break down.* So you bring it to the mechanic, right? Now, is it in the mechanic's interest to resolve the SOURCE of the problem (your choice of fuel)? Or does he give you the 'instant fix' you need to get the car going again for a little bit? After all, you are a busy person, you've got places to go, you're experiencing pain and you are 'immobilized'. You need this problem fixed as soon as possible. So that's what the mechanic offers you: a 'fix'. Better yet: an *instant* fix. The car gets going again… but it's not going to last.

Think about this carefully. What *should* you do? What is the *intelligent* thing to do? Keep taking the car to the mechanic, or clean the fuel tank and use a cleaner fuel?

For every health challenge out there, all you ever hear from the doctor (the 'mechanic') is: *take this drug or that drug.* Simply go to Dr. FeelGood and pop a pill to make yourself feel all better again. Sure… *take* drugs to make *the symptom* go away… But what about the *source* of the problem?

Why Are The Richest, Most Industrialized Societies The Most *Diseased?*

If you kill all the mosquitoes around a stale pond with DDT chemicals, you won't have mosquitoes for a little while. But since the SOURCE of the problem is still there – the stale pond where mosquitoes can feed and lay their eggs – mosquitoes will come back!

It's the same with your body! You need to eradicate THE SOURCE of your health problems. You see, ultimately, any ailment you experience comes from a breakdown within your body. Diseases are just warning signs of something inside of you is out of kilter. Something is unbalanced. Deepak Chopra refers to this as *"The violation of simple laws of nature that make our body function."*

The richest – *read: most industrialized, modern, far-from-natural* – societies have the highest incidence of Cancer, Diabetes, Heart Disease, Arthritis, Multiple Sclerosis, Multiple Sclerosis, Chronic Fatigue, Fibromyalgia… despite the billions spent on so-called 'cures' by the pharmaceutical industry.

Why? Because we live a 'far-from-natural' lifestyle. **There are on average over 600 synthetic chemicals present in our bodies, that were created by Industry in the last 100 years…** We are filled with toxins from the food, water, air, personal care products, and medication we ingest and use.

If the delicate balance of our body's systems is 'out of whack' because of our modern, unnatural lifestyle, we experience *dis-ease.* Our diseases are nothing but a *symptom* of this imbalance. Lead a healthy lifestyle and there is very little chance you'll ever suffer from these ailments. What you will soon discover through these pages is that those ailments are all lifestyle and nutrition-related.

This book was written to inform you of an alternative for treating – and curing – ailments and diseases than that espoused by the medical establishment. Please do your due diligence in regards to this information. It is meant to be a stepping-stone towards experiencing vibrant health throughout your life. What I want is to give you a second opinion. A *choice.* An alternative. Do your research, ask questions, and educate yourself. Don't just take my word for it. You don't have to take on board anything I say, but if you practice what I suggest for just 10 days... I promise you a transformation in your health and in the quality of your life beyond anything you previously thought possible.

I *know* this information will transform your life in the way it has countless others. My hope is that you will become *free*. Free from disinformation and cultural hypnosis, and free from the fear of getting ill, getting sick and getting old. It is my sincerest wish that you, the reader, will in turn educate others about these fundamental principles for vibrant health and energy.

If you adopt a healthy lifestyle as described in this book you *will* put your body back into balance – that's what holistic medicine is all about. And yet you'll rarely hear about this in the media.

A Note On How To Read This Book

Understanding what is happening to your health starts with freeing yourself from the disinformation and propaganda of the current 'Medical Establishment'. This is why reading **Part I** of this book in full ("Everything You Know About Health Is WRONG") is extremely important, instead of just skipping ahead to the specific **'How To Eliminate Huntington's Disease' advice contained in Chapters 4 to 9**.

By freeing yourself from the lies designed to sell you more drugs, a new reality emerges, one that empowers you to take control of your health.

Part III ("The New Biology") lays the foundation of how to regain your health and overcome Huntington's Disease, with topics such as 'The Quality of Your Health Depends On The Health of Your Cells', 'Disease Starts In The Mind', 'Good Health Begins Before Birth', and 'How To Live to 100'.

Part IV ("17 Things In Your House That May Be Killing You") explains the devastating effect that certain foods and chemical products have had on our health – including the onset of Huntington's Disease symptoms.

Part II and III lay the foundation to better understand and *implement* the 'How to' advice contained in this book. Again, I recommend you read this book in its entirety and in the proper sequence, rather than skip ahead to Chapters 4 to 9.

Part V of this book ("How To Experience Vibrant Health, Superhuman Energy, and Live Longer!") contains practical, step-by-step advice that anyone can take to transform their health and energy.

I recommend you read this book in its entirety, **with an open mind**. You may disagree with some passages, but that's only normal, considering how much disinformation is out there. The important thing is that you *get* the overall point I am making.

I am sharing with you **the truth** today, as unpalatable as it may be. You may not like it, but the truth is neither good nor bad; It is just the truth.

This book was written with the intention to help you. I do not have an 'agenda' or 'an axe to grind'; I only have your best interests at heart.

With that in mind… let's dive in.   :)

PART I

Everything You Know About Health Is WRONG

CHAPTER 1

The Truth About "The Sickness Industry"

We live in a cultural hypnosis that has taught us that we are *fragile*. We have been conditioned to believe that things are happening *to* us. We have been conditioned to feel "under attack" from 'bugs' and 'viruses'. We have been conditioned to believe that drugs are the answer to disease.

I'm here to remind you of the truth… YOU ARE *NOT* FRAGILE. The truth is that our natural state is one of Strength, Health, and Energy. We are genetically programmed to be utterly HEALTHY and to THRIVE. You are the end result of tens of thousands of generations of human beings, the pinnacle of evolutionary perfection… You are a 'genetic champion'!

Most of us believe that our bodies are constantly under attack by bugs, germs, viruses… Our society as a whole has been led to believe that most sickness and disease comes from external agents 'attacking' our body. This is simply not true. The truth is that health comes from *within*, and is also lost from within. The truth has been with us for thousands of years. It has been swept under the carpet, however, in the name of profit – *it is in certain people's interest that we feel vulnerable.*

You see, fear will make us buy and consume just about anything. Keeping people afraid SELLS! It sells medicine. It sells newspapers. It increases television ratings…

Television stations, radio stations, newspapers and magazines are paid *billions* in advertising to condition us a certain way. Do NOT believe ANYTHING the media tell you. For example, every other week it seems that I hear on the news how *this* drug company or *that* drug company is just about to discover a cure for cancer. Yup, the cure for cancer is just around the corner… and yet they never do. This charade has been going on for 70 years. It is simply *manipulation* (mind-control programming).

Remember: your 'dis-ease' is a *symptom* of something very fundamental happening within you. Drugs deal with the *short-term* effect, the *surface* cause of your discomfort, the *symptom*. The real source of the problem is the way you live your life. 99% of people out there are completely asleep. Ignorant. Oblivious to what is really going on. The truth is that pharmaceutical companies will *never* discover a cure for Cancer, AIDS, or Diabetes. Billions of dollars have been spent on finding treatments for

11

symptoms of diseases. They want us to keep applying an 'ointment' on the symptoms, but never deal with the *source* of the disease.

It is not in their interest at all to discover a cure for your disease. **They are raking in billions every year from selling you consumable products** to treat symptoms. Products that you have to buy over and over again every day until the day you die. You see, it's *much* more profitable this way…

The Sickness Industry

Western Medicine is completely backward. If the medical establishment was really about health, the whole system would be designed to keep people *healthy*. Instead, it operates on the basis of 'fixing people when they are sick'. Having lots of sick people creates jobs, and pumps out profits for pharmaceutical companies, taxes for governments, and fees for doctors. This is extremely worrying.

Cancer was allowed to reach epidemic proportions for no other reason than the billions of dollars the pharmaceutical industry is earning from it. A cancer cure would instantly wipe out billions in profits.

Our lives are being sacrificed so that the food and pharmaceutical industries may make more money. This is the most incredibly genocidal deception ever inflicted upon the unsuspecting public, and it is costing hundreds of billions of dollars and millions of human lives. Increased awareness, a healthy lifestyle, prevention, and natural remedies and cures mean bad business for the drug cartel. **In fact, the healthier you get, the less money the medico-pharmaceutical establishment makes.**

It gets worse – now, the Medical Establishment is doing everything in their power to discredit 3,000-year old science, even going as far as lobbying the European Commission to pass laws banning vitamins and supplements – Google 'Codex Alimentarius' – Our health is being taken hostage!

The noted economist Paul Zane Pilzer, in his excellent book *"The Next Trillion Dollar Economy"*, exposes and blames the processed food and pharmaceutical companies for the current sad state of affairs when it comes to America's health problems:

> "When I started looking at the packaged foods companies, I could start to see what the problem was. You see, it's much easier and cheaper to sell additional products to an existing customer than it is to sell to a <u>new</u> customer. So the packaged food companies follow the rule of "OK, how do we get our existing customers to consume more?"
>
> The food industry, by the way, is worth $1 trillion (the entire US economy = $10 trillion).

Hollywood actors and actresses know not to publicize their diet habits when they endorse these products. They don't want to damage their career. They don't eat this kind of junk, but who are the sponsors of all the TV shows you see? Fast food and packaged foods companies... They have enormous influence over TV channels' editorial choices.

I then started looking at the medical business, in the knowledge that the food business was causing the problem. The medical companies made the food companies look like Mother Theresa. They spend $1.3 trillion, and they target their own market: the physician. The reason is that doctors go to Med School, they learn all these wonderful things – half of which are obsolete by the time they're out of school!

So they're dependent on the medical/pharmaceutical companies to teach them new things. And they don't teach them openly, they teach them about the things they want to sell to them. There are two major problems with medicine today: the way R&D dollars are spent, and the fact we are spending 'other people's money' when it comes to healthcare.

If you sit on the board of one of these pharmaceutical companies, you're not there to help the world. Think about it! Somebody's entrusted you with their money to make the most return, ahead of your competitors. And you decide every day on where the Board is going to spend the money for R&D of new medical services and products.

You can make a product that cures a disease! Cost: $100. Or... you can make a product that treats a symptom of the disease for $1 a day for the rest of that person's life.

Where do you spend your money? They didn't hire you to be Mother Teresa! They hired you to sit on the Board and help the company make money. So you go for a <u>consumable</u> product. Virtually all R&D money goes into products that treat symptoms of a disease, for the rest of the life of a patient.

90% of our pharmaceutical sales are from "maintenance" drugs that you take for the rest of your life, as opposed to a drug that cures the disease. That applies to any treatment. So we've seen the entire medical business shift to treating symptoms versus curing diseases.

Our Health Insurance system is breaking down. Today people work 4-5 years in each company. Your company is interested in keeping you healthy and productive, but not over the long-term. People are spending other people's money on treatment and healthcare (government, insurance companies), which is why we spend $1.3 trillion on these. It's the fastest-growing segment of the US economy. At present rates of increase by 2050 it will surpass US GDP. Something is going to have to break in such a system.

Worst part of all: when it comes to going to your physician for weight loss, nutrition, stopping smoking, anything to do with "Wellness", it's not covered. They only cover "treating the disease". The entire medical business is what I call, **"The Sickness Business".**

No one voluntarily becomes a customer, no one wants to stay a customer. And yet we spend 1/7 of our economy on it and it is our fastest-growing sector. It's like a conspiracy. It's not like the medical companies and the food companies get together in a meeting. But the effect is 10 times worse, because this conspiracy is governed by the laws of economics. Each of us seeking our individual gains has caused a terrible collision here."

How The Present-Day Legal Drug Cartel Was Born

This eye-opening report by Hans Ruesch exposes the origins of the modern-day pharmaceutical industry set up by John D. Rockefeller from the profits of his monopolistic Standard Oil corporation. In 1901 he set up the Rockefeller Institute for Medical Research, and funded medical schools across the U.S. on the express proviso that they trained 'doctors' to sell his product – pharmaceutical drugs – to the public. His fortune at the time of his death would be equivalent to $253 billion in 2013 dollars, and it is interesting to note that the shares of most pharmaceutical companies around the world today are owned by financial interests linked to the Rockefeller family.

"In the 30's, Morris A. Bealle, a former city editor of the old Washington Times and Herald, was running a county seat newspaper, in which the local power company bought a large advertisement every week. This account took quite a lot of worry off Bealle's shoulders when the bills came due.

But according to Bealle's own story, one day the paper took up the cudgels for some of its readers that were being given poor service from the power company, and Morris Bealle received the dressing down of his life from the advertising agency which handled the power company's account. They told him that any more such 'stepping out of line' would result in the immediate cancellation not only of the advertising contract, but also of the gas company and the telephone company.

That's when Bealle's eyes were opened to the meaning of a 'free press', and he decided to get out of the newspaper business. Bealle used his professional experience to do some digging into the freedom-of-the-press situation and came up with two shattering exposés – *The Drug Story*, and *The House of Rockefeller*. In spite of his familiarity with the editorial world and many important personal contacts, he couldn't get his revelations into print until he founded his own company, The Columbia Publishing House, in 1949. This was just a prime example of the silent but adamant censorship in force in 'The Land of the Free'. Although *The Drug Story* is one of the most important books on health and politics ever to appear in the USA, it has never been admitted to a major bookstore nor reviewed by any establishment paper, and was sold exclusively by mail. Nevertheless, when we first got to read it, in the 1970s, it was already in its 33rd printing.

As Bealle pointed out, a business which makes 6% on its invested capital is considered a sound money maker. Sterling Drug, Inc., the main cog and largest holding company in the Rockefeller Drug Empire and its 68 subsidiaries, showed operating profits in 1961 of $23,463,719 after taxes, on net assets of $43,108,106 – a 54% profit. Squibb, another Rockefeller company, made 576% on the actual value of its property, in 1945.

That was during the luscious war years when the Army Surgeon General's Office and the Navy Bureau of Medicine and Surgery were not only acting as promoters for the Drug Trust, but were actually **forcing drug trust poisons into the blood streams of American soldiers**, sailors and marines, to the tune of over 200 million 'shots'.

'Is it any wonder,' asked Bealle, 'that the Rockefellers, and their stooges in the Food and Drug Administration, the U.S. Public Health Service, the Federal Trade Commission, the Better Business Bureau, the Army Medical Corps, the Navy Bureau of Medicine, and thousands of health officers all over the country, should combine to put out of business all forms of therapy that discourage the use of drugs?'

'The last annual report of the Rockefeller Foundation', reported Bealle, 'itemizes the gifts it has made to colleges and public agencies in the past 44 years, and they total somewhat over half a billion dollars. These colleges, of course, teach their students all the drug lore the Rockefeller pharmaceutical houses want taught. Otherwise there would be no more gifts, just as there are no gifts to any of the 30 odd colleges in the United States that don't use therapies based on drugs.

'Harvard, with its well-publicized medical school, has received $8,764,433 of Rockefeller's Drug Trust money, Yale got $7,927,800, Johns Hopkins $10,418,531, Washington University in St. Louis

$2,842,132, New York's Columbia University $5,424,371, Cornell University $1,709,072, etc., etc.'

While 'giving away' those huge sums to drug propagandizing colleges, the Rockefeller interests were growing to a world-wide web that no one could entirely explore. Already well over 30 years ago it was large enough for Bealle to demonstrate that the Rockefeller interests had created, built up and developed the most far-reaching industrial empire ever conceived in the mind of man. Standard Oil was of course the foundation upon which all of the other Rockefeller industries have been built. The story of Old John D., as ruthless an industrial pirate as ever came down the pike, is well known, but is being today conveniently ignored. The keystone of this mammoth industrial empire was the Chase National Bank.

Not the least of its holdings are in the drug business. The Rockefellers own the largest drug manufacturing combine in the world, and use all of their other interests to bring pressure to increase the sale of drugs. The fact that **most of the 12,000 separate drug items on the market are harmful** is of no concern to the Drug Trust...

The House of Rockefeller has had its own 'nominees' planted in all Federal agencies that have to do with health. So the stage was set for the 'education' of the American public, with a view to turning it into a population of drug and medico dependents, with the early help of the parents and the schools, then with direct advertising and, last but not least, the influence the advertising revenues had on the media makers.

A compilation of the magazine *Advertising Age* showed that as far back as 1948 the larger companies in America spent for advertising the sum total of $1,104,224,374.

Of this staggering sum the interlocking Rockefeller-Morgan interests controlled about 80 percent, and **utilized it to manipulate public information** on health and drug matters – then and even more recklessly now.

'Even the most independent newspapers are dependent on their press associations for their national news,' Bealle pointed out, *'and there is no reason for a news editor to suspect that a story coming over the wires of the Associated Press or the International News Service is censored when it concerns health matters. Yet this is what happens.'*

In fact, in the 1950s the Drug Trust had one of its directors on the directorate of the Associated Press. He was no less than Arthur Hays

Sulzberger, publisher of the New York Times and as such one of the most powerful Associated Press directors.

It was thus easy for the Rockefeller Trust to persuade the Associated Press Science Editor to adopt a policy which would not permit any medical news to clear that is not approved by the Drug Trust 'expert', and this censor is not going to approve any item that can in any way hurt the sale of drugs.

This accounts to this day for the many fake stories of medical cures and just-around-the-corner breakthrough victories over cancer, AIDS, diabetes, Multiple Sclerosis, which go out brazenly over the wires to all daily newspapers in America and abroad.

Emanuel M. Josephson, M.D., whom the Drug Trust has been unable to intimidate despite many attempts, pointed out that the National Association of Science Writers was 'persuaded' to adopt as part of its code of ethics the following chestnut: 'Science editors are incapable of judging the facts of phenomena involved in medical and scientific discovery. Therefore, they only report 'discoveries' approved by medical authorities, or those presented before a body of scientific peers.'

Thus newspapers continue to be fed with propaganda about drugs and their alleged value, although according to the Food and Drug Administration (FDA) **1.5 million people landed in hospitals in 1978 because of medication side effects** in the U.S. alone, and despite recurrent statements by courageous medical men that most pharmaceutical items are useless at best, but more often harmful or deadly in the long run.

The truth about cures without drugs is suppressed, unless it suits the purpose of the censor to garble it. Whether these cures are effected by Chiropractors, Naturopaths, Naprapaths, Osteopaths, Faith Healers, Spiritualists, Herbalists, or MDs who use the brains they have, you never read about it in the big newspapers.

To teach the Rockefeller drug ideology, it is necessary to teach that Nature didn't know what she was doing when she made the human body. But statistics issued by the Children's Bureau of the Federal Security Agency show that since the all-out drive of the Drug Trust for drugging and vaccinating the human system, the health of the American nation has sharply declined, especially among children. Children are now given 'shots' for this and 'shots' for that, when the only safeguard known to science is a pure bloodstream, which can be obtained only with clean air and wholesome food. Meaning by natural and inexpensive means – just what the Drug Trust most objects to.

When the FDA, whose officials have to be acceptable to Rockefeller Center before they are appointed, has to put an independent operator out of business, it goes all out to execute those orders. But the orders do not come directly from Standard Oil or a drug house director. The American Medical Association (AMA) is *the front* for the Drug Trust, and furnishes the quack doctors to testify that even when they know nothing of the product involved, it is their considered opinion that it has no therapeutic value.

Wrote Bealle: 'Financed by the taxpayers, these Drug Trust persecutions leave no stone unturned to destroy the victim. If he is a small operator, the resulting attorney's fees and court costs put him out of business. In one case, a Dr. Adolphus Hohensee, who had stated that vitamins were vital to good health, was taken to court for misbranding his product. The American Medical Association furnished ten medicos who reversed all known medical theories by testifying that 'vitamins are not necessary to the human body'. Confronted with government bulletins to the contrary, the medicos wiggled out of that one by declaring that these standard publications were outdated!'

In addition to the FDA, Bealle listed the following agencies having to do with 'health' – i.e., with the health of the Drug Trust to the detriment of the citizens – as being dependent on Rockefeller: U.S. Public Health Service, U.S. Veterans Administration, Federal Trade Commission, Surgeon General of the Air Force, Army Surgeon General's Office, Navy Bureau of Medicine & Surgery, National Health Research Institute, National Research Council, National Academy of Sciences.

The National Academy of Sciences in Washington is considered the all-wise body which investigates everything under the sun, especially in the field of health, and gives to a palpitating public the last word in that science. To the important post at the head of this agency, the Drug Trust had one of their own appointed. He was none other than Alfred N. Richards, one of the directors and largest stockholders of Merck & Company, which was making huge profits from its drug traffic. When Bealle revealed this fact, Richards resigned forthwith, and the Rockefellers appointed in his place the President of their own Rockefeller Institution, Detlev Bronk.

The medico drug cartel was summed up by J.W Hodge, M.D., of Niagara Falls, N.Y., in these words: 'The medical monopoly or medical trust, euphemistically called the American Medical Association, is not merely the meanest monopoly ever organized, but the most arrogant, dangerous and despotic organization which ever managed a free people in this or any other age. Any and all methods of healing the sick by means of safe, simple and natural remedies are sure to be assailed and denounced by the arrogant leaders of the AMA doctors' trust as fakes, frauds and humbugs. Every practitioner of the healing art who does not ally himself with the medical trust is denounced as a 'dangerous quack' and impostor by the predatory trust doctors. Every sanatorium who attempts to restore the sick to a state of health by natural means without resort to the knife or poisonous drugs, disease imparting serums, deadly toxins or vaccines, is at once pounced upon by these medical tyrants and fanatics, bitterly denounced, vilified and persecuted to the fullest extent.'

The Lincoln Chiropractic College in Indianapolis requires 4,496 hours in order to graduate, the Palmer Institute Chiropractic in Davenport a minimum of 4,000 60-minute classroom hours; the University of Natural Healing Arts in Denver five years of 1,000 hours each to qualify for a degree. The National College of Naprapathy in Chicago requires 4,326 classroom hours for graduation. Yet the medico drug cartel spreads the propaganda that the practitioners of these three 'heretic' sciences are poorly trained or not trained at all – **the real reason being that they cure their patients without the use of drugs**.

Rockefeller's various 'educational' activities had proved so profitable in the U S. that in 1927 the International Educational Board was launched, as Junior's own, personal charity. It was endowed with $21,000,000 for a starter, to be lavished on foreign universities and politicos, with all the usual strings attached. This Board undertook to export the 'new' Rockefeller image as a benefactor of mankind, as well as his business practices. Nobody informed the beneficiaries that every penny the Rockefellers were *throwing out the window* would come back, bearing substantial interest.

Medical colleges in China were instructed that if they wished to benefit from the Rockefeller largesse they had better convince 500 million Chinese to throw into the ashcan the safe and useful but inexpensive herbal remedies of their doctors (which had withstood the test of centuries), in favour of the expensive carcinogenic 'miracle' drugs Made in USA. All of which had to be replaced constantly with new ones, when the fatal side effects could no longer be concealed; and if they couldn't 'demonstrate' through large-scale animal experiments the effectiveness of *acupuncture*, this could not be recognized as having any 'scientific value'. Its millenarian effectiveness proven on human beings was of no concern to the Western wizards.

'No candid study of his career can lead to other conclusion than that he is victim of perhaps the ugliest of all passions, that for money, money as an end. It is not a pleasant picture.... this money maniac secretly, patiently, eternally plotting how he may add to his wealth.... He has turned commerce to war, and honeycombed it with cruel and corrupt practices.... And he calls his great organization a benefaction, and points to his church-going and charities as proof of his righteousness. This is supreme wrong-doing cloaked by religion. There is but one name for it – hypocrisy.'

This was the description Ida Tarbell made of John D. Rockefeller in her *'History of the Standard Oil Company'*, serialized in 1905. And that was several years before the Ludlow Massacre, so JDR was as yet far from having reached the apex of his disrepute. But after World War II it would have been hard to read, in America or abroad, a single criticism of JDR, nor of Junior, who had followed in his father's footsteps; nor of Junior's four sons who all endeavoured to emulate their illustrious forbears. Today's various encyclopaedias extant in public libraries of the Western world have nothing but praise for the Family. How was this achieved? Rockefeller Foundation had $100 million lying around for promotional purposes without knowing what to do with it. [They] donated large sums – none less than a million – to well-known colleges, hospitals, churches and benevolent organizations.

In the following years, not only newsmen, but whole newspapers were bought, financed or founded with Rockefeller money. So Time Magazine, which Henry Luce started in 1923, had been taken over by J.P. Morgan when the magazine got into financial difficulties. When Morgan died and his financial empire crumbled, the House of Rockefeller wasted no time in taking over this lush editorial plum also, together with its sisters Fortune and Life, and built for them an expensive 14-story home of their own in Rockefeller Center – the Time & Life Building. JDR must have been himself surprised to discover how easily the so-called intellectuals could be bought. By founding and lavishly endowing his Education Boards at home and abroad, Rockefeller won control not only of the governments and politicos but also of the intellectual and scientific community, starting with the Medical Power – the organization that forms those priests of the New Religion that are the modern medicine men. No Pulitzer or

Nobel or any similar prize endowed with money and prestige has ever been awarded to a declared foe of the Rockefeller system."

Source: Hans Ruesch, *The Truth About the Rockefeller Drug Empire*

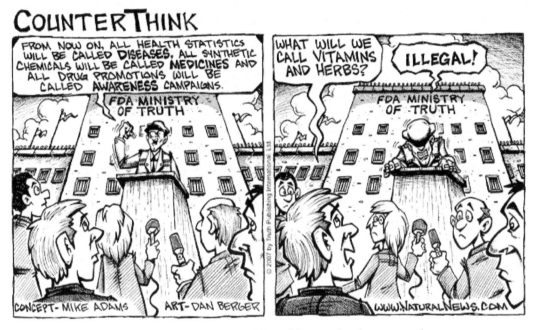

Thanks to Mike Adams and *www.NaturalNews.com* for the cartoon above.

The Inception Of The "Medical Mafia"

Ty Bollinger, in his excellent book *"Cancer: Step Outside The Box"*, adds the following to the Rockefeller story:

> "John D. Rockefeller's goal was to dominate the oil, chemical, and pharmaceutical markets, so his company (Standard Oil) purchased in 1910 a controlling interest in a huge German drug/chemical company called I.G. Farben. I.G. Farben later became the single largest donor to the election campaign of Adolph Hitler. […] The I.G. Farben cartel used the victims of the concentration camps as human guinea pigs. Tens of thousands of them died during human experiments such as the testing of new and vaccinations.
>
> In order to build his drug cartel, Rockefeller needed to 're-educate' the medical profession to prescribe more pharmaceutical drugs, so he hired Abraham Flexner to travel the country and assess the success of American medical schools. In reality, the results of his study were

predetermined. The gist of the report was that it was far too easy to start a medical school and that most medical schools were not teaching 'sound medicine'. In other words, they weren't pushing enough drugs.

Carnegie and Rockefeller commenced a major 'upgrade' in medical education by financing only those medical schools that taught what they wanted to be taught. In other words, they began to immediately shower hundreds of millions of dollars on those medical schools that were teaching "drug intensive" medicine. In return for the financing, the schools were required to continue teaching course material that was exclusively drug oriented, with no emphasis put on natural medicine. All accredited medical schools became heavily oriented toward drugs and drug research.

In 1913, the AMA went on the offensive even more strongly by their establishment of **the "Propaganda Department," which was dedicated to attacking any and all unconventional medical treatments** and anyone (M.D. or not) who practiced them. Medical schools that offered courses in natural therapies and homeopathy were told to either drop these courses from their curriculum or lose their accreditation.

Dr. Samuel Epstein chronicles in *The Politics of Cancer Revisited*, how, for monetary reasons, the Cancer Industry is suppressing mountains of information about environmental causes of cancer rather than making this information available to the public. Keeping the public ignorant about the causes of cancer results in more cancer patients, more sales of chemotherapy drugs, more radiation, and more surgery."

And finally, Dr. Henry Jones adds: "The medical monopoly also managed to outlaw or marginalize over 70 healthcare professions. 'Protection of the healthcare consumer' was, as always, the rationale for this power grab. Whether the object of destruction by the medical monopoly be homeopaths, midwives, or chiropractors, the purge is conducted in the same manner. No scientific proof or research data is offered to discredit these practitioners. The entire approach is one of character assassination…"

Pharmaceutical Companies Spend 19 Times More on Marketing than on Research

The medical profession has unfortunately been taken over by massive financial interests. It is patently obvious that pharmaceutical companies do not care one iota about people's health.

Prescription drugs are a massive market. In 2013 Americans spent $329 billion on prescription drugs. Drug companies spent more than $3 billion in 2012 marketing to consumers in the U.S. ($3.83 billion in 2013, and $4.53 billion in 2014). No television network or newspaper dare cross the Drug Cartel and risk them pulling out their advertising dollars.

While $4.53 billion is spent on advertising to consumers, an estimated $24 billion is spent by Big Pharma *marketing directly to health care professionals*. This means influencing the doctors who *prescribe* the drugs. Doctors are brainwashed at Corporate Drug School (Medical School), then influenced and bribed throughout their careers, through sales reps and Medical Conventions.

By some estimates, pharmaceutical companies spent 19 times more on self-promotion than basic research in 2013, with the biggest spender, Johnson & Johnson, spending $17.5 billion on sales and marketing and only $8.2 billion for R&D. Their focus is *profit*, rather than helping people get healthy.

Dr. John Virapen Reveals Astounding Levels of Corruption in The Pharmaceutical Industry

Dr. John Virapen worked for more than 35 years for the pharmaceutical industry, including in senior management positions at companies such as Eli-Lilly. Turned whistleblower, he revealed how pharmaceutical companies have a 'bribery' budget of €35,000 per physician per year, to get the physicians to prescribe their products. He went on to say that more than 75 percent of leading scientists in the field of medicine are paid for by the pharmaceutical industry, and in some cases outright corruption and bribery is used for the approval of drugs by government agencies.

The truth about the adverse side effects of Eli Lilly's pharmaceuticals – such as the role of Prozac in inducing suicide and homicide – were withheld and kept secret for decades. Evidence that Prozac induced violence and suicidality existed from the outset, when the drug was first tested in pre-marketing trials. The first week they commenced the clinical trial for Prozac in Sweden, two of the patients tried to commit suicide, but they swept this under the rug, and Virapen admitted he successfully bribed the Swedish government to approve Prozac for sale in Sweden!

John Virapen also revealed how new illnesses are *made up* by the pharmaceutical industry and specifically marketed to enhance sales and market shares for the companies in question. More worryingly still, pharmaceutical companies increasingly target *children*, the consumers of tomorrow.

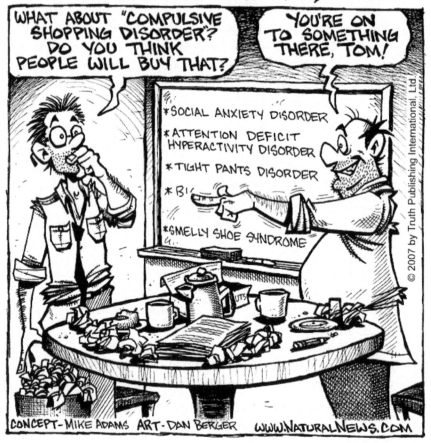

Thanks to Mike Adams and *www.NaturalNews.com* for the cartoon above.

During a speech in Germany, Virapen stated: "Pharmaceutical companies are not interested in curing any diseases. **They are more interested in creating new diseases**, that are symptomatic, like Diabetes, cardiomyopathy, rheumatoid arthritis... When have you ever heard of a pharmaceutical company coming up something that actually cured a disease? They don't cure anything. On the contrary, **their aim is to make you sick. Pharmaceutical companies kill more people than all the wars combined**, but they do it over the long-term. Eli Lilly sold a drug for schizophrenia to old people's homes, so that the patients would be easier to control, but a lot of people died of heart failure, kidney problems, and even got Diabetes... and who is the biggest diabetes drug company? Eli Lilly. [...] Doctors don't really know much. These days they don't really care about the patient... they're just thinking about how much they're going to get paid."

According to research by Dr. Joseph Mercola:

❑ 100,000 Americans die each year from *correctly* prescribed pharmaceutical medications.

❑ The medical profession and their pseudo-scientific dogma kill 250,000 Americans a year.

❑ Doctors and drug companies are the 3rd leading cause of death in the U.S.

❑ Over 50% of Americans ingest at least one pharmaceutical drug each day.

In *Cancer: Step Outside The Box*, Ty Bollinger reports:

❑ In August of 2012, Eli Lilly admitted to more than **$200 million worth of doctor payoffs**.

❑ In the first quarter of 2012, Eli Lilly agreed to pay $1.4 billion to settle criminal and civil allegations of promoting drugs for unapproved uses.

❑ Since Eli Lilly knew that **Zyprexa causes diabetes** and didn't let patients know this, they have already settled numerous 'failure to warn' lawsuits totalling 1.2 billion dollars.

❑ In 2012, Eli Lilly agreed to another $1.42 billion: $615 million to settle the Justice Department's criminal investigation and approximately $800 million to settle the civil investigations brought by the states for Medicaid fraud.

❑ In June of 2012, **an Italian Court ruled that Merck's MMR vaccine caused autism** in a now 10-year old boy. The court awarded the family a 15-year annuity totalling 174,000 Euros

❑ In July of 2012, two virologists filed a federal lawsuit against Merck (their former employer) alleging that **Merck had falsified test data** to fabricate a vaccine efficacy rate of 95%, spiked the blood test with animal antibodies in order to artificially inflate the appearance of immune system antibodies, pressured the two virologists to *"participate in the fraud and subsequent cover-up,"* used the falsified trial results to swindle the U.S. government out of *"hundreds of millions of dollars for a vaccine that does not provide adequate immunization,"* and intimidated the scientists, threatening them with jail unless they stayed silent.

❑ In July of 2012, in what is now the largest criminal fraud settlement ever to come out of the pharmaceutical industry, GlaxoSmithKline plead guilty to bribery, fraud, and other crimes and agreed to pay $1 billion in criminal fines and $2 billion in civil fines following a nine-year investigation into its activities. According to U.S. federal investigators, GlaxoSmithKline routinely bribed doctors with luxury vacations and paid speaking gigs, "fabricated" drug safety data, and lied to the FDA.

❑ **GSK has a "bribery network" of 49,000 doctors** who received financial kickbacks to prescribe more Glaxo pharmaceuticals to patients!

❑ In 2012, Pfizer agreed to pay $2.3 billion to settle criminal liability due to its illegal off-label promotion of Geodon, Zyvox, and Bextra (a painkiller already pulled from the market).

How the Medical Mafia Suppresses the Truth

Ty Bollinger adds the following, regarding disinformation and propaganda techniques used by the pharmaceutical companies to hide and *distort* the truth:

❑ The testimonies of people who heal themselves naturally are explained away as "unreliable" or "anecdotal". The alternative cancer treatments are ignored and suppressed.

❑ The patients are said to have undergone "spontaneous remission" unrelated to the alternative cancer treatment.

❑ The patients are said to have been cured from the "delayed effects of conventional cancer therapy" which was administered before the *alternative* cancer treatment

❑ The physicians who administer the alternative cancer treatment are persecuted.

Those few doctors that dare to question the status quo are frequently ostracized and blackballed. The FDA has a track record of raiding the offices of successful alternative practitioners and destroying their medical records. For instance, Dr. Stanislaw Burzynski of Houston, Texas **uses non-toxic 'antineoplastons' to successfully treat brain cancer, non-Hodgkin's lymphoma**, and many common cancers. The FDA's lawyers have spent tens of millions of dollars and 20 years trying to put Dr. Burzynski in jail, despite not having done anything wrong or illegal whatsoever and his patients begging the courts to let him continue with his treatments (I recommend you watch on YouTube the documentary *Burzynski: Cancer Is Serious Business*). The FDA won't tolerate any treatment that goes against Big Pharma's chemotherapy profits, especially one that is *actually getting results for patients.*

In 1953, the Fitzgerald Report, which was commissioned by a United States Senate committee, concluded that organized medicine had "conspired to suppress" the Hoxsey herbal cancer therapy that helped thousands of patients eliminate their cancer.

Royal Raymond Rife was able to show "pleomorphism" of cells (cells can change form and mutate if their environment becomes toxic), using his microscopes, and in one study, **he took 16 'terminal' cancer patients and achieved a 100% cure rate**. He did this by bombarding micro-organisms in the body with radio and audio frequencies, killing the microforms like bacteria, fungi, parasites, etc. that thrive in an acidic environment, and whose waste products contribute to making your bloodstream more toxic. Rife's lab was vandalized, his lab was burned down, and some of his supporters died under suspicious circumstances.

In 1944, Dr. Milbank Johnson arranged a press conference to announce a cure for cancer using Rife's machine. Mysteriously, the night before the press conference, Dr. Johnson suddenly died and all his notes were pronounced 'lost' by executors of his estate. The police illegally confiscated the remainder of his fifty years of research.

Dr. Jonathan Wright promoted natural treatments. One of his favourite treatments was using L-Tryptophan to treat depression but the FDA had outlawed this amino acid, just a few months before the FDA put a big push on Prozac as a treatment for depression.

How the Medical Establishment Distorts Cancer Data

- ❏ The Cancer Industry has defined the term "cure" to apply to a cancer patient who survives 5 years from the date of diagnosis. It does not mean 'healed' nor does it mean 'free of cancer'.

- ❏ Patients are living 'longer' from the point of diagnosis, since diagnosis happens earlier, not because of improvements in the cure rate.

- ❏ If a patient develops the same cancer again after the period is up, or if they drop dead two days after the period is up, they are still deemed to be "cured".

- ❏ The Cancer Industry typically omits certain groups of people from their statistics and includes certain groups based upon what will make their statistics look more favourable. For example, lung cancer patients are typically excluded from their statistics, despite the fact that lung cancer is the leading cause of cancer death.

- ❏ The Cancer Industry typically will remove a patient who dies during a conventional treatment protocol from the population of the sample.

- ❏ The Cancer Industry routinely ignores counting people who die from the effects of the treatments. For example, if you're on chemotherapy, and as a result of your newly compromised immune system, you catch pneumonia and die, your death will likely **not** be counted as a death from cancer.

❑ The Cancer Industry tells us that if a chemotherapy drug shrinks the size of a tumour, then it must be considered effective. Does it mean that the patient will live longer? No. It has been well documented that shrinkage of tumours has little to do with a longer survival rate (more on this later).

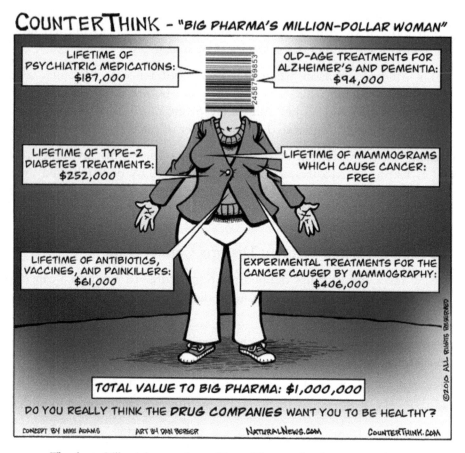

Thanks to Mike Adams and *www.NaturalNews.com* for the cartoon above.

Drug Company Lies and Disinformation Techniques Exposed

Sharyl Attkisson is an investigative journalist who was a correspondent for CBS News for twenty years. In a recent TED talk she explained how drug companies use propaganda agents to manipulate our views and opinions:

"Say you're watching the news and you see a story about a new study about a Cholesterol-lowering drug called Cholextra. The study says that Cholextra is so effective, that doctors should consider prescribing it to adults, and even children who don't yet have high cholesterol. You decide to do some of your own research. You do a Google search, you consult social media, you look at

Wikipedia, you look at WebMD, a 'non-profit' website, and you read the original study in a peer-review published medical journal. It all confirms how effective Cholextra is. You do run across a few negative comments about a potential link to cancer but you dismiss that because medical experts call the cancer link 'a myth' and say that those that do think there is a link there are 'quacks', and 'cranks', and 'nuts'. Finally, you learn that your own doctor attended a medical seminar. The lecture he attended confirmed how effective Cholextra is.

But what if all isn't as it seems? What if the reality you find was false? A carefully constructed narrative, by special interests, designed to manipulate your opinion?

Incredibly powerful propaganda and publicity forces mean we sometimes get little of the truth. Special interests have unlimited time and money to figure out new ways to spin us. There's an entire industry built around it in Washington. [...] Political, corporate or other special interests disguise themselves and publish blogs, start Facebook accounts, publish ads, letters to the editor or simply post comments online to try to fool you into thinking that an independent movement is speaking. The whole point is to try to [change] your opinion by making you feel as if you're an outlier, when you're not.

They seek to controversialize those who disagree with them. They attack news organizations that publish stories that they don't like, whistleblowers who tell the truth, politicians who dare to ask the tough questions, and journalists who have the audacity to report on all of it. Sometimes they shove intentionally so much confusing and conflicting information into the mix that you're left to throw up your hands and disregard all of it, including the truth.

And then there's Wikipedia. Built as the 'Free Encyclopaedia' that anyone can edit, the reality cannot be any different. Anonymous editors control and co-opt pages on behalf of special interests. They bid and reverse edits that go against their agenda. Wikipedia were caught offering a PR service to skew and edit information, on behalf of publicity-seeking clients.

It turns out the Facebook and Twitter accounts you found were actually written by paid professionals hired by the drug company to promote the drug. The Wikipedia page had been monitored by an agenda monitor, also paid by the drug company. The drug company also arranged to optimize Google Search Engine results. The non-profit was of course secretly founded and funded by the drug company. The drug company also funded that positive study, and it used its editorial control to omit any mention of cancer as a possible side-effect.

What's more, each and every doctor who publicly touted Cholextra, or who called the cancer link 'a myth', or ridiculed the critics as 'paranoids', 'cranks', and 'quacks', or served on the government advisory board who approved the drug, each of those doctors is actually a paid consultant for the drug company. As for your own doctor, the medical lecture he attended was in fact sponsored by the drug company. And the news report didn't mention any of that.

They use inflammatory language such as – crank, quack, nutty, lies, paranoid, pseudo, and conspiracy. They claim to "debunk myths" that aren't myths at all. Beware when interests attack an issue by controversializing or attacking the people, personalities, and organizations surrounding it rather than addressing the facts. And most of all, they tend to reserve all of their public scepticism for those exposing wrongdoing rather than the wrongdoers. In other words, <u>instead of questioning authority, they question those who question authority</u>."

Pharmaceutical Drugs Are Extremely Dangerous To Your Health

Your body is a delicately balanced organism. Injecting chemicals into it might have a short-term effect *somewhere* in your body, but it might create chemical imbalances in 4 or 5 *other* areas of your body. Pharmaceuticals are exceedingly dangerous, and are proven to be less and less effective. In fact, in some cases placebos are *more* effective than pharmaceuticals, and they don't cause side-effects. Drugs *never* cure any disease. They merely mask the symptoms of an illness. And what happens over time, since you are not addressing the root cause of your illness? It gets worse, so doctors prescribe you *yet more drugs!*

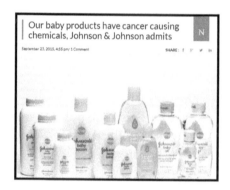

Our baby products have cancer causing chemicals, Johnson & Johnson admits

September 23, 2015, 4:55 pm/ 1 Comment   SHARE:

I came across the following story, just this week, in *The New York Times*: *"Johnson & Johnson Admit: Our Baby Products Contain Cancer-Causing Formaldehyde"*. Time Magazine actually wrote, *'This is just the tip of the toxic iceberg'*…

It is as if pharmaceutical companies like Johnson & Johnson *want* us to be poisoned and induced with cancer. As Virapen warned us, they are now targeting *children,* their 'consumers of tomorrow'.

Big Pharma Spends Millions on Political Contributions

How do these companies get away with it, you may ask? Pharmaceutical and healthcare companies spent $51 million on the 2012 federal elections and nearly $32 million on the 2014 elections, according to the Center for Responsive Politics (CRP) – and that's just the 'official' figures.

For every $1 the industry spent on contributions during the last election cycle, $7 were spent on *lobbying* senators, congressmen, and the government in 2014. And one can only wonder at how many tens of millions were spent on outright *bribes and corruption.*

"The pharmaceutical industry's lobbying expenditures steadily increased from 1998 to 2009, when spending hit a $273 million peak as Congress debated the Affordable Care Act, according to CRP. In 2014, drug companies and their lobbying groups spent $229 million influencing lawmakers, legislation and politicians.

The Pharmaceutical Research and Manufacturers of America (PhRMA), the industry's lead lobbying group, has spent nearly $150 million on lobbying since 2008, and ranks sixth among the nation's top lobbying spenders, outspending powerful interests like defense contractors and the oil and gas industry. Pfizer ranks among the top 25 lobbying spenders in the nation, with $94 million spent since 2008 and $8.5 million spent in 2014 alone."

Mike Ludwig, www.truth-out.org

But they also get away with it… because they have spent billions of dollars over the past six or seven decades to make sure *they own your mind.* You need to understand the power of "propaganda".

"To Control The Masses You Must Control Their Minds!"

As exposed in Adam Curtis's excellent documentary *The Century of Self*, at the turn of the twentieth century Austrian psychoanalyst Sigmund Freud claimed to have discovered that human beings had "primitive, sexual, and aggressive forces hidden deep inside their subconscious minds, which if not controlled could lead societies to chaos and destruction". The oligarchy and ruling class of that time saw this as proof that human beings could not be trusted to make rational decisions, and that mass democracy was not possible. Humans needed the iron hand of the elite to rule them, they rationalized.

In the 1920s Freud's nephew Edward Bernays brought his uncle's ideas to America, and put them to use for the benefit of US corporations. He had been impressed at how successfully propaganda had been used to entice American men to enlist and fight in Europe in the First World War. While the British abandoned propaganda in peace time, the Americans continued and expanded its use with the help of Bernays, who argued that American public opinion must be engineered from above to 'control the rabble'. He considered the average person to be *stupid, incapable of rational thinking.*

He couldn't use the term 'propaganda', as it had a negative connotation. Since the war, people had realised that propaganda had been used to deceive the public into acquiescing to the government's agenda. It was basically misleading, dishonest and exploitative. So Bernays called it 'Public Relations', creating a new industry in the process.

The political writer Walter Lippmann argued that "if human beings were driven by unconscious, irrational forces, then it was necessary to re-think democracy." The government needed to manage 'the bewildered herd' through psychological techniques that would control the unconscious feelings of the masses. Bernays put forward the following theory: "by stimulating people's inner desires and then sating them with consumer products you can manage the irrational force of the masses." They would sublimate their inner, primitive, sexual and aggressive forces through the consumption of goods. He called it *"The engineering of consent"*. Its aims would be achieved through clever, subtle, and pervasive propaganda aimed at controlling the minds of the unknowing public.

One of Bernays' first successes was in reengineering how women felt about smoking. George Washington Hill, president of the American Tobacco Company, hired Edward Bernays in 1928 to lead a campaign to entice more women to smoke in public. At that time there was a taboo against women smoking, because, in the minds of people, it was associated with prostitution. Psychoanalyst Abraham Brille told Bernays: "Cigarettes are a symbol of the penis and of male sexual power. If you can find a way to connect cigarettes with the idea of challenging male power, then women will smoke because then they would have their own penises."

Bernays decided to stage an event at the 1928 New York Easter day parade. He persuaded a group of rich, fashionable upper-class young women to hide cigarettes under their clothes, and light them up dramatically on his prompt. He had informed the press that suffragettes were protesting for the right to vote, by lighting up 'torches of freedom'... The pictures were all over the press across America the next day. Bernays managed to make women associate smoking with the idea that it made them more powerful and independent, a ridiculous idea that persists to this day.

Bernays also persuaded female film stars to smoke ostentatiously on screen, thus endorsing cigarettes as respectable and desirable. Thanks to his psychological mass mind control methods, he had successfully associated *smoking* with feelings of independence, power, glamour, and freedom. Women throughout the world began to smoke in their millions. **The idea that smoking actually *made* women freer, was complete nonsense, of course. It was irrational.** Women were just being exploited and made poorer and unhealthy by becoming addicts to cigarettes, enriching Big

Tobacco in the process. Tobacco use has killed over 100 million people in the 20th century, more than all deaths in World Wars I and II combined.

This experiment made Bernays realize that **it is possible to persuade people to behave irrationally** – *even do something that kills you* – **if you link a product to people's subconscious desires and feelings.** He had proven to American corporations that they could make people want things they didn't need, through psychological manipulation. This got them *very* interested indeed…

In the 1930s leading Wall Street banker Paul Mazer wrote: "We must shift America from a 'needs' to a 'desires' culture. People must be trained to desire, to want new things even before the old had been entirely consumed. We must shape a new mentality in America. Man's desires must overshadow his needs."

The New York banks funded the creation of chains of department stores across America, which would display the new consumer products, while **Bernays was tasked by the banks with creating a 'consumer culture',** through the promotion of fashion in women's magazines, press releases about new products, product placement in movies, celebrity endorsements, and many more of the mass consumer persuasion techniques that we see today.

They also tasked Bernays with **remaking the image of 'Big Business'**, seen up until then as the exploiters of the working class. Under the aegis of The National Association of Manufacturers, an organization consisting of all the major corporations in the US, a major PR campaign was launched on a grand scale (it is ongoing to this day), using every channel possible, and every technique possible, to program the population with the following concepts: corporations are inevitable and indispensable; corporations create jobs; corporations are much more efficient than governments; corporations are responsible for progress; corporations create the products that make your life better; corporate successes and domination are to be celebrated. Unfortunately, none of these statements are true.

They Mind-Control You Through Your Television

❏ The average child in America spends 1680 minutes a week watching television (28 hours a week, or 4 hours a day).

❏ By comparison, parents spend just 3.5 minutes a week, on average, in meaningful conversation with their children.

❏ The average American sees 3,000 advertisements a day. The average American child sees 20,000 TV commercials a year.

❏ Television ads *program* children to adopt a consumeristic, materialistic lifestyle.

❏ Television makes you feel miserable. "Heavy television watchers are more likely to be dissatisfied with their lives than light ones. Advertising executives freely admit that one of their main objectives is to create a sense of dissatisfaction with existing possessions so that consumers will want to buy new, 'better' ones." – British psychologist Oliver James, author of *Affluenza*

❏ If people believe their lives are 'empty and meaningless' (futile) they are much more likely to fill that void through mindless consumption...

"Most people in western nations have departed from old-time standards of religion and philosophy, and having failed to develop forceful views to take their places, hold to 'a philosophy of futility'. This concentrates human attention on the more superficial things that comprise much of fashionable consumption."

– Paul Nystrom, marketing professor at Columbia University, 1938

❏ Over 200 ads for junk-food are broadcast in the US during morning cartoons, conditioning children to eat "junk food". A study of 10,000 Chinese found that the more television they watched, the more likely they were to be obese.

The average 18-year-old in the US will be exposed to over 50,000 drug ads in their lifetime, conditioning them psychologically to consume pharmaceuticals.

CHAPTER 2

Conventional Medicine Kills 800,000 People A Year

Medical Schools are an incredibly de-humanising place. It is an *intentionally gruelling process*, designed to physically push the weaker students over the edge. They are given more work than they could possibly do, and they learn early on to be dependent on *chemicals* to stay up late to study... Medical students have no time to stop and ask themselves if what they are learning makes any sense to them. They just learn it all by heart. They are conditioned to think like drug-pushing robots, never questioning authority. If they don't give the correct answer (i.e. prescribe drugs or surgery in every instance), they're flunked out of medical school, thousands of dollars in debt.

Many doctors are wonderful people who got into this profession for all the right reasons. They want to help people. But are they doing the right thing? As I mentioned earlier, at least 100,000 Americans die each year from correctly prescribed pharmaceutical medications. The medical profession kills 250,000 Americans a year and are *the third leading cause of death in the U.S.*

We Are Being Medically Treated In A Way That Endangers Our Health.

In Detroit, Dr. Farid Fata was recently sentenced to 45 years in prison for misdiagnosing cancer and giving cancer treatment drugs to 553 patients who didn't need them and who DID NOT HAVE CANCER, destroying their health or killing them in the process. He collected $17.6 million from Medicare and private insurance companies for doing this; and this is not an isolated incident.

Health crusader Mike Adams writes in his website www.NaturalNews.com: "I recently heard of a case where a woman had a small cancer tumour removed from her breast and was told all the other surrounding tissue (including lymph nodes) tested negative for cancer. The cancer was 100% local and non-systemic, in other words. Yet for weeks after surgery, **she was hounded by the hospital's oncologist** who demanded to see her for a "treatment plan" that would involve exposing her to toxic chemotherapy chemicals while billing her insurance for hundreds of thousands of dollars. When she pointed out that there was no other cancer and asked what purpose chemotherapy could possibly play in a person who had no cancer, she was told -- get this -- that **chemotherapy works as a "preventive" measure against cancer**. You can't overstate the quackery and outright medical fraud in such a suggestion. The idea that chemotherapy is some sort of nutrient that prevents cancer is nothing more than the delusional wild fantasy of the very oncologists who profit from selling patients these toxic treatments. Yet these unscrupulous doctors disguise their for-profit sales calls as "medical consultations" -- all while wholly neglecting to mention their **outrageous financial conflicts of interest**. [...] these doctors engage in the most insidious scare tactics imaginable, telling patients things like, "You won't be alive in six months unless you agree to this treatment."

To maximize their income, **doctors are taught to spend less than ten minutes with each patient**. They have had almost no training in nutrition or in how to keep a human being *healthy*. They are trained to prescribe the 'right' drug, at the 'right' time, to 'treat' a patient, not heal them, to 'manage' a condition, not cure it. The maxim taught to medical students is: *"There aren't any healthy patients... only patients who haven't been diagnosed properly yet."* Another common maxim in medical schools is, ***"Hurry up and operate before the patient gets better.***

The more surgeries they perform, and the more drugs they administer, the more money they make. This is why caesareans are recommended to perfectly healthy women who can give birth naturally, despite studies that show that children born by C-section more often suffer from chronic disorders such as asthma, rheumatism, allergies, bowel disorders, and leukaemia than children born naturally.

Doctors particularly love to pluck out organs that are not needed for daily use, especially with women. They tell them they should remove their ovaries, uterus, thyroid, gall bladder, or breasts. All in the name of *profit*. Pretty soon there will be a lot of 'hollow' women walking around!

Psychiatrists love to put people on drugs. Every year the American Psychiatric Association get together and invent new 'social disorders' to justify prescribing more drugs. Have you heard of the latest one? It's called "Oppositional Defiance Disorder" (O.D.D.). If you don't agree with what the authorities say, you probably suffer from O.D.D. and need pharmaceutical drugs to 'get better'.

Stalin used this method, with his Soviet psychologists explaining that Communism is so perfect and good for the people, that anyone who *opposes* Communism is obviously mentally unwell. Thousands were condemned to mental institutions, where the drugs really *did* make them go crazy. The side-effects of psychiatric drugs are, very often, more horrendous than the mental condition itself. The fact that children are put on Ritalin in America is shocking to the rest of the world.

It takes a great deal of courage, and a knack for *'thinking outside the box'*, for a doctor to opt out of the conventional way of thinking and learn about alternatives. These traits are all but trained out of doctors by the time they leave medical school. It takes a long time for medical convention to accept anything 'holistic' or 'new' and doctors who stick their necks out publicly to examine or recommend anything 'unconventional' are risking their reputation. As a result, such doctors are rare.

Furthermore, according to the American Medical Association, the half-life of the current medical education is 4 years. This means that *half* of what a doctor learned is *obsolete* within 4 years. **With so many patients to see, doctors rarely have time to further their education.** How do doctors keep up-to-date? Doctors are primarily educated about new advances in medicine by the drug companies' salesmen. Similarly, we 'The Consumers' are constantly being told what to believe through billions spent on advertising by the pharmaceutical companies whose only interest is *selling their drugs!*

As doctors and patients, we have allowed these salespeople to become our Health Gurus even though they patently have other interests other than our wellbeing.

> "What if I told you your own medical profession holds back cures, refuses to approve alternative medicines and procedures because they threaten the very structure of the "healing" profession? Doctors in the West deny the healing efficacies of doctors in the East because to accept them, to admit that certain alternate modalities might just provide some healing, would be to tear at the very fabric of the institution as it has structured itself. ... because to those institutions it's a matter of survival. The profession doesn't do this because it is evil. It does it because it is scared."
>
> Neale Donald Walsch, *Conversations with God*

Conventional Medicine Is DEADLY

Did you know that prescription drugs **injure over two million Americans** each and every year? Since September 11, 2001, there have been *over one million deaths* in America from adverse drug reactions. Where is the *"War On Pharmaceutical Companies"*? Ah, yes, I forgot. They actually *own* the congressmen and senators, through multi-million dollar bribes.

A study by Harvard University professor Lucian Leape found that one million patients are injured by errors during hospital treatment annually, with some 120,000 deaths. He noted that *less than 10%* of medical mistakes are reported to hospital authorities. Professors Gary Null and Dorothy Smith published a report titled "Death By Medicine", where they revealed that America's leading cause of death isn't heart disease or cancer – **it is conventional medicine**. They found that 783,936 people a year die because of doctors and/or medical treatments. By comparison, there are only 31,940 deaths by firearms in the US each year, and 41,149 suicides a year.

Deaths per year	Cause
106,000	Correctly administered drugs (negative side-effects)
88,000	Hospital infections
98,000	Medical error
115,000	Bedsores
37,136	Unnecessary procedures
108,800	Malnutrition
199,000	Outpatients
32,000	Surgery-related

783,936	Total Deaths Per Year from Doctors and Medical Treatments

People Live Longer When Doctors Go On Strike!

The deadly nature of the **pseudoscientific "conventional medicine" is laid bare whenever there is a doctors' strike** – as the death rates in those areas *goes down*. In 1976 in Bogota, Columbia, doctors went on strike for 52 days, except for emergency care. The death rate went down 35%. There was another doctors' strike during 1976 in Los Angeles. The death rate dropped 18%. During 1973, there was a doctors' strike in Israel. According to statistics from the Jerusalem Burial Society, the death rate dropped 50%

The Helsinki Businessmen Study conducted over a 15-year period (1974 – 1989) showed that the death rate for the group that was medically treated more was 4 times higher! That's right! According to this study, if you go to a hospital or take pharmaceutical drugs more diligently than the average person, you are 400% more likely *to die!* In his book "Diabetes", Dr. Bernard E. Lowenstein, M.D. reported that the death rate from Diabetes among doctors was 35% higher than the general population. He theorized that doctors are more likely to follow the conventional treatment programs they prescribe *more strictly*, and therefore manifest more intensely their negative side-effects.

Listen, I'm not saying that "all doctors are bad". In many instances they truly perform miracles in the operating room. And drugs might be a necessary last-gasp solution for alleviating pain. But most patients would not reach that point in the first place *had they been empowered through education.*

The Drugs Don't Work... And They Don't Make Us "Healthier"!

If prescription drugs are so good for us, then where are all the 'healthy' people on drugs? Shouldn't the millions of people on prescription drugs be mentally sharp, physically fit, bursting with energy? In reality, typically, when you meet someone who is taking multiple prescription drugs, they are mentally fuzzy, sickly in appearance, chronically fatigued, and emotionally unstable and depressed.

Don't statin drugs lower LDL cholesterol, though? While statin drugs may positively affect *one* marker, they disrupt the body's physiology in many other ways. There are over 900 studies proving the adverse effects of statin drugs, including cancer, chronic fatigue, liver dysfunction, thyroid disruption, Parkinson's, Alzheimer's, and even Diabetes! Not to mention that "high cholesterol" is a scam that is killing millions of people!

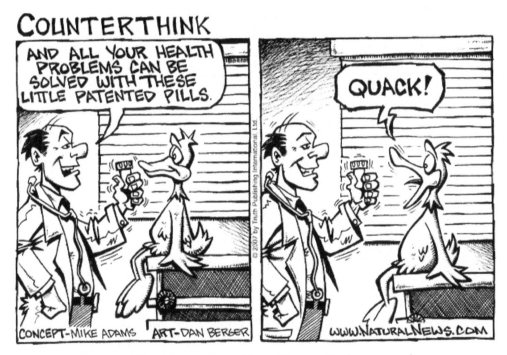

Thanks to Mike Adams and *www.NaturalNews.com* for the cartoon above.

In truth, cholesterol is a necessary ingredient that is required to be regularly delivered around the body for the efficient healthy development, maintenance, and functioning of our cells. It is vital for good health. Perhaps most importantly, cholesterol is an essential component in the machinery that triggers the release of neurotransmitters in the brain. That's right. Cholesterol is not the 'bad guy' that the Medical Mafia claims, and elevated cholesterol is not the cause of heart disease!

According to recent research at Harvard, the primary causes of atherosclerosis (hardening of the arteries which leads to heart disease) are lesions and plaque in the arteries caused by **sugar** which causes insulin to be released. Insulin causes lesions in the endothelium of the arteries. These arteries then become clogged with cholesterol. So, cholesterol gets the blame, but the real culprit is *sugar!* Cholesterol is actually your body's 'repair mechanism' to correct the arterial damage resulting from excess sugar. Remove sugar from your diet, and you shouldn't have any issue with heart disease nor cholesterol.

When patients begin to have additional problems which are *caused* by prescription drugs, what do they do? They head back to the doctor's office where their doctor diagnoses them with *another* disease or disorder. And then, they give them another prescription drug to help 'fix' the problem caused by the first drug.

CHAPTER 3

The Drugs Don't Work

Adverse reactions from pharmaceutical drugs kill and injure millions of patients a year. In the US alone an estimated 2,216,000 hospitalized patients have serious adverse drug reactions each year, whilst 106,000 die because of them; and that is only the figure from *correctly prescribed and administered drugs*. The real figure is much higher still. As I reported in the previous chapter, deaths caused by conventional medical treatment in the US stand at 783,936 a year.

In the UK, one million hospital admissions a year are known to be the result of an adverse reaction to a pharmaceutical drug. The UK's National Health Service is spending a whopping £2 billion a year treating these patients who have had an adverse reaction to drugs *prescribed to them by their doctor!* In Europe, pharmaceutical drugs are the fifth biggest cause of death in hospital.

Side-effects from taking pharmaceutical drugs can be devastating:

❑ Pharmaceutical drugs can cause birth defects and miscarriages.

❑ At least 800,000 deaths and 500,000 major strokes worldwide have been caused by beta-blockers (drugs used to supposedly cut the risk of a heart attack after surgery).

❑ Antibiotics alone put 142,000 US patients into emergency rooms each year.

❑ Avandia, a diabetes drug manufactured by GlaxoSmithKline, has been estimated to have caused as many as 205,000 heart attacks and strokes (and deaths) between 1999 and 2006.

❑ When you take drugs for Type II Diabetes they may lower your glucose levels... but you die early. A 14% reduction of glucose results in a 43% increase in cardiovascular death.

❑ Medications can cause mental decline. Drugs that can cause Dementia include: anticonvulsants, corticosteroids, sedatives, antidepressants, antihistamines, anti-Parkinson's drugs, anti-anxiety medications, and cardiovascular drug.

❑ Non-steroidal anti-inflammatory drugs and COX-2 inhibitors linked to Dementia include: Tylenol, Panadol, Codeine, OxyContin, MS Contin, Fentanyl Skin patch, Oxycodone, Percocet, Percodan, Tramadol, Vicodin.

❑ An FDA scientist admitted Vioxx alone may have caused as many as 150,000 deaths.

❑ Lipitor (statins) is the bestselling drug in the world because every adult with high LDL is on it, as well as 2.8 million children. But the many side effects include weakness, dizziness, muscle breakdown, pain and arthritis. *"My older patients literally do without food so that they can buy these medicines that make them sicker, feel bad, and do nothing to improve life,"* says an ophthalmologist from Tennessee. Statins actually act as cellular poisons that *accelerate ageing*, they deactivate DNA repair, they promote diabetes, muscle fatigue and memory loss, and they actually *increase* heart disease!

❑ The Yaz (or "Yasmin") birth control pill was released in 2006. But then 18-year-olds started coming down with blood clots, gall bladder disease, heart attacks and even strokes. One fifteen-year-old had to have her gallbladder removed. Another had a stroke and part of her skull removed. Another still collapsed and died of a pulmonary thromboembolism.

❑ Lyrica, Topamax and Lamictal – epilepsy seizure drugs administered for pain relief. These drugs can make you lose your memory. They cause hair loss. They also can cause aseptic meningitis (brain inflammation), and increase the risk of suicidal behaviours. Seizure drugs were linked to 801 attempted suicides and 41 violent deaths over a five-year period.

❑ Humira, Prolia – made from genetically engineered hamster cells, they actually suppress your immune system. Supposedly used for treating Crohn's disease, rheumatoid arthritis, psoriatic arthritis, postmenopausal Multiple Sclerosis. Side-effects include possibly lethal infections, new or worsening psoriasis (a condition it is supposed to treat!), melanoma, lymphoma and "unusual cancers in children and teenagers".

❑ The antismoking drug Chantix was linked to 227 suicides, angioedema, serious skin reactions, visual impairment, dizziness, muscle spasms, seizures and loss of consciousness.

❑ The breast cancer drug Tamoxifen actually *causes* cancer, birth defects, and is a chemical cousin of organochlorine pesticides.

❑ Pfizer's hormone drugs Prempro and Premarin cause a 26% increase in breast cancer, 41% more strokes, 29% more heart attacks, 22% increase in cardiovascular disease, 100% more blood clots and links to deafness, urinary incontinence, cataracts, gout, joint degeneration, asthma, lupus, scleroderma, dementia, Alzheimer's disease and lung, ovarian, breast, endometrial, gall bladder and melanoma cancers. The cancer rate in the U.S. and Canada *fell* when women quit hormone therapy in 2002, as did the number of heart attacks in women.

❑ Pharmaceutical drugs deplete your nutrients. Oral contraceptives, cholesterol-lowering statins, and antibiotics are particularly deleterious in this regard. Medications can interfere with your body's ability to absorb or make use of certain nutrients, leading to deficiency-related health problems!

❑ Proton pump inhibitors PPIs used to treat gastric cancer actually *increase* Adenocarcinomas!

❑ The chemotherapy drug Adriamycin is killing people so effectively it is referred to in hospitals as "Red Death". The chemotherapy drug "5FU" is so lethal it is nicknamed "five feet under".

❑ The AIDS drug AZT is in fact **1,000 times more toxic** than the manufacturer claims it to be, and it *destroys* a patient's immune system – ironically *causing* *"acquired immune-deficiency syndrome"* in patients. That's right. The AIDS drug AZT *causes* AIDS.

❑ The anti-depression drug Zoloft causes dementia.

❑ Antidepressants cause children to be twice as likely to commit suicide.

❑ Harvard health scientists conducted a study that showed how high doses of brain-altering chemicals marketed as "anti-depressants" actually *increase* the likelihood of self-harm.

❑ Another recent study found that pregnant mothers that take antidepressants are more likely to have babies with brain defects.

❑ Young people taking antidepressants are more likely to commit violent crimes.

❑ Research suggests the use of antidepressant drugs may actually result in *more relapses* back into depression in the long run, turning depression into a more chronic condition.

❑ People who are the most prone to getting cancer are those who have taken the most non-prescription and prescription drugs and who have eaten the most fast-food.

❑ The New York Times reports that Johnson & Johnson's popular treatment for congestive heart failure, Natrecor, has now been shown to reduce kidney function.

❑ The common acne drug Accutane causes severe birth defects and miscarriages.

❑ Prescription drugs are killing more people than the diseases they are supposed to be curing.

Pharmaceuticals are *so dangerous and deadly* they should be called "**HARMaceuticals**".

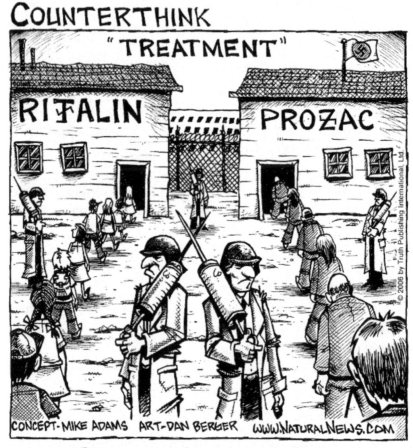

Thanks to Mike Adams and *www.NaturalNews.com* for the cartoon above.

The 'Cholesterol Scam' That Is Killing Millions

According to the American microbiologist Dr. Robert O. Young, author of *The pH Miracle*, the main reason you may get more cholesterol in your body than you need is because your bloodstream is overly acidic (it should remain slightly alkaline, at a pH of

7.365). Acid is corrosive, and an overly acidic bloodstream would damage your blood vessels. To stop this from happening, your body secretes cholesterol and places it on your arteries' walls – *to protect them.* So cholesterol is a *good* thing, up to a point. It's your body trying to defend itself. If you keep getting more and more acidic, your body keeps producing cholesterol and lining your arteries with it, until pretty soon there's no room for the blood to flow through. By getting more alkaline, your body doesn't *need* the cholesterol anymore. You will simply release it out of your system naturally.

According to Dr. Leonard Coldwell, author of *The Only Answer To Cancer,* one of the main culprits for high cholesterol levels is table salt – and all the added salt you find hidden in processed foods and snacks. According to Dr. Coldwell, most commercially-available salt is **one third glass, one third sand, and only one third *actual* salt.** They claim the sand and glass is there for 'anti-caking' purposes, but what it actually does is scrape the arteries and makes them bleed. The body produces cholesterol *to plug those holes* and save your life. Like I mentioned above, cholesterol is part of your body's defence mechanism! According to Dr. Coldwell we need to have a combined cholesterol level of 250. By advertising the arbitrary numbers of "your cholesterol level should be 170 to 200", the pharmaceutical industry is creating a massive market for its ultimately useless – and deadly – 'statin' and beta-blocker drugs.

One study reported that <u>Beta-Blockers killed 800,000 people in Europe</u> over a 5-year period, and over one million Americans. An October 2013 study done in New York found that beta-blocker use *increased* the odds of having an acute coronary event. In fact, researchers were so concerned by what they found that they commented: *"The results from this study become especially important in view of the fact that beta-blockers are currently recommended by the American College of Cardiology/American Heart guidelines regarding cardiac risk and management".* In 2015, the US government did a U-turn on their warnings, finally acknowledging that cholesterol is not *'a nutrient of concern',* but not before Big Pharma made over 1.5 TRILLION dollars from selling cholesterol-lowering drugs to gullible consumers over a 40-year period, killing millions of people in the process.

Attempting to control cholesterol is a very dangerous practice. Ironically, Statin drugs actually *increase* Heart Disease, and the majority of people that have heart attacks have normal cholesterol levels. The truth is the majority of the experts who created the lower guidelines have multiple financial ties to pharmaceutical companies. Dr. George V. Mann M.D. states: *"Saturated fats and cholesterol in the diet are not the cause of coronary heart disease. That myth is the greatest deception of the century, perhaps of any century".*

"Cholesterol guidelines have been created to increase pharmaceutical profits, not to improve peoples' health. I know from my experience as a pharmaceutical sales representative for a statin drug. Statins do not prevent heart disease, but that is the myth that the drug companies have made billions of dollars from for more than 20 years. The lower guidelines simply created a larger lasso to rope more people into buying statin drugs," wrote K.L. Carlson, in his article *The Great Cholesterol Scam.*

COUNTERTHINK

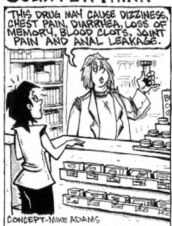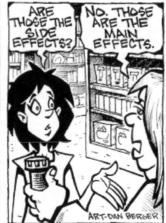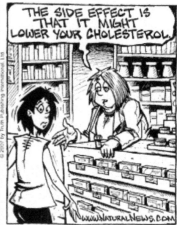

Thanks to Mike Adams and *www.NaturalNews.com* for the cartoon above.

They've been warning us to stay away from high-cholesterol foods to avoid heart disease and clogged arteries, when in fact it is the ***sugar*** in processed foods and highly toxic chemicals in our water/air/food/products that have been causing an epidemic of over-acidity in our blood and putting our arteries under attack. You *should* be eating healthy fats such as avocadoes, organic eggs, nuts, coconut oil, organic meat and wild salmon, for example *(see Chapter 27 on Superfoods and Outstanding Nutrition).*

FACT:

The more pharmaceutical drugs a person takes, and the longer they take them, the more rapidly their health deteriorates.

CHAPTER 4

33 Facts Vaccine Companies Don't Want You To Know

Fact #1: Vaccines Enrich Pharmaceutical Companies To The Tune of $25 Billion a Year

Vaccines sales translate into big profits for vaccine manufacturers. Merck Pharmaceuticals alone made $5.72bn in 2012 from the sale of its vaccines. But the real profits, worth hundreds of billions a year, come from promoting vaccines that ultimately *destroy* the immune systems of millions of people (children) who then become 'patients for life'. That is the *real* purpose of vaccination programs, behind all the rhetoric, propaganda, and false assurances that *'vaccines are safe…'*.

Fact #2: Vaccinated Children Are Five Times More Prone To Disease

In some Western countries, more than 50 doses of 14 different vaccines are administered to children before they reach kindergarten age, including 26 doses in their first year. Do they actually keep your children healthy? In a groundbreaking study conducted in Germany and released in 2012, it was revealed that **children who have been vaccinated are five times more likely to contract a preventable disease** on average than children who developed their own immune systems naturally without vaccines. In other words, vaccines destroy the immune system of young children.

The survey included data on 8,000 unvaccinated children. It revealed:

❏ Vaccinated children are about two-and-a-half times as likely (250% more) to develop a pattern of **migraine headaches** compared to unvaccinated children

❏ Vaccinated children are eight times more likely (800% more) to develop **asthma** and **chronic bronchitis** (respiratory problems) than unvaccinated children.

❏ Vaccinated children are also three times more likely (300% more) to develop **hyperactivity**, four times more likely (400% more) to suffer from **hay fever**, and a shocking 17 times more likely (1,700% more) to experience **thyroid disease**, compared to unvaccinated children.

❑ Vaccinated children are 22 times more likely (2,200% more) to develop **ear infections**.

❑ Vaccinated children are about **19 times more likely to develop severe autism** compared to unvaccinated children.

You might also be interested to know that…

❑ Less than 10% of unvaccinated children suffer from allergies. This compares with 40% of vaccinated children in the USA ages 3-17.

❑ A study in *The Lancet* reported that Crohn's disease and ulcerative colitis were far more prevalent in vaccinated individuals than non-vaccinated ones.

❑ There is a **94 times greater risk (9,400% more) of dying from the DPT vaccine** than from whooping cough itself. There is also a **3,000 times greater risk** of acquiring long-term damage from the DPT vaccine than from whooping cough itself.

❑ The long-term **adverse effects of vaccines include autism, hyperactivity, ADD, allergies, cancer**, and many other conditions that barely existed before vaccination programs began.

In a 1992 study conducted in New Zealand they found that vaccinated children were:

❑ 500% more likely to develop Asthma (20 children vs only 4)

❑ 1,000% more likely to display Hyperactivity and "Attention Deficit Disorder"

❑ 268% more likely to develop Eczema or rashes (43 children vs only 16)

❑ 325% more likely to develop Chronic otitis (26 children vs only 8)

❑ 367% more likely to experience recurrent tonsillitis (11 vs only 3)

❑ 450% more likely to die from "Sudden infant death syndrome" (9 vs only 2)

Fact #3: Vaccinated Children Are 19 Times More Likely to Develop Autism

In 1983 there were 10 vaccines given to children in America, and the autism rate was 1 in 10,000. By 2013 that number has risen to 44 vaccines, and the autism rate has exploded to just 1 in 88 children. 1,082,353 cases of autism were reported in 2014, a condition that barely existed at the turn of the twentieth century.

As mentioned above, <u>vaccinated children are 19 times more likely to develop **severe autism** compared to unvaccinated children</u>. One in every 100 vaccinated children develops autism (1%), while only 4 out of the 8,000 unvaccinated children in the study did (0.05%), and those four tested very high for metals such as *mercury* (which causes inflammation in the brain, among other damaging consequences). And yet, despite overwhelming evidence, the medical establishment vehemently denies any link between vaccines and the *surge* in cases of autism.

Many researchers have found evidence of vaccines causing autism, but they are dismissed, ostracized, or destroyed professionally, with PR companies paying media outlets to portray their research as being 'controversial' or 'discredited', when in fact *it is simply the truth – a truth that is highly inconvenient for pharmaceutical companies.*

For example, Dr. Mary Megson's research has shown total deficiency of vitamin A in almost all autistic children. She found that the MMR vaccination depletes the body of vitamin A.

Dr. John O'Leary, a world class researcher and molecular biologist from Ireland, showed how he had found measles virus in the gut of 96% of autistic children, compared to 6.6% of normal children. Interestingly, this virus did not come from the natural disease; it came *from the measles vaccine.*

Dr. V. Singh, an autism specialist from Utah, found that in over 400 cases of autism, the children had experienced an 'autoimmune' episode, in which their own body has been made to attack the lining of the nervous system, in response to the measles virus present in the vaccine. He reported that 55% of families have stated that autism appeared <u>soon after the MMR vaccine</u>, and 33% of families said it appeared soon after the DPT vaccination. (source: www.thedoctorwithin.com)

Incredibly, whistleblower Dr. William Thompson admitted in 2014 that a CDC study published ten years earlier was falsified to remove a link between MMR vaccine and autism. I recommend you watch the documentary *"Vaxxed"* to hear the full story (visit www.vaxxedthemovie.com). Since 2002 the Center for Disease Control has paid Dr. Poul Thorsen $14.6 million to publish studies that *disprove* the links between vaccinations and autism, despite the fact that investigations uncovered research fraud in his previous studies! It is clear that the CDC hierarchy works for Big Pharma.

Over and over again I have come across families who have cured their children of autism by cleansing their children's bodies of **heavy metals**. In one story by a mother, from *Cancer: Step Outside The Box*:

"I was fortunate enough to find a doctor that was able to run the proper lab test and discovered the core of his health problems not just the symptoms. He found that my son was toxic, under-nourished, and had a weakened immune and metabolic system. We focused on all four issues for the next 12 months and slowly started to see improvements. [...] I found a diet that his body responded to, which included fresh juices daily. We removed the toxins through chelation. And by restoring his metabolic and immune system, his body was able to heal. Today, my son is fully recovered. At six years old, he is in a mainstream first grade classroom and involved in baseball, swimming, and tennis, and is indistinguishable from his peers."

Fact #4: The Vaccine Industry Refuses To Conduct Scientific Tests on Unvaccinated Children

The vaccine industry *refuses* to conduct scientific tests on the health of vaccinated children compared to unvaccinated children. Is it any surprise when you consider the results of the studies mentioned in this chapter? Our neighbours' and friends' children seem to be going in and out of doctors' offices every week. *These children were all vaccinated.* Isn't it even *a bit* suspicious that the most heavily-vaccinated kids are the ones who get sick all the time? Isn't it worth researching why groups like the Amish, who largely refuse to vaccinate their children, have near-zero rates of autism?

Our nieces are ten months old, and the staff at the local hospital found it hard to believe they hadn't experienced a single health issue yet. This was out of the ordinary. But this was not a surprise to us: they had never been poisoned by vaccines and their immune systems were fine.

Just this week, one of our neighbours told us that their 8-month-old child had high fever and a rash all over his body. The doctor called it 'Roseola', or 'Sixth Disease', supposedly a 'viral illness'. He's been in-and-out of the doctor's office the past few months. When my wife enquired whether their child had been vaccinated, they answered, *'Oh yes, just three months ago.'* But they completely failed to see any link, so trusting were they of their doctor and the medical establishment.

Fact #5: Vaccines Kill Children

Vaccinated children are much more likely to die young. An alarming medical study has found a direct statistical link between higher vaccine doses and infant mortality rates (*'Infant mortality rates regressed against number of vaccine doses routinely given'*, by Neil Z. Miller and Gary S. Goldman, published in *the Human and Experimental Toxicology journal*). In other words, **the more infants are vaccinated, the more likely they are to *die.***

Japan and Sweden, which require the **fewest** vaccinations, have the **lowest** mortality rates of infants in the developed world (2 per 1000 live births). The USA, which administers **more** childhood vaccines than any other country in the developed world (26), also has the **highest** number of infant deaths per 1000 births in the developed world (6.22 per 1000 live births, or 311% *more* than Japan or Sweden).

Many people now believe that 'sudden infant death syndrome' (SIDS) is related to vaccinations. The peak incidence of SIDS in the US occurs between the ages of 2 and 4 months: precisely when the first two routine immunizations are given. But hospitals and doctors routinely label these deaths as "Sudden Death Syndrome" rather than

"Adverse Reaction To Vaccination" … One study found that 3,000 children die within four days of vaccination each year in America.

The internet is full of stories of children who've died right after being administered a vaccine, such as this tragic message posted online: *"Our beautiful daughter was born on February 14 and died on April 17. What was unusual was that earlier on the day she died I had taken her to the Military Base hospital for her two-month check-up. The doctor told me that she was just perfect. Then the doctor said that she needed four shots…".*

Dr. Archie Kalokerinos was a physician who began routinely vaccinating aboriginal children in Australia during the late 1960s. Shortly after he began vaccinations, he noticed that extremely high numbers of these children became very ill or died. Kalokerinos also noted that <u>children experiencing adverse reactions would recover after receiving large doses of vitamin C</u> and the numbers of children who suffered adverse reactions declined dramatically when only healthy children who had taken large doses of vitamin C received vaccinations. *"One would have expected, of course, that the authorities would take an interest in these observations…. But instead of taking an interest, their reaction was one of extreme hostility.* **I found that the whole vaccine business was a hoax.** *Most doctors are convinced that they are useful, but if you look at the proper statistics and study the instance of these diseases you will realize that this is not so",* he stated in 1995.

Fact #6: There Is No Evidence That Vaccines Actually Work. None.

We are told that vaccines have made the world a healthier place. This is disinformation, pure and simple. <u>Studies show a decrease in diseases across the world at the same rate for countries that did not introduce vaccines</u>. Vaccines are not responsible for decreasing diseases after their introduction. Access to sanitation and clean water, as well as access to better nutrition, is what dramatically reduced human mortality and the spread of infectious diseases over the past 150 years.

According to the *British Association for the Advancement of Science,* childhood diseases decreased 90% between 1850 and 1940, paralleling improved sanitation and hygienic practices, well before mandatory vaccination programs. Deaths from infections disease in the USA and England declined steadily by an average of about 80% during the same period. What actually stopped most of the diseases in the 1900s was sanitation, sewage control, refrigeration, and central heat.

Not only do vaccines *not* work, in many cases they actually *create epidemics of the disease they are supposedly eliminating,* thereby increasing public demand for more vaccines which cause more outbreaks! Ty Bollinger writes: *"Once smallpox vaccination became mandatory in England, massive epidemics began to occur. Between 1857 and 1859, there were over 14,000 deaths from smallpox. Then, between 1863 and 1865, there were over 20,000 smallpox deaths. A few years later, there were almost 45,000 smallpox deaths between 1870 and 1872…".*

Furthermore, the majority of the children affected by an infectious outbreak *have already been vaccinated against the virus!* This is yet more proof that vaccines do not confer immunity. A CNN report stated recently that 77% of the children who caught mumps in New Jersey had already been vaccinated against mumps. It would not surprise me to find out that it was the vaccinated children who *caused* this outbreak of mumps, since they were infected with the virus in the first place.

Fact #7: Highly Potent Neurotoxic Chemicals Are Injected Into Children's Bloodstream

Vaccines are not natural. As listed on their packaging (which is never shown to parents), they contain Thimerosal, Aluminium, Formaldehyde, and *live viruses*. Parents are rarely – if ever – told of their potentially devastating side-effects. <u>Doctors are not told what is in vaccines</u>. Most doctors are surprised to find that vaccines contain mercury. They are simply trained to administer them, without asking any questions. <u>Doctors take at face value what the pharmaceutical sales reps are telling them</u>.

Fact #8: Thimerosal in Vaccines Can Cause Learning Disabilities and Mental Retardation

Thimerosal is a mercury compound, which can be particularly hazardous for pregnant women and small children. Even in low doses, mercury may affect a child's development, delaying walking and talking, shortening attention span, and causing learning disabilities. High dose prenatal and infant exposure to mercury can cause mental retardation, cerebral palsy, deafness and blindness. In adults, mercury poisoning can adversely affect fertility, and blood pressure regulation; can cause memory loss, tremors, vision loss, numbness of fingers. It may also lead to heart disease and kidney failure.

Flu vaccines contain Thimerosal. Some contain as much as 25 micrograms of mercury per dose, or 250 times the EPA's safety limit! Dr. Boyd Haley states: *"If you inject thimerosal into an animal, its brain will sicken. If you apply it to living tissue, the cells die. Put it in a petri dish, the culture dies."*

Fact #9: Aluminium in Vaccines May Lead To Auto-Immune Disorders and Brain Inflammation

Aluminium is a known neuro-toxin. It may lead to auto-immunity disorders, long-term brain inflammation and associated neurological complications, and thus may have profound and widespread adverse health consequences. According to a new study published in Current Medical Chemistry, children up to 6 months of age receive 14 to 49 times more aluminium from vaccines than the U.S. Food and Drug Administration (FDA) safety limits allow.

Fact #10: Formaldehyde Causes Cancer, Childhood Leukaemia, Organ Failure, and Even Death

Formaldehyde is a known carcinogen, which can lead to cancer, organ failure, and even death. Ingestion of formaldehyde leads to damage of the liver, kidney, spleen, pancreas, brain, and central nervous system. It causes significant inflammation in the human body. Some see a link between formaldehyde in vaccines and childhood cancers including leukaemia, which is a blood cell cancer, and cancers of the brain and central nervous system, which account for over *half* of the new cases of childhood cancer. And yet this substance is routinely injected into the bloodstream of babies!

Fact #11: The Live Viruses in the MMR Vaccine Cause Brain Damage

The MMR vaccine contains three live viruses: measles, mumps, and rubella. Live viruses have been shown to cause brain damage over prolonged periods of time. Mike Adams of NaturalNews.com writes: "Injecting mercury into a human being should be considered a criminal act. There is no safe level of mercury for injecting into a human child. There is NO evidence of safety for mercury at any dose whatsoever. Any doctor who says the level of mercury in a vaccine is "safe" to inject into a child is only demonstrating their outrageous ignorance of scientific facts. Mercury is arguably the most neurotoxic element on the entire Table of Elements. It is used in vaccines for the convenience of the vaccine manufacturer at the expense of the safety of the child. Any doctor who injects mercury into a child at any dose should be immediately stripped of their medical license. [...] All of these substances are toxic to human biology when injected. All of them are still listed on the CDC website as vaccine additives. There is no rational doctor or scientist in the world who can say they believe injecting infants and children with mercury, formaldehyde, MSG and aluminum is somehow "safe," yet doctors inject children with these substances every single day in the form of vaccines. Doctors who inject children with vaccines are practicing a medical holocaust against humanity while fraudulently calling it "immunization." For the record, vaccination does not equal immunization."

Fact #12: The Flu Vaccine Caused 84,000 Adverse Reactions and 1,000+ Deaths in 2012

In reality, only about 2.7 in every 100 adults get the flu in the first place. A large-scale, systematic review of 51 studies involving over 260,000 children in 2006 found *no evidence* that the flu vaccine is any more effective than a placebo in children under the age of two years. **Zero percent effective!**

At the end of 2012, there were more than 84,000 reports of reactions, hospitalizations, injuries and deaths following influenza vaccinations, including over 1,000 related deaths and over 1,600 cases of GBS (Guillain-Barré syndrome). The vaccine seems to be *much more dangerous than the virus!*

53

Fact #13: Vaccines Cause Cancer

<u>60 lab studies now confirm vaccines are linked to cancer</u>. In 2002, the journal Lancet published compelling evidence that the polio vaccine, which contained the SV40 cancer-causing virus, was responsible for half of the 55,000 non-Hodgkin's lymphoma cases that were occurring each year.

A top Merck vaccine scientist named Maurice Hilleman, one of the most prominent vaccine scientists in the history of the vaccine industry, revealed in a video interview prior to his death that polio vaccines injected into tens of millions of people over *decades* **were contaminated with leukaemia and cancer viruses**. When these vaccines were injected into hamsters, they developed tumours – *and Merck Pharmaceuticals knew this*. Up to 98 million Americans were exposed to **up to 40 different cancer viruses in polio vaccines**. Dr. Hilleman was the developer of Merck's vaccine program. He developed over three dozen vaccines, more than any other scientist in history. He was a member of the U.S. National Academy of Science, the Institute of Medicine, the American Academy of Arts and Sciences and the American Philosophical Society. He even received a special lifetime achievement award from the World Health Organization…

Dr. W.B. Clark said in a New York Times interview in 1909: *"Cancer was practically unknown until the cowpox vaccination began to be introduced… <u>I have seen 200 cases of cancer, and never saw a case in an unvaccinated person.</u>"* Could *vaccines* be the primary reason for the massive surge in cancers throughout the Western world? Are vaccines compromising our immune system?

Cancer has *exploded* in the US since the introduction of these vaccines. Just before they released the new Salk polio vaccine in 1955, Bernice Eddy, a bacteriologist at the National Institute of Health (NIH), was told to safety-test it. When she tried it on her test monkeys, they became paralysed. She tried to delay the release of the vaccine, but a handful of prominent doctors stepped in to throw their weight on the side of the vaccine.

Dr. Alton Ochsner was a stockholder in one of the laboratories that produced the polio vaccine, and he was one of the past presidents of the American Cancer Society. He was so adamant about vaccinating the entire US population that he decided to publicly inoculate his own grandchildren with the vaccine in front of the faculty of Tulane Medical School. Ochsner's grandson died of polio within 48 hours and his granddaughter was crippled by it. Despite this tragedy, the mass inoculation proceeded on schedule and within days children fell sick from polio, some became crippled, and some died. It was the biggest fiasco in US medical history. A huge lawsuit erupted, the director of the NIH resigned, and the Secretary of Health, Education and Welfare stepped down.

In 1956 Bernice Eddy was taken off polio research and transferred to the influenza section. In 1959, confronted with overwhelming evidence, Eddy came to the conclusion: They had just inoculated AN ENTIRE GENERATION OF AMERICANS with cancer-causing monkey viruses! **She was the first to predict an epidemic of cancer in the future.**

This information was deemed CLASSIFIED by the US government. No information was to be given to the public about the cancer-causing viruses given to 200 million Americans…

In October 1960, Bernice Eddy gave a talk to the New York Cancer Society and, without warning the NIH in advance, announced that **she had examined monkey kidney cells in which the polio virus had grown, and found they were infected with cancer causing viruses,** *including* SV-40. She went on to forecast the coming cancer epidemic, to her stunned audience.

The suggestion that cancer-causing viruses were in the polio vaccine was NOT welcomed at the NIH. They crushed her professionally. They took away her lab, destroyed her animals, put her under a gag order, and delayed publication of her scientific papers.

Despite federal regulations ordering to remove SV-40 from vaccines in 1961, contaminated vaccines with SV-40 were administered to children and adults until they were used up… in 1965.

When scientists injected young hamsters with SV-40, over 80% developed brain cancers.

According to an article in *The Lancet,* **"SV-40 virus has been found in 43% of tumours from patients with non-Hodgkin's lymphoma.** *It has also been linked to brain, bone, and lung cancer."*

In a 1979 paper by doctors Farwell, Dohrmann, Marrett, and Meigs, they reported a substantial increase in childhood brain tumours, especially medullo-blastoma, when the mothers had been inoculated with vaccines containing SV-40.

SV-40 is repeatedly extracted from several types of tumours, including brain, bone, lung, and previously rare chest cancers. **20,000 children a year die from brain tumours that are found to contain the SV-40 virus**… People rarely exhibited brain tumours a hundred years ago.

Soft tissue Cancers started skyrocketing after the introduction of the Polio vaccine, increasing by 50% on average over a 16-year period: Lung cancer, Breast cancer, Prostate cancer, Lymphoma, Brain cancer, and Melanoma. Skin cancer increased 70%, Lymphoma 60%, Prostate 60%, Breast cancer 34%. Breast cancer cases in women jumped from 130,000 a year in 1978 to 180,000 a year in 1987. Men born between 1948 and 1957 have three times as much cancer as their parents.

Vaccines have been a major factor in what has caused all these cancers, but doctors can't talk about this because it constitutes *a crime against humanity perpetrated by the Medical Establishment.*

> "In the 1950s, SV40 was one of several dozen viruses that contaminated the original Salk and Sabin polio vaccines administered to children in the US and Europe."
>
> Journal of the National Cancer Institute, 1997

Fact #14: Vaccines Are Used to Covertly Depopulate Countries

A depopulation exercise was run in Mexico in 1974. The US *National Security Study Memorandum 200* highlighted the global population problem and urged governments to find ways to reduce the global population. **Depopulation was planned for 13 key countries, including India, Bangladesh, Pakistan, Nigeria, Mexico, Indonesia, Brazil, the Philippines, Thailand, Egypt, Turkey, Ethiopia and Colombia.** The document read, *"Perhaps the most significant population trend from the viewpoint of the United States is the prospect that Mexico's population will increase from 50 million in 1970 to over 130 million by the year 2000"* (note: it currently stands at 122 million, with a further 33 million in the US). To combat this problem, medical "sterilization teams" began injecting women all across Mexico with anti-fertility drugs disguised as vaccines. Anyone who pointed this out was immediately labelled "anti-science" and derided as ignorant. The same propaganda tactics are used today.

Fact #15: The Tetanus Vaccine Contains Sterilization a Chemical That Causes Miscarriages

Tetanus vaccines given to millions of young women in Kenya have been confirmed by laboratories to contain a sterilization chemical (HCG antigen) that causes miscarriages, reports the Kenya Catholic Doctors Association, a *pro*-vaccine organization. 2.3 million young girls and women were in the process of being given the vaccine, *pushed by UNICEF and the World Health Organization* (*note:* two thirds of the funding for the WHO comes from pharmaceutical companies).

The World Health Organization and its subsidiaries have been actively researching and funding the development of anti-fertility vaccines that prevent full-term pregnancies to take place, for over 20 years. There's even a Task Force on Birth Control Vaccines of the WHO! HCG-containing anti-fertility vaccines have been an aim of the Indian National Institute of Immunology and *The Population Council* of the Rockefeller

University for more than 20 years. A massive and suspicious mandatory vaccination program has also been carried out in Brazil, recently. The program is similar to other vaccination programs in recent years that have included a hidden sterilizing agent. The campaign mandates rubella vaccinations for all women ages 12 to 49, and 12 to 39 for men; a total of 70 million people, despite the fact that only 17 Brazilian children per year suffer from the disease...

Fact #16: Vaccines Cause Infertility

GlaxoSmithKline's Fluarix swine flu vaccine, among others, contains Polysorbate 80. A study done in Slovakia on female rats found that when newborn rats were injected with the substance within a week of birth, they developed hormonal changes, ovarian deformities, damage to the uterine lining, and infertility. The package insert for Fluarix mentions that the manufacturer cannot guarantee your fertility will be unharmed... *Would you feel comfortable being injected with a vaccine that contains a substance that has been strongly linked to infertility?* The Gardasil HPV vaccine has produced over 9,000 reports of problems since the vaccine's introduction in 2006, which include at least 28 spontaneous abortions, and 27 deaths. Between 2009 and 2010 flu vaccines increased foetal death reports by 4,250% in pregnant women.

Fact #17: Merck Insider Reveals Company Routinely Fabricated Lab Results to Fake Efficacy

Top virologists working for Merck have blown the whistle and gone public with shocking revelations that claim the company routinely fabricated lab results to claim a 95% efficacy rate of its mumps vaccine in order to continue receiving government contracts on a vaccine that didn't work.

The claimed **history of vaccine "successes" against polio and other diseases is a pure fabrication**. This is discussed and exposed in great detail in the powerful new book, *"Dissolving Illusions"* by Dr. Suzanne Humphries. Most of the so-called "reliable" research on vaccines is outright deception. In many cases, the same companies that *test* vaccines for safety... are the ones who sell them and make billions of dollars in profit each year! Talk about a conflict of interest...

Fact #18: Bill Gates' Polio Vaccine Program Caused 47,500 Cases of Paralysis and Death in 2011

Bill Gates, heavily invested in Monsanto's infertility-causing GMOs, hired the most beloved of Indian actors, Amitabh Bachchan, to promote the oral polio vaccine. The Oral Polio Vaccines were given to Indian children, and caused 47,500 cases of paralysis and deaths in 2011 alone. The CDC dropped the OPV from its vaccine schedule in the US because it was *causing* polio.

Fact #19: Bill Gates Has Publicly Stated That Vaccinations Can Lower The Global Population

It is interesting to note that Bill Gates' father was a leading proponent of the Eugenics movement that the Nazis espoused (promoting the sterilization of 'lesser races'). Bill Gates has said publicly that *'the world needs fewer people'* (he even gave a TED talk on the subject). He is heavily invested in GMO-producing and poison-producing Monsanto Corporation, he has recommended using vaccinations to lower the global population, and he is spending billions of dollars to that end.

His quote at TED: "The world today has 6.8 billion people... that's headed up to about 9 billion. Now **if we do a really great job on new vaccines [...] we could lower that by perhaps 10 or 15 percent**." He goes on to say: "If you gave me only one wish for the next 50 years -- ...I could pick a vaccine, which is something I love... -- this is the wish I would pick."

He is paying millions of dollars directly to magazines and newspapers to have them write positive articles about him and his foundation, and of course *omit* the truth about his vaccination programs.

Fact #20: Mercury-Filled Flu Shots Can Cause Alzheimer's

According to Hugh Fudenberg, MD, if an individual has had 5 consecutive flu shots between 1970 and 1980, their chances of getting Alzheimer's Disease is **10 times** higher than if they only had one, two, or no shots. Flu shots contain 25 micrograms of mercury, 250 times the EPA's safety limit.

Fact #21: The Rich & Informed Do Not Vaccinate Their Children; The Poor and Uneducated Do

Perhaps it is unsurprising that the highest rates of *unvaccinated* people are among the *rich and informed.* Conversely, the poorest and most uneducated segments of society are the most heavily vaccinated. Mississippi has the highest vaccination rate in the US, and perhaps unsurprisingly it also has the highest child mortality rate.

Fact #22: Deadly Peanut Allergies Are Caused By Vaccines

Have you ever wondered why so many kids these days are allergic to peanuts, when this was unheard of just a few decades ago? More than 1.5 million children in the US are allergic to peanuts.

'Peanut allergy' has suddenly emerged as the #1 cause of death from food reactions.

Injecting foreign protein in the blood is a universal trigger for allergic reaction. Many doctors in the early 1900s were dead set against vaccines because of the 'mass hypersensitivity' this produces.

According to Tim O'Shea in his article *Vaccines and The Peanut Allergy Epidemic*, it was soon found that additives called 'excipients' were necessary to prolong the effect of the antibiotic injected into the body. Without excipients, they found that penicillin's effect would only last about 2 hours. Refined oils worked best, acting as time-release capsules for the antibiotic.

Peanut oil became the favourite, because it worked well, and was available and inexpensive. Peanut oils were introduced as vaccine excipients in the mid-1960s. A newly patented ingredient containing peanut oil was added as an adjuvant to a new flu vaccine, in order to prolong the "immunity."

The first study of peanut allergies was not undertaken until 1973. It was a study of peanut excipients in vaccines. Soon afterwards, and as a result of the attention from that study, manufacturers were no longer required to disclose all the ingredients in vaccines – a blatant cover-up.

Following the enormous increase in vaccines on the Mandated Schedule in the US after 2001 (68 recommended vaccines), the peanut allergy soon reached epidemic proportions. Instead of researching the link between vaccines and peanut allergies, the media talk of how *"researchers are looking for a 'genetic link' to the dangerous childhood peanut allergy epidemic..."* (there is no genetic link – this is merely disinformation and propaganda).

Fact #23: The Polio Vaccine *Causes* Polio!

Didn't the polio vaccine save millions? History shows polio was caused by **pesticide exposure**, and was eradicated by the decline in DDT use – *NOT by the use of the polio vaccine.*

The population of New York in 1950 was fifteen million, and there were 13 polio cases and one polio death per 100,000 inhabitants. Hardly an epidemic. But Dr. Jonas Salk convinced the government to inoculate 97% of the American population with a culture grown in dead green monkeys from Africa. As the Salk vaccine program expanded, cases of paralytic polio began to increase. In 1959, more than 5,000 paralytic polio cases occurred. That's 50% *more* than in 1958, and 100% more than in 1957. This trend developed in spite of 300 million doses of Salk vaccine being administered in the US by the end of 1969. Six New England states reported increases in polio one year *after* the Salk vaccine.

In 1977, 20 years after the first polio inoculations, Salk testified before a Senate subcommittee that all polio outbreaks since 1961 were **caused** by the oral polio vaccine. In 1985, the CDC reported that 87% of the cases of polio in the USA between 1973 and 1983 *were caused by the vaccine* and most of the reported cases occurred in fully immunized individuals. Alarmingly, the CDC has admitted that the polio vaccine is the only known cause of polio in the USA today.

Recently, **GlaxoSmithKline was caught dumping 12 gallons of live, concentrated polio virus into a Belgian river!** That's the same company, by the way, that in 2012 was found guilty of conducting illegal vaccine trials in Argentina that led to the deaths of 14 babies.

Pesticide-contaminated milk was also responsible for polio outbreaks. Interestingly, milk-induced disease outbreaks were responsible for the later creation of milk pasteurization mandates. But it was the *pesticides* and their tolerance of polio virus, not the fact that milk was raw, that was responsible for spreading disease. And yet the belief that raw milk is dangerous is still prevalent today.

Fact #24: The 1918 'Spanish Influenza' Outbreak That Killed Millions Was Caused By Vaccines

Researchers recently uncovered a frightening truth regarding the 'Spanish influenza' outbreak of 1918 that killed more than 21 million people: the widespread disease was **the result of *forced vaccinations of millions of soldiers*** rather than an unfortunate incidence of contact with the Spaniards it was blamed on. The book *Swine Flu Exposé*, written by Eleanora McBean, Ph.D., covers the event in detail. The epidemic began in the barracks. Only one country, Greece, refused to accept these vaccinations, and no fatality was recorded in the country as a result.

Fact #25: The HPV Vaccine Doesn't Work *and* Accelerates Cancer

Researchers have reported that there is a lack of evidence that HPV vaccines prevent cervical cancer and there has been no evaluation of health risks associated with the vaccines. Furthermore, HPV has never been proven as a pathogen for any disease. As a matter of fact, studies show that over 90% of women have some form of HPV and in almost all those cases, **it goes away by itself.** Even the CDC's own website states, *"In most cases HPV goes away by itself before it causes any health problems."*

According to the National Vaccine Information Center, *"after Gardasil was licensed and three doses recommended for 11-12 year old girls and teenagers, there were thousands of reports of sudden collapse with unconsciousness within 24 hours, seizures, muscle pain and weakness, disabling fatigue, Guillain-Barré syndrome, facial paralysis, brain inflammation, rheumatoid arthritis, lupus, blood clots, optic neuritis, Multiple Sclerosis, strokes, heart and other serious health problems, including death, following receipt of Gardasil vaccine."*

It is likely that there have been close to 300,000 adverse reactions and over 1,000 deaths. 10% of Canadian females receiving HPV vaccines are sent to Emergency

Rooms following HPV vaccine injections. It turns out that studies actually show that not only does HPV *not* cause cervical cancer, the HPV vaccine itself *does*. Are you ready for this? Gardasil appears to **increase** cancer by 44.6% in folks who were already carriers of the same HPV strains used in the vaccine. The vaccine, in other words, may accelerate the development of cancer.

Fact #26: Vaccine-Induced 'Herd Immunity' Is a Lie Used to Frighten Doctors and The Public

Vaccination does NOT equal immunization, it does NOT lead to 'Herd Immunity', and in fact it *causes* many outbreaks. And yet repeatedly people tell me that doctors, teachers, and *other parents* coerce them into vaccinating their children, even if they don't want to. They bow down to peer pressure. Threats are made of *'social services taking away'* their kids if they don't vaccinate them. Some schools won't accept unvaccinated children. In Australia, those who refuse to vaccinate their kids will be denied as much as $11,000 in childcare rebates and welfare under new rules by the Federal Government. In the US, paediatricians might refuse to tend to your child if they are not vaccinated.

Dr. Russell Blaylock MD says: *"Vaccine-induced herd immunity is a lie used to frighten doctors, public-health officials, other medical personnel, and the public into accepting vaccinations."*

Fact #27: Vaccinations Cause Mini-Strokes in Children

Dr. Andrew Moulden quit his medical career in 2007, despite his sizable $500,000-a-year salary, stating **"vaccines produced the most profound damage to humankind in the history of humanity."** He died, and was likely murdered, in 2013, prior to a class-action suit against vaccine manufacturers going ahead. Dr. Moulden discovered the link between vaccines and a wide variety of serious health conditions including autism, which he showed are caused by cranial mini-strokes that produce abnormal facial features clearly visible after vaccination. He asserted: *"All vaccines cause harm."*

Fact #28: The Hepatitis B Vaccine Is Linked To Multiple Sclerosis, Arthritis, and Guillain-Barré

The Hepatitis B vaccine is associated with an increased risk of Multiple Sclerosis, according to the medical journal *Neurology* (2004 September 14). This vaccination is associated with the rare autoimmune neurological condition *transverse myelitis*. Hepatitis B vaccinations significantly increases the risk of a wide range of autoimmune diseases, according to the medical journal *Autoimmunity* (June 2005). Adult rubella and adult Hepatitis B vaccines were linked to chronic arthritis. In the US, the highest numbers of cases of Guillain-Barré syndrome are associated with Flu and Hepatitis B vaccines (Journal of Clinical Neuromusculature, Sept. 2009). There were also 69 reports of the

Guillain-Barré Syndrome after the Gardasil HPV vaccinations that occurred in the US between 2006 and 2009.

Fact #29: Vaccines May Be Causing The 'Autoimmune' Disease Epidemic

Autoimmune diseases include Lupus, Multiple Sclerosis, Type 1 Diabetes, Arthritis, Parkinson's, Fibromyalgia, Chronic Fatigue Syndrome, Celiac disease, Addison's disease, Crohn's disease, Ulcerative colitis, Endometriosis, Graves Disease, Lyme disease, Sjogren's disease, Kawasaki syndrome, Ankylosing spondylitis, Autism, and nearly 100 other diseases.

Dr. John Bergman blames vaccines for this 'autoimmune' epidemic. He says: *"With 69 different vaccines injected into children... well, we now see a response in our bodies and a massive rise in inflammatory brain disorders like encephalitis and autism, or inflammatory lung disorders, like Asthma; inflammatory sinus issues like sinusitis; inflammatory gut reactions like colitis and IBS, etc.".* The *Journal of Autoimmunity* (February 2000) states: *"Even though the data regarding the relation between vaccination and autoimmune disease is conflicting, some autoimmune phenomena are clearly related to immunisation."*

Fact #30: The AIDS Epidemic Was Created By Man-Made Vaccines

In 1978-1981 the gay population of New York and a specific area in Western Africa – coincidentally two locations where bioweapons manufacturers Litton Bionetics have laboratories – were given vaccines against the Hepatitis B virus, containing mutated simian viruses. Shortly thereafter, those people who had been vaccinated experienced a dramatic collapse of their immune system. Robert Gallo – a former researcher at Litton Bionetics, who later worked for the CDC – claimed it was a new virus and named the disease 'AIDS'. Dr. Len Horowitz has revealed government documents showing that 'HIV' was a bioweapon developed for the US military *(Google his name for the full story!).*

Fact #31: High Ranking Members of Medical Establishment Warn Their Friends NOT To Vaccinate

A member of the Czech government, who deals with the heads of hospitals and leading doctors in his country, recently told me: *"High-level directors of hospitals and doctors tell me all the time: 'DON'T vaccinate your children. We are telling YOU this, but we can't tell this to the public'."* They tell lies to the public, to protect themselves from legal repercussions.

Fact #32: At Least 30% of Vaccines Are Contaminated With Autism-Causing Retroviruses

In 2011, Dr. Judy Mikovits, a biochemist and molecular biologist with more than 33 years of experience, who served as the director of the lab of Antiviral Drug Mechanisms at the National Cancer Institute, found that at least 30% of vaccines are contaminated with gammaretroviruses. These retroviruses are known to cause **autism**, **chronic fatigue syndrome**, **Parkinson's**, **Lou Gehrig's disease**, and **Alzheimer's**. She was threatened and told to destroy her data; she refused. She was fired, arrested, and issued with a gag order! She has been released, and is now revealing the truth.

Fact #33: The Truth About Vaccines is Suppressed in The Media

The mainstream media receives billions of dollars a year in advertising revenue from the drug companies selling you vaccines. If they were to even *mention* stories of children hurt or killed by vaccines those advertising dollars would be withdrawn. They have a massive financial incentive in covering up this holocaust that is harming millions of children around the world. Ask yourself, *"Why don't these vaccine failures regularly make the news?"*

* * * * * * * * * * * * * * * * * * *

Note: I highly recommend you watch the documentary *'Vaxxed'*. **Do not believe doctors who tell you that** *"the science on vaccines has been settled"* **or that** *"vaccines are safe"* or that these facts are "anti-science". This is propaganda from pharmaceutical companies – *who routinely fabricate test data and routinely bribe government officials* – that doctors are merely repeating verbatim without questioning the source of their information. The smartest and wealthiest people do not vaccinate their children without being highly circumspect first. They definitely do not vaccinate from a young age (before the immune system has a chance to develop), or with vaccine "cocktails" (e.g. the MMR vaccine), or with multiple vaccines in a short timespan, or with vaccines known to cause major health problems, or with vaccines containing mercury! For example, the Tetanus shot is probably safe, but make sure you read the insert to check that it does not contain Thimerosal, mercury, or formaldehyde, and make sure your child gets a major dose of Vitamin C beforehand.

Recap – The Truth About Vaccinations:

❑ Better sanitation and living conditions improved people's health in the 1900s, *not* vaccines.

❑ Vaccines do *not* confer immunity. They don't work. Vaccine-induced 'Herd Immunity' is a lie. Vaccinated children are *not* immunized against that particular disease. On the contrary, vaccines often *cause* infectious outbreaks.

❑ Pharmaceutical companies routinely fabricate lab results to fake efficacy, and routinely bribe officials to get drugs approved for sale. This is actually the norm, rather than the exception.

❑ Vaccines *harm* children's immune system. Vaccinated children are 5 times more likely to contract a disease than unvaccinated children.

❑ Vaccinated children are 19 times more likely to develop autism than unvaccinated children.

❑ Many vaccines are designed *to cause cancer* later in life.

❑ Vaccinations routinely kill children, but this is suppressed by the media. The truth about vaccines is suppressed by the media, who depend on the pharmaceutical industry's advertising dollars.

❑ Vaccinated children have a much higher infant mortality rate.

❑ Mercury in vaccines causes brain damage, mental retardation, and Alzheimer's.

❑ Vaccines are used for 'national security' purposes to covertly sterilize millions of women in Third World countries, to 'reduce the global population'.

❑ Vaccines cause infertility and miscarriages in the Developed World as well.

❑ The handful of media conglomerates are owned by the same families that own the pharmaceutical conglomerates.

❑ Pharmaceutical companies pay millions of dollars a year to online 'PR & disinformation agents' so that positive articles about their vaccines are at the top of search engines, and so that people sharing the truth about vaccines are discredited, attacked, and 'neutralized' by character-assassination techniques.

❑ Vaccines generate $25 billion a year in profits for the pharmaceutical industry.

❑ The main purpose of vaccination programs is to wipe out people's immune system, who then become Big Pharma's 'patients for life'. The secondary purpose of vaccination programs is to reduce the global population, through lowered fertility and reduced lifespans.

CHAPTER 5

The Truth About "Autoimmune" Disorders

Autoimmune diseases include Lupus, Multiple Sclerosis, Type 1 Diabetes, Rheumatoid Arthritis, Parkinson's, Fibromyalgia, Chronic Fatigue Syndrome, Celiac disease, Addison's disease, Crohn's disease, Ulcerative colitis, Dermatitis, Endometriosis, Graves Disease, Lyme disease, Sjogren's disease, Kawasaki syndrome, Ankylosing spondylitis, Autism spectrum disorders, and nearly 100 other known diseases. It affects one in twelve people in the US (some 24 million Americans). Women are eight times more likely to have an "autoimmune" disease than breast cancer, for example. Rates of Type 1 Diabetes have increased 5-fold in the past 40 years.

Wikipedia informs us that *"Autoimmune diseases arise from an abnormal immune response of the body against substances and tissues normally present in the body"*. The only problem is… that this is hogwash. A lie. Total and complete fabrication. "Autoimmune" is pure propaganda designed to hide the truth. The body is *not* attacking itself nor is it having an "abnormal" response against substances "normally present" in the body. In truth, the body is literally *fighting for its life* against the toxic man-made substances that are wreaking havoc on our health. Calling it "autoimmune" puts the blame on *you* rather than on Big Pharma and Big Industry, and gives the Medical Mafia a perfect excuse to sell you more drugs while never addressing the real underlying issue.

The "Autoimmune disease" phenomenon is spreading so fast in <u>industrialised</u> nations that scientists have dubbed it *"The Western disease"*. But "autoimmune" diseases were incredibly rare before 1940. So why have they been skyrocketing since then? What has changed?

According to Dr. John Bergman, the body is <u>responding appropriately to environmental stimuli</u>. Environmental factors are the key to understanding the "autoimmune diseases" phenomenon.

This is what has changed dramatically since the 1940s:

- ❑ 69 different vaccines are now injected into children
- ❑ Thousands of new pharmaceutical drugs are now prescribed, with deadly side-effects. Even *children* are now given antidepressants.

- ❏ Genetically Modified Foods (GMO), untested on humans, are now in our food supply.

- ❏ Thousands of toxic pesticides are used on our crops.

- ❏ Thousands of toxic additives and chemicals are present in processed foods.

- ❏ Antibiotics, sex hormones, rBGH growth hormones, etc. are found in our meat and our water!

- ❏ Thousands of toxic chemicals are found in our beauty and personal care products.

- ❏ More recently, depleted Uranium used in the Middle East, Fukushima radiation in Japan, etc.

But interestingly enough, **governments are not looking into environmental factors**. Why? Because it is not to the benefit of Big Pharma, Big Food, and Big Industry, whose interests the governments *actually* serve and protect. The result is a disease holocaust that brings more and more patients to the medical establishment and more profits to the pharmaceutical companies.

It is particularly interesting to note that vaccines are designed to trigger an *inflammatory* response in the body. That is how they are *supposed* to work. Dr. Bergman puts the blame for the "autoimmune" epidemic squarely on the shoulders of the Vaccine industry: *"With 69 different vaccines injected into children... well, we now see a response in our bodies and a massive rise in* **inflammatory brain disorders** *like encephalitis and autism. Or inflammatory lung disorders, like Asthma, and inflammatory sinus issues like sinusitis, and inflammatory gut reactions like colitis and IBS, etc."*

Dr. John Bergman also points out that *obesity* is an inflammatory response as well, and vaccines might explain the massive surge in obesity in America. The body is retaining water to dilute this toxicity and is storing away the excess toxicity in *fat tissue*. This protects the cells in the rest of the body from inflammation, irritation, mutation, and eventually death.

He states that red meat, fats including butter, margarine, and oil, fried foods, sugary foods, highly processed foods and pre-packaged foods also cause inflammation in the body.

Dr. Bergman gives the example of a 14-year-old girl that came in to see him with her mom. She had been diagnosed with rheumatoid arthritis and fibromyalgia, and her mother wanted to put her on disability. She had received the full schedule of vaccinations; her diet was the "Standard American Diet" (SAD); her mother had nutritional deficiencies when the girl was in the womb; and finally, Pitocin was used at birth, to induce labour, and this chemical damaged the child further.

It is these kinds of factors that result in us having **the sickest generation of children ever**. In fact, the overall health of American children has been declining for more than fifty years:

- ❏ 97% of children were healthy in the late 1960s
- ❏ 94% of children were healthy in the late 1970s
- ❏ 88% of children were healthy in 1994
- ❏ 74% of children were healthy in 2006
- ❏ 26% of American children will suffer at least *one* chronic illness over their lifetime
- ❏ Since the mid-1990s America's infant mortality has *increased* and life span has *plummeted*.

Strengthening the immune system is a better approach than looking to using drugs. Dr. Bergman concludes his lecture with the following list of things that *weaken* our immune system and therefore make us more susceptible to disease:

What Makes Your Immune System Weak

- ❏ Overuse of antibiotics
- ❏ Vaccinations / Immunizations
- ❏ Radiation
- ❏ Blood Transfusions
- ❏ Pharmaceutical drugs, e.g. Ibuprofen, etc.
- ❏ Poisoned air, poisoned water, and poisoned food
- ❏ Prolonged stress
- ❏ Toxic cosmetics
- ❏ Toxic living environments; toxic work environments (e.g. hairdressing salon)
- ❏ Fear
- ❏ Toxic family members
- ❏ The treatment against "autoimmune" diseases! The treatment of autoimmune diseases is typically with immunosuppression—medication that *decreases* the immune response!

How To Eliminate 97% Of All Diseases – Dr. John Bergman

❑ Get deep, restful sleep every night; Go to sleep early.

❑ Change your diet to one of whole, organic foods.

❑ Consume good Omega 3 fats.

❑ Consume high antioxidant foods, e.g. organic blueberries, cranberries, blackberries, raspberries, strawberries, cherries, beans, and artichokes.

❑ Consume resveratrol – it is present in red wine, whole grape skins, grape seeds, raspberries, mulberries.

❑ Use Coconut oil.

❑ Do NOT consume GMOs.

❑ Do NOT consume Non-Organic Grains and Wheat.

❑ Do NOT consume Commercial Dairy.

❑ Get lots of Vitamin D3 (at least 3000 IUs per 100lbs of weight)

❑ Get Lugol's Iodine.

❑ Get Vitamin C with Bioflavinoids.

❑ Get lots of fresh organic veggie juice.

❑ Exercise regularly

❑ Eliminate chemicals and toxins from your life, e.g. toxic household cleaners, soaps, air fresheners, bug sprays, lawn pesticides, insecticides, etc.

❑ Avoid pharmaceutical drugs – these drugs kill thousands of people every year.

❑ Avoid chargrilling or frying your food. Instead, use moist heat, boil or steam, use lower temperatures to cook, use crock pots, and eat raw fruits, vegetables, and whole grains. Dry heat promotes Advanced Glycation End-product formation (which causes inflammation) by more than 10 to 100-fold above uncooked foods.

I encourage you to watch Dr. John Bergman's lectures online, and also encourage you to watch Dr. Randall E. Tent's lecture titled *"The Exploding Autoimmune Epidemic".* He also agrees that *vaccinations* are to blame for this "Autoimmune Epidemic". He reveals the history of how **new pathogens were created in bioweapon laboratories in America and then injected into tens of millions of people in the US and around the world under the guise of vaccination to test their efficacy.** It is these live pathogens, he claims, that are causing diseases and therefore normal immune responses in our bodies. However, because governments can *never* admit to this – they would lose any and all trust from the people – they have to call it an "autoimmune" disorder. In other words, they must convince you that *your body is messing up for no good reason.*

CHAPTER 6

The Quality of Your Health Depends On The Health of Your Cells

Your body is truly a divine miracle of self-healing technology. Your body originated from *a single cell* (the fertilized egg cell), and your *adult* body consists of **100 trillion cells**, working together in perfect harmony every second of the day without you even having to *think* about it. Every second three million cells die in your body... and that same second three million *new* cells are created!

Your cells are the tiny building blocks of life: these tiny powerhouses are what keep us energized and alive, and they must be *nurtured*. Cells are very sensitive little devices protected by an extremely fragile outer membrane, and they weaken and break down when exposed to toxic chemicals, pollutants, pesticides, pharmaceutical drugs, and electromagnetic interference (power lines, cell phones, Wi-Fi, electronic devices). Stress, fear, resentment, and depression also weaken them.

Understand *this*: **as the health of your *cells* go, *you* go.** If you want to be healthy, the key question you should be asking yourself is: *"What do I need to do to ensure optimum health at a cellular level?"*

To remain healthy and strong, **your cells need oxygen and nutrients**, which they use to produce the Adenosine Triphosphate (ATP) that powers your body, like tiny little power plants. Your cells also fulfil their specific function within the body. For example, red blood cells carry oxygen; nerve cells carry nerve impulses to different parts of the body; female reproductive cells (egg) join with the male cell and provide food for the new cell that is being formed; white blood cells (leukocyte) are part of your immune system and protect the body against infectious disease and foreign invaders; etc.

These *trillions* of chemical reactions within your body (using oxygen and nutrients as fuel) create *waste*, and therefore, to remain healthy, **your cells require the ability to eliminate their own waste**. Otherwise, this toxicity would build up in your body, pollute your bloodstream, slow down the flow of oxygen, attract an excess of bacteria, fungi, parasites, and other microforms, and weaken your cells. Microforms like bacteria and 'viruses' *thrive* in an acidic environment. They multiply, they feed on your waste, and contribute to creating *even more* toxic waste in your system. So your cells need oxygen and nutrients, and the ability to eliminate their own waste. Your bloodstream – the 'river of life' – **carries oxygen and nutrients to every cell in your body**, while your lymphatic system *drains* the waste that is produced. Your body then *eliminates* toxicity through your colon and urinary tract, your lungs and respiratory tract (phlegm, throwing up), and your largest eliminatory organ: the skin (sweat, acne, etc.). While your bloodstream has a pump (the heart) the lymphatic system does not, and requires physical movement to get it flowing. This is why exercising daily cleanses your body and helps keep you healthy.

The Germ Theory Fallacy

We've been taught that germs cause disease. That is false. The truth is, you *need* germs. In fact, you are filled with millions of them right now! Germs are scavengers; you will find germs any place you can find a tremendous amount of *waste*, **because they are nature's way of 'cleaning up'.**

Louis Pasteur came up with the *theory of germs* in the 1800s. He had noticed with his microscope that when you opened up dead people, there were plenty of germs and micro-organisms inside of them. So he concluded, *"There's the cause of disease! Germs!"* From then on conventional medicine has operated on the mistaken supposition that germs and viruses *cause* disease. The entire medical and pharmaceutical establishment is based on this erroneous theory. Pasteur had made a classic scientific error: *'correlation is not causation'*. Just because two things occur together, it does not mean that one *caused* the other. Even Pasteur, on his deathbed, admitted that he was wrong about germs *causing* illness, stating **"the microbe is nothing, the terrain is everything,"** but by then it was too late. The germ theory had taken hold and moved into mainstream science.

If you put rats in a clean place where there is no food... they won't be sticking around for long. Rats are attracted to a certain place only when there's 'junk' there for them to feed on! They then grow, multiply, and add to the filth by creating their own waste. The same happens with your inner terrain. You must make sure that you do not have a compromised (read: 'dirty', 'toxic') inner terrain. Germs feed on the dead matter that we create in our bodies through our modern *unnatural* way of living.

Germs *do* play a role in your *"dis-ease"*, but they cannot do it on their own. If your body no longer has much energy, you don't detoxify regularly, and you create an environment where germs proliferate to a tipping point of imbalance, then it is only natural that you experience 'dis-ease'.

You really don't have to be afraid of *"bugs"*. **If you want to be afraid of something, then fear an unhealthy lifestyle!** A lot of people have germs and viruses inside of them, but nothing ever happens to them. Since there is no such thing in science as a cause without an effect, germs *cannot* be the cause of disease. And yet I guarantee you that when you open your newspaper on January 1ˢᵗ – after the Christmas and New Year excesses you've subjected your body to – you are going to hear again about that dangerous 'flu virus' coming to get you, and how you should get your flu shots...

Let's think about this rationally. If you took *a poison* and put it into your bloodstream, your body would do whatever it takes to get it *out* of the body in the fastest way possible, right? It would use any elimination channel available, to preserve the integrity of your system. It might resort to fever (increasing your body temperature to sweat out the poison), acne, diarrhoea, throwing up, etc.

In fact, your body will use up every ounce of energy to *fight* the poison. Your body would shut down your digestive system, to focus all your energy towards getting rid of the poison. Your body might restrict blood flow to your brain to avoid the toxicity reaching that delicate and vital organ. As a result, you might experience headaches. You might also experience low energy, fatigue, joint pains, inability to sleep, kidney problems, convulsions, burping, irritations, etc. Right?

Now... do you know of any disease that does *not* have these symptoms?

A lot of so-called diseases are nothing more than your body dealing with *how toxic* your lifestyle has made it. But there's no money in educating people about having a healthier lifestyle. It is infinitely more profitable for pharmaceutical companies to spend billions of dollars in advertising and PR, to convince you that you are fragile, weak, and under attack from 'bugs', 'germs', and exotic 'viruses'.

"Yep, that 'flu season' is coming. Ain't nothing to do with your *lifestyle*, it's that 'bug' coming to get you. Because, if it's your lifestyle, then you might have to be 'responsible'. Plus, we can't sell you anything if it's your lifestyle. In fact, you might not even buy some of the things we have... if that were true! So we must continue to make sure you feel fragile and remind you that it is not you or your lifestyle, it's these *bugs* coming to get you..."

Anthony Robbins, *Living Health*

The True Cause of Disease: A Deficiency of Force

Dr. Isaac Jennings was a famous allopathic medical doctor in the late 1890s. Faced with a shortage of drugs in his city one day, all he could do was tell his patients to go home, rest, and drink lots of fluids. *Miracle of miracles, these people got well, without any medicine!* This caused him to question his beliefs and his medical education. He begun to ask new questions, which drove him to look at other possibilities. He had been fortunate enough to escape his 'conditioning'.

He decided to conduct an experiment. He was going to treat people just with some instructions about their lifestyle, and placebos. He had began to notice that his patients were just *'run down'* (they lacked energy), so he simply told his patients to do things that would allow them to build up some nerve energy: *get some rest, exercise, and drink lots of water to cleanse your system.*

According to Jennings, disease is due to a "Deficiency of Force". In other words, lowered *energy.*

Dr. Jenning's results with his patients were simply astounding. *Without* the use of medicine. Yet, instead of winning a Nobel Prize for his discoveries, Dr. Jennings was violently attacked, sued, and ridiculed by the pharmaceutical industry-funded "Medical Establishment".

Now, we *ALL* know that **our body heals itself.** But we have been *programmed* to rush to the doctor and inject a load of toxic chemicals into our bloodstream whenever we feel unwell...

> "Twenty-five years in which I used prescribed drugs, and 33 years in which I have not used prescribed drugs, should make my belief that drugs are unnecessary and in most cases injurious, worth something to those who care to know the truth."
>
> John H. Tilden, M.D. (1940)

This is how disease occurs: You work hard, over-exert yourself, eat junk food (with no nutritional value), and as a result you develop a lowered level of resistance *("enervation")*. Your body does not have enough energy to make everything work (a "Deficiency of Force"). But no matter what, it *must* constantly make your heart pump and your blood flow, so it shuts down your process of elimination. When you are not eliminating efficiently, waste builds up inside of you. Your nerve energy drops, and your toxin levels build up. *At this point the body's integrity is being challenged. Your body has to*

74

react or else you are not going to survive. Your body does whatever it can to get rid of the toxicity (this is what most people term 'disease', when in fact it is the *cure* to *the real underlying problem!)*

Because we've bought into the current 'cultural hypnosis', we ingest *more* chemical toxins and we try to stop these poisons from coming out of our body. We try to stop the fever. We try to stop the mucus coming out of our nose… Your body is ejecting poisons out of you, and you're pushing them back in! Not allowing that toxicity out of the body only results in one thing: more enervation, more build-up of toxins and eventually… *a major health problem!*

Most of us mistakenly think that the symptom IS the illness. **What you *truly* need to examine is *THE SOURCE* of the disease.** Your 'disease' is nothing but a *symptom* – a warning sign. Jennings found that when the natural strength of the body is depleted, it no longer has the energy to protect and heal itself. What *really* causes us to become ill is therefore the fact that you lack the energy to defend yourself from disease. Therefore, to be truly healthy you need plenty of ENERGY, and to have plenty of energy, you need to take really good care of… your cells!

The Importance of Alkalinity (The pH Miracle)

Since all metabolic reactions and nerve signals are dependent on the pH level of your blood, your bloodstream **must remain at a pH of 7.36**, which is slightly alkaline. At this level the blood is also ideally supplied with oxygen. <u>In order to survive, your body will do whatever it takes to maintain the proper acid/alkaline (pH) balance.</u>

The American microbiologist Robert O. Young, Ph.D. is the author of the best-selling book *The pH Miracle: Balance Your Diet, Reclaim Your Health.* Dr. Young's scientific findings have led him to a philosophy known as *The New Biology.* Simply put, the New Biology states that there is only **One Sickness and One Disease**, and that "this one 'sickness' is the over-acidification of the body due primarily to an inverted way of living, thinking, and eating."

This over-acidification leads to "the over-growth in our body of micro-organisms (such as yeast and fungi) whose poisons produce the symptomologies that medical science refers to as *'disease'.*"

Dr. Young has found that when the body is in a healthy alkaline balance, toxic micro-organisms – such as germs, bacteria, viruses, yeasts, fungi, moulds – are unable to get a foothold.

An over-abundance of these toxic microorganisms leads to the *symptoms* we view as disease: fever, throwing up, acne, sweat, diarrhoea, headaches, low energy, joint pains, inability to sleep, fatigue, kidney problems, convulsions, burping, irritations, etc.

What's great is that *you have the power* to stop these symptoms in a matter of days, by alkalizing and cleansing your inner environment.

UNHEALTHY BLOOD   **HEALTHY BLOOD**

Live Blood microscopy conducted by Dr. Robert O. Young; notice how red blood cells slam into each other when they find themselves in an acidic environment (top left picture), impeding the flow of oxygen and nutrients.

Alkalinity Maintains Your Inner Electro-Magnetic Conductivity

Electro-magnetic current is what actually runs our body. It is through tiny electro-magnetic pulses that nerve signals are sent through your body and nutrients are passed on to every cell in your body. Our pH balance of 7.36 allows for the conductivity of electro-magnetic power throughout our body. That electrical power is created by our internal biochemistry. This is a very delicate balance, and *acid* coursing through our system breaks it down completely. *In order to maintain this powerful electric current inside of us, our body MUST maintain a pH of 7.36 constantly.* In fact, this is so important, that if this were to change by just a couple of points, it would alter your chemistry so radically that **your entire system would simply shut down**. You would die instantly.

76

An Acidic Inner Terrain Destroys Your Energy Levels

Your blood is your *'river of life'*, bringing oxygen and nutrients to every cell in your body. It *must* remain at a pH of 7.36 in order to be able to continue doing so. You see, it is your red blood cells that carry the oxygen through your body, and the outside of each blood cell has a negative (-) electrical charge. This keeps the blood cells from sticking together (they constantly repel one another).

An acidic environment *strips* these negative electrical charges from your red blood cells and as a result **the blood cells start to slam into each other, clumping together** (see picture above), moving slower and ripping apart (remember, cells are very sensitive little devices). With the blood cells sticking together, they now go through the bloodstream more slowly and less oxygen and nutrients flow through your body. As a result, **your energy goes through the floor**.

An Acidic Inner Terrain Leads to Inflammation, Arthritis, Multiple Sclerosis, Diabetes, and Obesity

Since your survival depends on your blood maintaining a pH of 7.36, your body will do *whatever it takes* to maintain this balance. First, it will use up your stores of alkalinity – 'Alkaline buffers' – to neutralise the acids. But it takes 10 parts of alkalinity to neutralise 1 part of acid, and you will soon use up these reserves if you keep putting in more 'acid' than your body can deal with. Once you've depleted your reserves, you are at risk of developing a major *"dis-ease"* in your body.

Your body also takes the acids out of the bloodstream and away from the vital organs of the body by storing it in fatty tissues. This leads to **weight gain**. Your body will also *leach the alkaline calcium and magnesium* from your bones to bind it to the acid. This leads to **Multiple Sclerosis**. Your body also coats your arteries with **cholesterol** *to protect them* from the excess acidity coursing through your veins.

When your cells are constantly exposed to a toxic environment, they first get irritated, then they weaken, and eventually they die. If this occurs in your joints, and you start feeling pain, doctors label this 'arthritis'. By the way, whenever you see a medical condition that ends in '-itis' it simply means 'inflammation'. And *'árthron'* means 'joint' in Greek. So a doctor notices that you have pain in your joints, and he labels this… *"inflammation of the joints!"* Well, heck, that's a great name, doc, but what is *causing* this inflammation? *"We don't know"* is their answer. What is the cure? *"We don't know, but here are some drugs so that you don't feel the pain!"* That's brilliant, doc!

It is the same with **Colitis** (inflammation of the colon), **Sinusitis** (inflamed sinuses), **Meningitis** (the membranes that line the skull), **Cystitis, Bronchitis, Dermatitis, Gastritis, Hepatitis**, Mastitis, Poliomyelitis, etc. Doctors are seeing an inflammation of your cells in a particular part of your body, and instead of asking *why* is there inflammation in your body in the first place – **what is the source of the toxicity that**

is causing this inflammation? – they give it a Greek name which makes it sound vaguely scientific and gives the patient the *illusion* that the doctor knows what's going on. But nothing could be further from the truth! These words are used by doctors to **give a label** to a disease. This way, it is much easier to prescribe pharmaceutical drugs to an unquestioning patient…

An Acidic Inner Terrain Leads To The Destruction Of Your Cells

As the environment becomes more and more acidic, your cells weaken and die, releasing their waste into the bloodstream. This compounds the problem. Cells are now being destroyed more rapidly, and as all that acid builds up, your inner environment gets more and more polluted and compromised. Germs start to multiply rapidly – bacteria, yeast, fungus, and moulds – because you have created a feeding ground for them. This deteriorates until pretty soon you start experiencing pains and aches.

You are well on your way to experiencing debilitating diseases and ageing…

If, after continued irritation and inflammation, your cells die *en masse*, they are collected into little 'sacks' by your white blood cells, until the body has enough energy to break them down and eliminate them naturally. Conventional (Western) medicine labels this 'cancer'.

Keiichi Morishita writes in his book *Hidden Truth of Cancer* that as blood starts to become acidic, cells in your body weaken and die. However, some of these cells may adapt to that environment by *mutating* into 'abnormal' cells. Doctors label these as being 'malignant cells' – also known as *'cancer'.*

Since we now know that cancer cells thrive in an acidic bloodstream that is low in oxygen (because toxicity turns your blood to an acidic 'sludge' that strips it of oxygen), it stands to reason that the opposite conditions (an alkaline pH and oxygen) reverses the condition.

According to Dr. Robert Young, *"A chronically over-acidic body pH corrodes body tissue,* **slowly eating into the 60,000 miles of our veins and arteries like acid eating into marble.** *If left unchecked, it will interrupt all cellular activities and functions, from the beating of your heart to the neural firing of your brain. Over-acidification interferes with life itself, leading to all sickness and disease."*

Dr. Robert O. Young also explains in his lectures how…

❑ **Diabetes** is due to the breakdown of the pancreas by an over-acidification of your system. You "do" Diabetes with your lifestyle, and can reverse this condition in 90 to 120 days.

- ❑ **Psoriasis**, **Dermatitis**, and **Eczema** are simply acid coming out directly through your skin.

- ❑ Inflammation of the cells of your digestive tract leads to **Colitis, Crohn's Disease**, and '*Irritable Bowel Syndrome*'.

- ❑ **Multiple Sclerosis** is a symptom of acidity attacking your myelin sheaths *(the insulating envelope of myelin that surrounds the core of a nerve fiber)*.

- ❑ **Allergies** are due to acid irritating your tissues, making them sensitive to dust, pollen, etc.

- ❑ Most **"genetic diseases"** are not genetic at all. In most instances we simply adopt the same values and duplicate the lifestyles and dietary habit of the people we grew up with.

What Creates an Over-Acidic Inner Terrain?

Pollution, pharmaceutical drugs, recreational drugs, sugar (sugar metabolizes into acid), coffee, alcohol, tobacco, refined carbohydrates (bread, pasta, rice, potatoes, white flour, etc.), all processed foods, fruit juices, soft drinks, peanut butter, dairy products (milk, cheese, ice cream), meat products, eggs, cooked oils, all metabolize into acid in the body.

You *alkalize* your inner terrain by cutting out these acid-forming habits and foods, and eating a lot more organic **green vegetables** and salads. The general rule of thumb is to eat 20% acid foods and 80% alkaline foods. Some excellent alkaline-forming foods are: lemon juice (although acidic to the taste, it metabolizes to an alkaline 'ash'), most raw vegetables and fruits, wheatgrass, barley grass, figs, lima beans, olive oil, honey, miso, green tea, most herbs, sprouted grains, and sprouts (see full list of alkaline foods here: www.rense.com/1.mpicons/acidalka.htm).

CHAPTER 7

Disease Starts In The Mind

The British health researcher Richard Moat spent two decades compiling his 'Encyclopaedia' of psychoneuroimmunology, listing the specific psychological and emotional states that manifest outwardly as diseases and illnesses. I attended a seminar of his in 2005. When he took to the stage, after introducing himself and explaining a bit about his work, he asked the audience if anyone there was suffering from a serious health condition. A few people put their hand up. He pointed to a lady in the front row, and asked her about her condition. She informed him that she had breast cancer.

Breast Cancer Revealed Where She Had Not Been Loving

"Which breast?" he enquired. "The left one" she replied. He paused for a moment, thinking it over, and then proceeded to ask her: *"Which significant **female** person in your family did you have a major falling out with… approximately two years ago?"*

The woman was taken aback. "How did you… how could you know…" she said, stuttering. "I had a huge argument with my mother two years ago, and we haven't spoken since!".

Richard's research points to the fact that breast cancer emanates from – or begins with – a mind pattern of anger, inter-family feuding, separation, low self-worth, self-devaluing, putting others first, unfulfillment, sexual shame, and conflicted feelings. This mind pattern leads to a specific weakness in a woman's body, which in time may manifest itself as *breast cancer*. Clear the mind-pattern, using love, forgiveness, and understanding… and you don't need to express that outcome anymore. The breast cancer may be a way for your body's innate intelligence (your soul, the Universe…) to communicate to you where you have not being loving in your life.

The modern medical establishment would advise chemotherapy or surgery to 'cut out the cancer'. This is often ineffective. Why? Because even if you successfully 'remove' the 'cancer', <u>unless you change your mind-pattern the cancer comes back <i>stronger than before</i></u> within 2-3 years, until you've learned the lesson you are here to learn. You must show more love, forgiveness, and understanding, towards yourself, for starters.

Stewart Swerdlow writes: "Anger is usually accompanied by frustration, violent behaviour, high blood pressure, digestion problems. Anger ultimately leads to physical and mental illness. It always results in relationship difficulties. Suppressed anger and frustration are one cause of cancer in the body."

He Developed Multiple Sclerosis After Seeing His Father Hang Himself

In 2012, I met a Greek woman in Melbourne, Australia. We spoke of her family, and she mentioned her husband, who suffered from Multiple Sclerosis. I told her "Hold on one minute", as I looked up Richard Moat's research on the subject. "Ah, there it is! Richard contests that the psycho-emotional patterns that manifest themselves as MS are: feeling trapped, inflexibility, stubbornness, feeling unsupported, suppressed emotions, polite exterior hiding bitterness, hardened or desensitised in order to avoid emotional suffering."

She broke down in tears. "How… could he have known… this describes my husband perfectly…"

At the age of six, her husband had witnessed his father commit suicide by hanging himself. The little boy had to rush into the house to call his mother and grandmother to help bring his father down…

All those decades of suppressed emotions, hardening himself to avoid the emotional pain of what he had witnessed, combined with the decision that he is 'all alone in the world, unsupported' – since the grownups can't provide safety even for themselves – manifested itself as this terrible disease.

Multiple Sclerosis is the label doctors give to the collection of symptoms that arise when the insulating covers of nerve cells in the brain and spinal cord fray away. That repeated mind pattern literally and physically *frays your nerves*.

Over and over again I was presented with proof about the validity of Richard's research. We are manifesting diseases and illnesses through our mind-patterns (check out www.richardmoat.com).

Fear of Childbirth and Female Sexuality Results in Endometriosis

One of my friends has suffered from Endometriosis, as well as Cystitis, since her teenage years. Of course, doctors have no idea what causes these conditions. She has been in constant pain recently. She tried everything. At the behest of her doctors, she has had a series of surgeries. Each time it only made the condition *worse*. They even wanted to *remove her uterus altogether*.

I then shared with her that according to Richard Moat, the psycho-emotional root causes of Endometriosis are likely to be one or more of: 'Wanting to have children but fearing the consequences of childbirth, maybe even fear dying in the process.

Significant males in your life (past or present) cause you to feel anguish about your sexuality or ability as a woman to be a Mum" (these are just *some* of the themes associated with Endometriosis, according to Richard's work).

We discussed this for a while, and suddenly she remembered something. Her grandmother had died at childbirth, in India, more than 60 years ago, when her father was only three years old. She described how "a million times" during her childhood, growing up in England, her father had told her, "*I don't want to lose you. I don't want to lose you.*" Traumatized as a child, his highly charged *fear of women dying at childbirth* had been seared into his daughter's subconscious from the moment she was born. And what better way *to make sure* you don't get pregnant, than to have Endometriosis (the main symptoms are pelvic pain and infertility), Cystitis, and a host of related conditions in your female organs, that affect your sex life, your relationships, and your ability to have children.

A *"significant male in her life"* – her father – had caused her to feel anguish about her sexuality and her ability to become a mother, out of his love for her and his *fear* of losing her to childbirth.

Dr. John Demartini states: "Whatever you disown in yourself you attract into your life in one form or another. You marry your disowned parts, have children that represent your disowned parts, become business partners with them, and attract them as clients and friends. Whatever you don't want to see or appreciate in yourself, you keep attracting into your life until you learn to love it."

Her father needed to come to terms with what happened to his mother, accept it, and even *'learn to love it'*. That is why his daughter is in his life – to help him *learn that lesson* and overcome that pain. I believe they will both be able to heal and move on, once this has been achieved.

It is interesting to note that some health websites state that "Pregnancy is the only thing that reliably cures Endometriosis, and it still provides relief even in those rare cases when endometriosis is not completely cured. The condition always stops when menopause begins." Well *duh!* Of course pregnancy or menopause "cures" the condition, since it implies coming to terms – or eliminating altogether – one's fear of getting pregnant! Some people even report that receiving the male ejaculate can lessen the symptoms... Again, no surprise there, as that act would imply this particular woman is less prone to *"anguish about her sexuality and her ability to become a mother"!*

Get It Off Your Chest!

One of my cousins was diagnosed at the age of 30 with a thymoma tumour the size of a grapefruit, in the center of his chest. We weren't close, and all I knew of his life was that he still lived with his parents, he had never held a job, and his mother had prevented him from taking one abroad, as per his wish, since him 'leaving her' to go abroad *"would have killed her"*.

I invited him over, and I explained *how we manifest health problems*, and what we can do to resolve health issues. I warned him that going ahead with the surgery, without *first* changing the mind pattern that had *caused the issue in the first place*, was not the answer. I feared that 2-3 years down the line, the 'message' would come in sharper focus, for example with a tumour that was not benign. I shared with him Richard Moat's insight into chest problems, specifically: *"a conflicted sense of identity, lack of self-expression and 'not getting something off your chest'."*

He listened politely for two hours, and thanked me for my concern, but I could tell that I had not gotten through to him. His sister told me that he is too stubborn and stuck in his ways to change. I hope that he does, for his sake. At the time of writing, his operation led to complications, and he is in a lot of pain. Hopefully it will all go well in the end.

At one point I asked him, "Did doctors tell you *what* caused your tumour in your chest?" He seemed very perplexed, and had to concede that no, in fact, they hadn't. *"These things just happen"* seemed to be the brilliant scientific explanation from the medical establishment. And yet we accept their explanations – or lack thereof – without question, and submit ourselves to their operating table.

Stomach Ulcers are a Result of Festering Anger

One of my neighbours recently told me of her stomach ulcers. The medical establishment tells us that stomach ulcers occur when "the thick layer of mucus that protects your stomach from digestive juices is reduced", thus enabling the digestive acids to eat away at the lining tissues of the stomach. Ah, but *why* does this happen? *"We don't know"*, they reply. So how do you *cure* it, one might ask. *"We don't know, but here's some drugs to 'treat' it"*.

The psychological and emotional root causes of stomach ulcers, according to Richard Moat, in case you are interested: *"Festering anger, feeling powerless, difficulty coping, something is wearing you down, worry due to over-extending yourself."* Similarly, suppressed anger, festering thoughts, and a desire for revenge leads to *abscesses*.

It is endlessly fascinating to me how <u>the medical establishment cannot point to the source of any disease, and yet are keen to push drugs and surgery upon us</u>. Surely they should be more *informed* as to what is really happening in the human body, before they go in there and upset the body's delicate systems and chemical balances with drugs and surgeries?

Here are a few more examples of Richard Moat's brilliant work:

- ❏ **Acne** = stems from low self-esteem, not accepting self, life seeming unfair, avoiding contact with others, buried feelings, guilt, difficulty facing up to something.

- ❏ **Addictions** = stems from feeling emptiness, wanting to hide, avoiding problems, not trusting life's flow, lacking self-love; (addictions are an attempt to avoid or self-medicate our feelings).

- ❏ **Allergies** = stems from intolerance and irritation of a particular person or behaviour in others, internal conflict, over-sensitive, feeling easily intimidated, craving attention.

- ❏ **Alzheimer's Disease** = stems from reality-avoidance tendencies, fear of the future, wishing to be cared for, thoughts of revenge, need to control others.

- ❏ **Anal problems** = stems from repressed anger, unwillingness to let go, need for control, holding things back.

- ❏ **Arthritis** = stems from having a critical nature, anger and bitterness, feeling unloved, low self-worth, fearing change, being inflexible and blame-oriented, stubborn, non-trusting.

- ❏ **Asthma** = stems from having unclear boundaries, feeling inadequate, seeking control, excessive mother's love, feeling stifled, suppressing sadness, approval-seeking, fear of rejection, feeling unworthy.

- ❏ **Back problems** = stems from feeling overloaded, carrying other's burdens, feeling held back, feeling unsupported, financial worries, concerns for one's survival.

- ❏ **Baldness** = stems from feeling a sense of loss, protective of others, low self-worth, opinionated and controlling, frustration and worry.

- ❏ **Bladder Disorders** = stems from bottling up feelings, feeling irritated and frustrated, fear of loss, holding on.

- ❏ **Bulimia** = stems from guilt and low self-esteem, lacking unconditional love, rejecting yourself, challenging relationship with mother, desperate to control own feelings, longing to be free.

- ❏ **Cancer** = stems from unexpressed anger, self-deprecation, deep hurt or long-standing resentment, lacking self-love, unforgiving. *(note: depending on the location of the Cancer, other issues could be at play. e.g. Kidney cancer = feeling like an outcast, alone and abandoned, fear for own survival).*

- ❑ **Diabetes** = stems from a need for control, missing feeling loved or smothered with love, lack of ability to experience joy.

- ❑ **Eczema** = stems from irritation and anger, a frustration continues unresolved, low in confidence, missing or longing for someone, boundaries not being respected.

- ❑ **Fibromyalgia** = stems from chronic guilt, rigid and inflexible thinking and attitude, a 'victim' mentality, lacking confidence and creativity.

- ❑ **Headaches** = stem from being self-critical, over-intellectualizing, restriction of self-expression, narrow-minded, fear of failure, controlling, not flowing with life, perfection-seeking, feeling under pressure to deliver, unexpressed strong feelings are surfacing, feeling continuously disappointed and let down.

- ❑ **Heart Attack** = stem from materialistic tendencies, achievement-oriented, unforgiving, struggling to cope, emotionally detached, demanding high standards.

- ❑ **Infertility** = can stem from unresolved early-years trauma, uncertainty around partner or parenting, fear of life change, underlying reluctance, responsibility aversion. *(Richard told me he has worked with 8 couples with infertility issues, and all of them got pregnant!)*

- ❑ **Kidney Stones** = stems from holding on to long-standing thoughts, feelings, and attitudes that today serve no purpose, still living with past hurts; unshed tears that have calcified...

- ❑ **Liver Disorders** = anger at injustices, powerlessness, judgemental and demanding of others, fault-finder, overly-corrosive emotional suppression.

- ❑ **Hyperthyroidism** = always expending energy usually for others rather than yourself, feeling responsible (feeling obliged to engineer the lives of your loved ones), acting hastily, holding high expectations, fearing missing out.

- ❑ **Uterine Disorders** = stems from feelings of fear or a guilt hangover, uncertainty, lack of self-acceptance, feeling pressured.

- ❑ **Pain** = feeling deserving of punishment, guilt just under the surface, a longing to feel loved, self-critical, judgemental; an intelligent attempt by the body to avoid emotional pain.

This is just a tiny sample of his work, which goes into much more detail, and covers hundreds of diseases and illnesses. You can find out more at www.RichardMoat.com.

Many authors concur with Richard's findings. Dr. John Demartini states that a stroke represents a loss of the will to go on living. He writes in *The Breakthrough Experience*: "I sat down with a doctor a few days after his stroke, which psychosomatically represented a state of futility, a loss of will to push on, and no more details left within his life vision", He goes on to say: "Disease and illness are the signs and symptoms that the body uses to reveal to us where we are not loving. <u>Your body's signs and symptoms are a feedback mechanism to help you be true to yourself.</u>"

Louise Hay is the author of *"You Can Heal Your Life"*. She reveals that she was raped at the age of five, and describes how fifty years later, in 1977, she was diagnosed with 'incurable' cervical cancer. She came to the conclusion that by holding on to her resentment for her childhood abuse and rape she had contributed to its onset. She refused conventional medical treatment, and began a regime of forgiveness, coupled with therapy, nutrition, reflexology and a thorough 'detox'. She successfully rid herself of the cancer. *Love, understanding, and compassion* were the answer.

Stewart Swerdlow, explains in his book *'Stewart Says'*: "The mind produces the physical effects based upon the electromagnetic qualities of thought. <u>Everyone is given a chance to correct a mind-pattern. When you do not, the negative thought degenerates into an emotional condition.</u> If you do not correct it then, it becomes a physical manifestation as an illness in the body or mind. Each part of the body represents a thought, or a thought-band, that coalesces into an energy center. Whenever you have an illness, you can determine the mind-pattern from the part of the body that is affected. For example, the legs and feet represent stepping into the future as well as the future support structure. When you have deep emotional issues that you do not release, the heart and lungs are affected. When you do not feel supported in life, the spinal column suffers, and so on with other sections of the body."

Most people would never accept responsibility for their illness. They prefer to take on the role of 'victim' to this 'terrible thing' that is happening *'to'* them. The medical establishment definitely plays to people's victimization mind-pattern, by reinforcing the message that illnesses are things that *'just happen'* to people, for which the only answer is drugs – rather than *taking responsibility and changing their lifestyle!*

Swerdlow writes: "<u>The issues of this lifetime are being re-played, if they weren't dealt with then</u>. You're going through the same experiences because you haven't fixed it. All of us know people who at some point have had cancer. They have surgery, beat the cancer. Then a few years later, they have cancer again, so severely, that they pass away. Why? Because they **didn't** cure the cancer. They kept the mind pattern of it! Because they didn't correct the mind-pattern, it re-organized in a more intense way so that they get the lesson. Ultimately it is down to that person to do and affect the healing."

It is the same with plastic surgery: "One of my clients is a plastic surgeon. He told me that in 100% of his clients, whatever work they had done, they must get it done again within 4-6 years. Why? Because they didn't change their mind-pattern!"

Stewart Swerdlow goes on to say: "Your DNA is created by atomic structure forming around the electromagnetic energies of your thought streams or mind-patterns. Literally, you are what you think! Your health, or lack of it, is a direct result of your thoughts. You must take responsibility for yourself. The environment, accidents, germs, and toxins are tools that the mind uses to create dis-ease."

Dr. Patrick Quillin also agrees that we need to focus on the **cause** of disease rather than merely treating the symptoms: "Mrs Jones might be suffering from metastatic breast cancer because, in her case, she is still hurting from a hateful divorce of 2 years ago, which drives her catecholamines into a stress mode and depresses her immune system; she goes to bed on a box of high-sugar cookies each night; she has a deficiency of fish oil, zinc, and vitamin E; and she has an imbalance of estrogen and progesterone in her body. Her oncologist may remove the breasts, give her Tamoxifen, administer chemo and radiation; but none of these therapies deals with the underlying causes of the disease. And it will come back unless these driving forces for the disease are reversed."

My Thyroid Swelled Up to The Size of a Golf Ball

In 2014, my thyroid unexpectedly swelled up, on the left side of my neck. It was pressing on my oesophagus, making speaking and swallowing food difficult. Everyone was telling me that I needed to immediately go to a doctor, take pharmaceutical drugs, and even contemplate surgery. But I knew better. I understood that there was a *message* in this for me. So I did a bit of research into the meaning of thyroid issues – in this case, having an enlarged thyroid.

I found out that Louise Hay believes thyroid issues stem from feeling like you never get to do what you want to do. Her affirmation for that issue is *"I move beyond old limitations and now allow myself to express freely and creatively."* Also: *"I Confidently Do What I Truly Want To Do And What I Am Meant To Do!"*

Stewart Swerdlow was kind enough to email me the following advice: "The mind-pattern for the thyroid is about speaking up for yourself in a proper manner. When it swells, there are issues you are suppressing or holding back from expressing. Always speak up tactfully and honestly." He recommended visualizing the colour ice blue in my throat chakra area, taking myrrh gum and arnica, and putting warm castor oil packs over the throat for 30 minutes a day.

I also spoke with Richard Moat over the phone, who confirmed the relevance of self-expression to this issue. "This is about who you were born to be and the gift you are meant to bring to the world... You have been finding out what it is that makes your heart sing... and it is now singing a different song from the one you've become so familiar with."

He added: "The universe is inviting you to take a deeper look at who and how you are being in the world, and attempting (albeit subtly and indirectly at times) to get you to attend to re-connecting with what makes your heart sing (as opposed to what bores you to tears!). Your conflict is most likely to be related to the fear of what it will mean to change your relationship with the lucrative business you have so successfully created... change is always scary because of the uncertainty that goes with it. However, I know you as someone who is personally very aware and committed, so I sense it won't take much... the key is to establish exactly what it will take to align you with your heart's calling. Yes, stress will be present and a direct symptom of your inner conflict. And the thyroid thing will be an intelligent but veiled message from your body as to what needs your attention first. However, neither of these things – stress or thyroid – is the issue... they are just the end result (hence symptoms) of a series of behaviours and beliefs that have become so unconsciously ingrained you do them without thought. By shifting your focus, I believe you'll still harness that ability but channel it into a more flowing, harmonious and peaceful way of being in the world, meaning that stress and symptoms become a thing of the past."

In the days prior to this happening, I had delivered more than twenty talks in a row, on topics that I believed would be commercially profitable and of interest to my clients, but that bored me. I was ready to move on with my business and my life.

The Universe had sent me a message. *"It's time to be ON PURPOSE!"* I started writing about health and about more *spiritual* matters. I started feeling happy again. I used the Louise Hay affirmations. I decided to focus on *contribution* and *expressing love*. Within a week the swelling vanished as suddenly as it had appeared. No drugs needed.

Moving from the old paradigm to the "new" me was scary. How would people respond to this new message? What would happen to my business?

One night as I was falling asleep, a strong feeling of reassurance washed over me. I cannot put it in words. I have never experienced anything quite like it. It flooded my body as I telepathically received the message, *"Ewan... it is OK to let go of CONTROL. Relax, have FAITH, and TRUST that you are taken care of.... You always have been...".* It was the first time *in ten years* that I had felt like I could relax. No matter what happens... I will be OK. Was it from my spirit guides?

When you let go of your need for control, you allow miracles to come into your life.

During our call, Richard shared with me some more of his wisdom. He said:

> **"Our #1 goal in life is to live an authentic life**. To live life according to our internal guidance system. It gets screwed up by the well-meaning intentions of parents, teachers, society.... <u>Failed relationships, health problems, unfulfilling careers are veiled messages for us... to get us back on track.</u> They are the end result of how we are in the world, that dishonours

our AUTHENTICITY. Are you not communicating what you really want to say? Do you find yourself saying yes when you want to say no? Did you let people violate your boundaries without expressing it to them at the time? At the heart of who we really are is our AUTHENTIC self. FEAR-FREE, heroic, warrior-like, integrated, whole, balanced, and at peace. That is our blueprint. It means that inside of us we have a memory of that. And it is the memory of that, that gets us all to constantly be looking for something better, which actually translates as a return to that way of being. The most significant barrier to this: FEAR. Everyone needs to be willing to address, master, and work through their FEARS in order to access their authentic self."

How Our Thoughts Control Our DNA: Bruce Lipton's *Biology of Belief*

We were told that The Human Genome Project would usher in a new era of pharmaceuticals that would help us turn on healing genes and more. Why have we not heard anything about it for the past few years?

The truth is that DNA sequencing and The Human Genome Project were a massive (and expensive) failure. Scientists expected to find at least 100,000 genes in the human genome, one for each of the 70,000+ proteins and the 30,000+ regulatory genes found in a human. But the Genome project revealed that there are only about 34,000 genes in the human genome. Two thirds of the anticipated genes do not exist! Even more humiliating for the dogma of 'genetic determinacy' is the fact that the tiny roundworm is comprised of almost as many genes (nearly 20,000).

Once again the dogma of mainstream "medicine" is proven to be nothing more than propaganda based on falsehoods. It is our beliefs and our perception of our environment that switches our genes on or off. Bruce Lipton writes in his groundbreaking book *The Biology of Belief*:

"The common idea that DNA determines so much of who we are—not only our eye or hair color, for example, but also our addictions, disorders, or susceptibility to cancer—is a misconception. [...] A person's perception, not genetic programming, is what spurs all action in the body: It's actually our beliefs that select our genes, that select our behavior."

What Would Love Do Now?

In the book *Conversations With God*, 'God' reveals to the author: *"In highest Truth, love is all there is, all there was, and all there ever will be. You are, at the core of your wonderful Self, that aspect of divinity called love."* If love is our true essence, the 'truth of us', it would make sense that balance, peace, order, and *good health*, would flow from such a state. Move away from your natural state of love, and chaos and disorganization ensues.

The spiritual channeller Barbara Marciniak states that *love* is what returns people to a state of health. She says: "Understand that ill people are looking for love. There isn't enough love in their lives. It is LOVE that brings them back." Since everything is *energy*, and we are all vibrating at different frequencies, one can imagine that there is a particular *frequency of health*, and conversely there must exist a vibrational frequency of 'disease'. Marciniak hints at the intriguing possibility that a vibrational device could be invented, that restores health to people's bodies: "Are there devices that can reproduce the LOVE FREQUENCY? When you can develop machines that can have frequencies adjusted so that they remind the body of its health and to restore the vibration of health, that CAN bring people back. Then they have to deal with the question 'Am I loved or am I **not** loved'?"

Dr. John Demartini confirms the healing power of *love* in this passage from his book The Breakthrough Experience: "I've worked with terminal cancer patients who had spontaneous remissions, and in each case, some form of love and gratitude came into their lives and shifted them. A spiritual experience transformed their illness. Even watching a movie about love has been shown to increase the levels of immunoglobulin A in the saliva, the body's first line of immunological defence. **We get ill to teach us to love**. It's not a punishment or a mistake. It's a gift."

He adds: "Illness is your body's way of telling you that you're lying about life. Every symptom and sign in your physical body is designed to reveal to you what you're lying about." If you are angry and have festering thoughts of anger, it is a lie. You are angry with that part you recognize within *yourself*. Your soul is revealing something to you about *yourself*. If you are miserable because you work in a job that you hate, you are *living a lie*. You are being fearful. That job is *not* the truth of you; you are not being authentic to who you really are and *what you really want to do*.

Your abandonment issues are a lie, because in truth nothing in this Universe could ever abandon you. You are one with your Oversoul family and God-Mind, at all times. If you are bottling up your feelings, not expressing how you really feel or what you really want to say... *that* is a lie. The truth of you is that you are here to powerfully *express* yourself, in every way. If you don't accept yourself or love yourself, and have feelings of low self-worth, well, that is the *biggest lie*, since who you are is a part of the Divine, a powerful creator, and the *essence* of you is love and light.

Anger, fear, low self-worth, feelings of guilt, lack of self-expression, abandonment issues, and many other negative emotions manifest themselves as dis-ease in the body, as we have seen repeatedly.

"All Illness Is Self-Created"

"All illness is self-created. Even conventional medical doctors are now seeing how people make themselves sick. Most people move through life unconsciously. People smoke and wonder why they get cancer. People stay angry all their lives and wonder why they get heart attacks. People compete with other people – mercilessly and under incredible stress – and wonder why they have strokes.

The not-so-obvious truth is that most people worry themselves to death. Worry is just about the worst form of mental activity there is – next to hate, which is deeply self-destructive. Worry is pointless. It is wasted mental energy. It also creates bio-chemical reactions which harm the body. Health will improve almost at once when worrying ends."

[...] "Hatred is the most severely damaging mental condition. It poisons the body, and its effects are virtually irreversible. Fear is the opposite of everything you are, and so has an effect of opposition to your mental and physical health. Fear is worry magnified. Worry, hate, fear – together with their offshoots: anxiety, bitterness, impatience, avarice, unkindness, judgmentalness, and condemnation – all attack the body at the cellular level. It is impossible to have a healthy body under these conditions. All illness is created first in the mind. [...] Nothing occurs in your life – nothing – which is not first a thought. You can "solve some of the health problems," by solving the problems in your thinking."

[...] "For God's sake, take better care of yourself. You take rotten care of your body, paying it little attention at all until you suspect something's going wrong with it. You take better care of your car than you do of your body – and that's not saying much. [...] You do not exercise it, so it weak from non-use. You do not nourish it properly, thereby weakening it further. Then you fill it with toxins and poisons and the most absurd substances posing as food. And still it runs for you, this marvellous engine; still it chugs along, bravely pushing on in the face of this onslaught. It's horrible. The conditions under which you ask your body to survive are horrible. But you will do little or nothing about them.

You will read this, nod your head in regretful agreement, and go right back to the mistreatment. **And do you know why? Because you have no will to live.** [...] If you ever lit a cigarette in your life you have very little will to live. You don't care what you do to your body. And if you've ever taken alcohol into your body, you have very little will to live."

Neale Donald Walsch, Conversations With God

PART II

EVERYTHING YOU KNOW ABOUT COLON CANCER IS <u>WRONG</u>

CHAPTER 8

Everything You Know About Cancer Is Wrong

What exactly *is* 'cancer'? According to the National Cancer Institute, "Cancer is the name given to a collection of related diseases. Some of the body's cells begin to divide without stopping and spread into surrounding tissues. Normally, human cells grow and divide to form new cells as the body needs them, but when cancer develops, this orderly process breaks down. Many cancers form solid tumours, which are masses of tissue. Cancerous tumours are malignant, which means they can spread into, or invade, nearby tissues. In addition, some cancer cells can 'break off and travel to distant places in the body through the blood or the lymph system and form new tumours'."

Right. The only problem is… **this is complete nonsense and disinformation.** This "Mutational Theory" of cancer has provided the prevailing explanation for the cause of cancer, where, *supposedly*, accumulated mutations within our cells lead a few susceptible ones to '*go berserk*', and these '*rogue*' cells '*replicate incessantly*' and form a tumour which grows and grows.

But then, paradoxically, these 'rogue' cells start expressing *highly organized behaviour*. They are capable of building their own blood supply (angiogenesis), are able to defend themselves, alter their metabolism to survive in low-oxygen, high-sugar and acidic environments, and know how to alter their proteins proteins to avoid being detected by white blood cells. This seems to be far from 'random'. Why exactly are these cells acting this way? It looks to me as if **these cells are desperately trying to survive**.

Ask a doctor "Why do people get cancer?" and you'll often get a vague, "*Uhmm… it's random mutations. 'Bad genes' run in your family… these things 'just happen' with age…*". The truth is, the theory they base their understanding of 'cancer' on is patently false.

Understanding What Your Body Needs on a Cellular Level

First of all, some basic biology: Your body consists of trillions of cells. Your bloodstream – *your 'river of life'* – flows oxygen and nutrients to every cell in your body. Without this, your cells would weaken and die. Your cells use the oxygen and nutrients to create Adenosine Triphosphate (ATP, the energy that powers your body) and to complete whatever other specific function that cell is designed to do.

Your lymphatic system drains your body of the *waste* produced by these cellular chemical reactions, by collecting this waste and disposing of it through your natural elimination processes (sweat, urine, phlegm, faeces). If your bloodstream is too polluted with waste, toxicity starts accumulating in your tissues and bloodstream (imagine your bloodstream becoming a viscous, sludge-like toxic wasteland…), making it harder for your cells to get the oxygen and nutrients they need to survive.

In the mid-1800s the French chemist and biologist Antoine Béchamp put forward his theory of *pleomorphism* (from the Greek for 'many forms') – the idea that <u>cells have the ability to alter their shape or size in response to environmental conditions</u>. But the work of his rival Louis Pasteur (*'You are being attacked by germs!'*) caught on instead and Béchamp's work was all but ignored.

In the early 2000s I attended a talk given by the American microbiologist Dr. Robert O. Young. He had achieved remarkable results with his patients, helping them overcome diabetes, cancer, arthritis, fibromyalgia, and a host of other diseases in a matter of *weeks*, by simply changing their diets and helping them detoxify their bodies.

During this lecture, he proceeded to show the audience how new, powerful microscopes revealed what happens when a live, healthy red blood cell finds itself moving from healthy blood to an environment of highly acidic and 'toxic' blood: <u>the cell actually *mutates* and expands, in an all-out attempt at surviving in this toxic, low-oxygen wasteland</u>. Remember the opening sequence of *The Simpsons,* when the fish in the pond mutate because of Mr. Burns dumping toxic waste into that environment…? Or the story of Godzilla being borne out of exposure to nuclear radiation off the coast of Japan? You get the idea: **life forms mutate to adapt to a toxic environment!**

If that mutated cell flows into a 'cleaner' part of the body, where it gets plenty of oxygen and nutrients, *it reverts back to being a healthy red blood cell.* But if the environment *remains* toxic, the cell will display inflammation, irritation, will weaken, and eventually die. And when these cells die *en masse* in that specific part of the body, the 'clean-up crew' (your white blood cells) comes along and collects these dead cells into a little 'sack' (doctors call this a 'tumour') to isolate this toxicity from the rest of the body, until the body has enough energy to break it down and dispose of it. *The tumour is actually your body's way of protecting you! Cancer is not a disease; it is a survival mechanism!*

Cancer Is Not A Disease – It Is a Survival Mechanism

Despite the fact that oncologists are successfully able to shrink tumours, the cancer patient still dies in the majority of cases. Why? The reason is the tumour size has nothing to do with curing cancer, and furthermore, patients are dying from the toxic chemotherapy treatments. '*Orthodox medicine, with its focus on the highly profitable tumour, has* **brainwashed the public into thinking that the tumour is the cancer**" says cancer expert Webster Kehr. The tumour *is not* the cancer. The tumour is your body's way of telling you that you are really, *really* toxic, and it doesn't have enough *energy* to break down and eliminate all that excess waste.

Your body has to maintain enough energy to run your heart, your brain, your nervous system, your digestive system, your liver, your lymphatic system, etc. AND deal with the *poisons* you ingest numerous times a day in the form of coffee, sugar, alcohol, pesticides, pollution, pharmaceutical drugs, chemicals in household cleaning products, chemicals in toiletries, perfumes, and skincare products. Your body can heal itself. *But not if it is under constant assault and not provided with the nutrients and minerals it needs to survive!*

Cancer is happening in your body – on a cellular level – <u>because you are too *toxic*</u>. But doctors don't label this as such, and they don't recommend what we now know cures cancer naturally: cleansing and alkalizing your bloodstream, exercise, rest, and healthy nutrition. Instead, they label it 'Cancer' and they recommend the most toxic chemical cocktail possible, that destroys your immune system! And then for good measure they cut your body open, creating even more stress on the body.

As a result, many people who "die from cancer" *actually* die from the conventional treatments long before they would have actually died from the cancer itself. The American author Anthony Robbins begins his "Living Health" seminars by sharing the story of how, many years ago, his friend came to him in tears, because her mother had been diagnosed with Cancer. She had tumours the size of a *baseball* on her shoulders and in her female organs. The doctor gave her 9 weeks to live.

Robbins said to his friend: "Look, hundreds of thousands of people have had cancer and beaten it. I know you don't hear much about it, but it's a fact. <u>All we've got to do is find people who got cancer and beat it, find out exactly what they did and what they had in common, and model that</u>. If we model what most people do, we'll get what most people get."

He gave this woman a couple of books to read, and within a few days she started detoxifying her body – essentially, <u>getting rid of the poisons that were *in* her body</u>. Waste and toxins started streaming out of her system. Within 4 weeks she lost 28 pounds. After just 8 weeks, she was feeling amazing, she is in the best fitness of her life, the best health of her life, and she doesn't feel any sense of 'dis-ease' in her body. The doctors still insisted on performing an exploratory operation. So they opened her up, and found... nothing. No tumours. In her whole body. In 9 weeks. The doctors couldn't understand how that was possible. They said: *"It's a miracle!"* She tried to explain to them what she did, but they just repeated: *"No! It's a miracle!"*

Dr. Leonard Coldwell states that all cancer, along with *'all other kinds of immune diseases',* are based on emotional and mental stress and can be cured in less than 12 weeks through holistic cancer remedies (*see Chapter 16, 'Disease Starts In The Mind'*). In addition, Dr. Coldwell lists several cancer-curing treatments that are being suppressed by Big Pharma, including sodium bicarbonate (baking soda), apricot kernels, Rife machines, and colloidal silver.

Dr. Leonard Coldwell's "Shocking" Views on Cancer

- ❑ In the last 20 years, nobody has died of cancer, they have died from the side effects of the treatment. Chemotherapy and radiation cause cells to mutate.

- ❑ The medical profession is the #1 cause of death in the Western world.

- ❑ Cancer is the biggest money maker in history for the pharmaceutical industry.

- ❑ Cancer is a $60 billion a year industry, while cancer protection and the early intervention of cancer brings in an additional $162 billion each year.

- ❑ There are 300+ natural cancer cures that have no side-effects and a nearly 100% cure rate.

- ❑ The medical profession has a cancer cure rate of only 2%.

- ❑ If you do nothing, you have a 27% chance of recovery from cancer.

- ❑ Our immune system gets rid of 'cancerous' cells naturally.

- ❑ The only cause for illness is lack of energy. The main cause for lack of energy is physical stress, and emotional stress from bad relationships.

- ❑ 86% of all doctor visits and illnesses, statistically, are based on stress or are stress related. According to a Stanford University study, 95% of all illness is due to stress.

Dr. Leonard Coldwell also believes that <u>radiation and chemotherapy *cause* cancer, while surgery spreads the cancer *"like an explosion through the entire body."*</u> According to Dr. Coldwell, the causes of cancer include: living in constant worries, doubts and fears, lack of self-love, lack of self-respect, lack of hope for the future, and the biggest reason of all, **making a constant compromise against yourself.** He adds: *"That is why when you live in a relationship that you know is toxic and it's killing you, you need to get out of it or it will literally kill you. If you go to a job that you cannot bear anymore, this job will kill you. That's why most deadly heart attacks on Monday morning between 8 and 9am."*

Conventional Medicine's Measly 2% Cure Rate

I highly recommend Ty Bollinger's book *Cancer: Step Outside The Box*, for an in-depth understanding of the cancer industry and the natural cures available today (visit www.TheTruthAboutCancer.com). Here are some startling facts about cancer from his groundbreaking book:

❑ "Human cancer is primarily attributable to chemical pollutants, horrible eating habits, and unhealthy lifestyles, not genetics." – Karolinska Institute of Stockholm, Sweden

❑ "The cause of cancer is clear: poor diet, lifestyle and poor mental attitude result in toxic build-up which overloads the self-cleansing mechanism. Cancer is manifestation of long term nutritional and environmental irritation, resulting in cellular oxygen starvation, leading to uncontrolled cell replication." – Dr. Saul Pressman

❑ "Everyone should know that the 'war on cancer' is largely a fraud. Most cancer research is largely a fraud, and the major cancer research organizations are derelict in their duties." – Dr. Linus Pauling (two time Nobel Prize winner)

❑ "If a patient with a tumour is receiving radiation or chemotherapy, the only question that is asked is, 'How is the tumour doing?' No one ever asks how the patient is doing. [...] In primary cancer, with only a few exceptions, the tumour is neither health-endangering nor life-threatening. What is health-endangering is the spread of that disease through the rest of the body. [...] The survival time of the cancer patient today is no greater than it was fifty years ago. What does this mean? It obviously means that we are treating the wrong thing!" – Dr. Philip Binzel, *Alive and Well*

❑ "A true cure rate of 90% or more can easily be achieved by cancer patients who avoid orthodox medicine, go with alternative medicine first, and do their homework. The true cure rate of orthodox medicine is 3% or less. 95% of cancer patients who go with alternative cancer treatments have previously had the full orthodox treatment and have been sent home to die, meaning alternative medicine is handed a large number of cancer patients already in critical condition. For those who wait to go with alternative cancer treatments until after they have been sent home to die, only a handful of the 300 or more alternative cancer treatments are strong enough to give them a chance of survival (of about 50%). In other words, if you go with alternative medicine first, your chance of survival is 90% or more, if you do your homework. If you go with orthodox medicine first, and then alternative medicine second, you will have years of suffering, and if you are lucky, you will then have a 50% chance of survival." – Webster Kehr

❑ "Most people think that cancer is caused by DNA damage and that orthodox medicine is frantically searching for a cure for cancer. Both beliefs are complete nonsense and come from the propaganda and deceptions of television. Cancer is not caused by DNA damage. The definition of a cancer cell is a cell with low ATP energy. [...] Yet the media glorifies all of the "cancer researchers" who are diligently trying to "fix" the DNA damage of cancer cells. It is all a scam to make sure that cures for cancer are never found! The 5-year cure rate of orthodox medicine (e.g. oncologists) is 2.1%. In other words, in 97.9% of the cases, their cancer patients are dead within 5 years of diagnosis." – Webster Kehr

❑ "Diseases such as cancer are NOT caused by defective genes, as claimed by mainstream geneticists, but rather by non-genetic factors. In fact, diseases are not senseless "disorders" but in reality meaningful biological processes trying to **save** an organism rather than to destroy it." – Dr. Joseph Mercola

❑ According to a 2004 report by Morgan, Ward, and Barton: "The contribution of cytotoxic chemotherapy to 5-year survival in adult malignancies... <u>survival in adults was estimated to be 2.3% in Australia and 2.1% in the USA</u>."

❑ "Western medicine has failed our people. Today, even while prescription drugs are more frequently consumed than ever before in the history of civilization, our nation has skyrocketing rates of obesity and chronic disease. [...] <u>Western medicine simply does not work. It is an outmoded system of medicine dominated by the financial interests of pharmaceutical companies</u>, power-hungry officials at the FDA, and old-school doctors whose myopic view of health prevents them from exploring the true causes of healing. Modern medical schools don't even teach healing or nutrition. **No practitioner of western medicine has ever taught me a single thing about being healthy**." – Mike Adams, www.NaturalNews.com

❑ "<u>Surgery is oftentimes responsible for the spread of the cancer</u>, since a minute miscue or careless handling of the tumour tissue by the surgeon can literally spill millions of cancer cells into the cancer patient's bloodstream."

❑ Biopsies can also result in the spread of cancer: "Often while making a biopsy the malignant tumour is cut across, which tends to spread or accelerate the growth. Needle biopsies can accomplish the same tragic results." – Dr. Donald Kelley, *One Answer to Cancer*

❑ "<u>Cancer cells cannot thrive in an oxygenated environment</u>. Exercising daily, and deep breathing help to get more oxygen down to the cellular level. Oxygen therapy is another means employed to destroy cancer cells." – Johns Hopkins hospital

❑ In 1957, P.G. Seeger who was twice nominated for the Nobel Prize, successfully changed normal cells into cancer cells within a few days by introducing chemicals that blocked the respiratory chain. He discovered that certain nutrients, including the B vitamin inositol, have the ability to restore cellular respiration in cancer cells, thus transforming them back into normal cells. In other words, cancer is reversible.

❑ Dr. Otto Warburg, a cancer biochemist and the 1931 Nobel Laureate in Medicine, discovered that **cancer occurs whenever any cell is denied 60% of its oxygen requirements**, and showed that cancer cells exhibit anaerobic respiration. His thesis was that cancer is a fermentative disease caused by cells which have *mutated from aerobic respiration to anaerobic respiration*, resulting in glucose fermentation and uncontrolled cellular growth. He theorized that **tumours are nothing more than walled-off toxic waste dumps inside the body sustained by fermenting sugar**. According to Warburg, most, if not all degenerative diseases, are a result of lack of oxygen at the cellular level. [Remember what I told you about Dr. Robert O. Young's research? Cells mutate when they don't get enough oxygen. It stands to reason that cleansing the body and doing things that bring oxygen to the cells helps patients regain their health…]

❑ "In primary cancer (with only a few exceptions) <u>the tumour is neither health endangering nor life threatening</u>. What is health endangering and life threatening is the spread of cancer through the rest of the body. <u>Surgery, chemotherapy, and radiation, do not prevent the spread of cancer</u>. On the contrary, it accelerates it." – Dr. Philip Binzel, *Alive and Well*

❑ "The most startling fact about 2002 is that the combined profits for the ten drug companies in the Fortune 500 ($35.9 billion) were more than the profits for all the other 490 businesses put together ($33.7 billion)." – Dr. Marcia Angell, *The Truth About The Drug Companies*

❑ "You might think that chemotherapy is designed to stop the spread of cancer. Chemotherapy does not target cancer cells. It kills fast growing cells, whether cancerous or non-cancerous. Chemotherapy can only slow down the cancer; it cannot stop it from spreading and killing the patient. <u>Every chemotherapy drug they have ever approved is virtually worthless or does more harm than good</u>. […] <u>Chemotherapy is toxic, carcinogenic (causes cancer), destroys red blood cells, devastates the immune system, and kills vital organs</u>. How toxic is it? Your hair falls out, your immune system is destroyed, you are constantly nauseated, you get sick and vomit, you are frequently dizzy, and you have severe headaches. Are these signs that maybe this stuff is poison and doesn't belong in your body?" – Ty Bollinger

❑ "In 1953, a US Senate Investigation reported that a conspiracy existed to suppress effective cancer treatments. The Senator in charge of the investigation conveniently died. The investigation was halted. It was neither the first nor the last of a number of strange deaths involving people in positions to do damage to those running the nation's cancer program." – Barry Lynes – *The Healing Of Cancer*

❑ "The medical establishment works closely with the drug multinationals whose main objective is profits, and whose worst nightmare would be an epidemic of good health. Lots of drugs MUST be sold. In order to achieve this, anything goes: lies, fraud, and kickbacks. Doctors are the principal salespeople of the drug companies. They are rewarded with research grants, gifts, and lavish perks. The principal buyers are the public – from infants to the elderly – who MUST be thoroughly medicated and vaccinated… at any cost! Why do the authorities forbid alternative medicine? Because they are serving the industry, and the industry cannot make money with herbs, vitamins, and homeopathy. They cannot patent natural remedies. They control medicine, and that is why they are able to tell medical schools what they can and cannot teach." – Dr. Guylaine Lanctot, *The Medical Mafia*

❑ "94% of the information contained in promotional literature sent to doctors by Big Pharma has absolutely no scientific basis." – Study carried out by the Institute of Evidence-Based Medicine in Germany (19 out of 20 statements made by drug companies in their marketing literature are false, unsubstantiated and unsupported by scientific evidence)

❑ "Young physicians are offered research grants by drug companies. Medical schools are given large sums of money for clinical trials and basic pharmaceutical research. Drug companies regularly host lavish dinner and cocktail parties for groups of physicians. They provide funding for the establishment of hospital buildings, medical school buildings, and 'independent' research institutes… practicing physicians are intimidated into using treatment regimes which they know do not work. One glaring example is cancer chemotherapy." – Dr. Alan Levin, *Dissent in Medicine – Nine Doctors Speak Out*

❑ "With billions of dollars spent each year in research, with additional billions taken in from the cancer-related sale of drugs, and with vote-hungry politicians promising ever-increasing government programs, we find that, today, there are more people making a living from cancer than dying from it. If the riddle were to be solved by a simple vitamin, this gigantic commercial and political industry could be wiped out overnight." – Edward Griffin, *World Without Cancer*

❑ "In 1974, I began working at Memorial Sloan-Kettering Cancer Center, the world's leading cancer treatment hospital. [...] A big part of my job as Assistant Director of Public Affairs was to write press releases for the media about cancer news and to write the in-hospital newsletter. I began interviewing <u>Dr. Kanematsu Sugiura, who had repeatedly gotten positive results shrinking tumours in mice studies with a natural substance called amygdalin</u> (a.k.a. 'laetrile' or Vitamin B17 found in apricot seeds and apple seeds). I told my "discovery" of Sugiura's work to the Public Affairs Director and other superiors, and laid out my plans for an article about it. Then I got the shock of my life. They insisted that I stop working on this story immediately and never pick it up again. Why? They said that Dr. Sugiura's work was invalid and totally meaningless. But I had seen the results with my own eyes. And I knew Dr. Sugiura was a true scientist and an ethical person. My bosses told me to lie. They ordered me to write an article and press releases for all the major news stations emphatically stating that all amygdalin studies were negative and that the substance was worthless for cancer treatment. I later discovered that <u>the CEOs of top pharmaceutical companies that produced cancer drugs dominated the board at Memorial Sloan-Kettering, including the chairman of Bristol-Myers Squibb, the world's leading producer of chemotherapy</u>. Not surprisingly, profits from chemotherapy drugs were skyrocketing." – Dr. Ralph Moss, *The Cancer Industry*

❑ "Jason Vale was handed a death sentence by his doctors in the mid-1990s when it was discovered that he had terminal cancer. Through extensive research, he discovered that people who once had cancer found healing properties in something as simple as the seeds of apples and apricots. It turned out that these seeds contain natural substances that kill cancer cells (Vitamin B17 or 'laetrile'). Jason immediately began to feel better by eating apple seeds. Within a short period of time, Jason's cancer literally disappeared. [...] In 2001, Jason was coerced by the FDA into signing a Consent Decree that <u>would prevent him from sharing his story</u>. Despite the fact that he had not broken any law, the FDA brought criminal charges against Jason for distributing apricot seeds." – Ty Bollinger, *Cancer: Step Outside The Box*

❑ "Experimental studies performed in 1906 suggest that leukaemia (cancer of the blood) could be caused by exposure to the radioactive element radium. [...] By 1922 over 100 radiologists had died from X-ray-induced cancer... I had a brain cancer specialist sit in my living room and tell me that he would **never** take radiation if he had a brain tumour. And I asked him, 'But, do you send people for radiation? And he said, 'Of course. I'd be drummed out of the hospital if I didn't'." – Dr. Ralph Moss, *The Cancer Industry*

❑ "Why is there 'no official scientific evidence' for alternative treatments? Because they are not highly profitable to Big Pharma. It is impossible, by law, for a substance to be considered to have 'scientific evidence' unless Big Pharma submits it to the FDA, and they will only submit things that are very, very profitable to them. Thus, thousands of studies of natural substances that have cured or treated cancer are not 'scientific evidence' and they are ignored by our government, because they were not done under the control of Big Pharma." – Webster Kehr

❑ "Secondary cancers are known complications of chemotherapy and irradiation used to treat Hodgkin's and non-Hodgkin's lymphomas and other primary cancers." – The New England Journal of Medicine, September 21, 1989

Thanks to Mike Adams and *www.NaturalNews.com* for the cartoon above.

❑ "Several studies have shown that cancer patients who undergo radiation therapy are more likely to have their cancer metastasize to other sites in their bodies. The radioactivity used to kill cancer cells also triggers the process of

DNA mutation that creates new cancer cells of other types." – Dr. Lucian Israel, *Conquering Cancer*

❑ "Complications following high-dose radiotherapy for breast cancer are: fibrous, shrunken breasts, rib fractures, pleural and/or lung scarring, nerve damage, scarring around the heart… suppression of all blood cells, immune suppression. Many radiation complications do not occur for several years after treatment, giving the therapist and the patient a false sense of security for a year or two following therapy. The bone marrow, in which blood cells are made, is largely obliterated in the field of irradiation… This is an irreversible effect." – Dr. Robert F. Jones, The Seattle Times, July 27, 1980

❑ "When chemotherapy and radiation are given together, secondary tumours are 25 times more likely to occur than the normal rate." – Dr. John Laszlo, *Understanding Cancer*

❑ "Most cancer patients in this country die of chemotherapy. Chemotherapy does not eliminate breast, colon, or lung cancers. This fact has been documented for over a decade, yet doctors still use chemotherapy for these tumours." – Dr. Allen Levin, *The Healing of Cancer*

❑ "In a trial on a chemotherapy drug tested for leukaemia, 42% of the patients died directly from the toxicity of the chemotherapy." – Kenny Ausubel, *When Healing Becomes a Crime*

❑ "The amount of toxic chemicals needed to kill every last cancer cell was found to kill the patient long before it eliminated the tumour… I remembered the story of a celebrated Sloan Kettering chemotherapist who, when he found out that he had advanced cancer, told his colleagues, 'Do anything you want – but no chemotherapy.' It was an open secret that an official of Sloan Kettering sent his mother to Germany for alternative treatment… Perhaps the strangest thing about chemotherapy is that many of these drugs themselves are carcinogenic. This may seem astonishing to the average reader – that cancer-fighting drugs themselves cause cancer. Yet this is an undeniable fact." – Dr. Ralph Moss, *Questioning Chemotherapy*

❑ "A study of over 10,000 patients shows clearly that chemo's supposedly strong track record with Hodgkin's disease (lymphoma) is actually a lie. **Patients who underwent chemotherapy were 14 times more likely to develop leukaemia and 6 times more likely to develop cancers** of the bones, joints, and soft tissues than those patients who did not undergo chemotherapy." – Dr. John Diamond (NCI Journal 87:10).

❑ "Children who are successfully treated [by conventional medicine] for Hodgkin's disease are 18 times more likely later to develop secondary malignant tumours. Girls face a 35% chance of developing breast cancer by the time they are 40 – which is 75 times greater than the average." – The New England Journal of Medicine, March 21, 1996

❑ "58 out of 64 oncologists surveyed by The McGill Cancer Center in Montreal said that chemotherapy was unacceptable to them and their family members due to the fact that the drugs don't work and are toxic to one's system. **91% of the oncologists would not take chemotherapy themselves**." – Philip Day, *Cancer: Why We're Still Dying To Know The Truth*

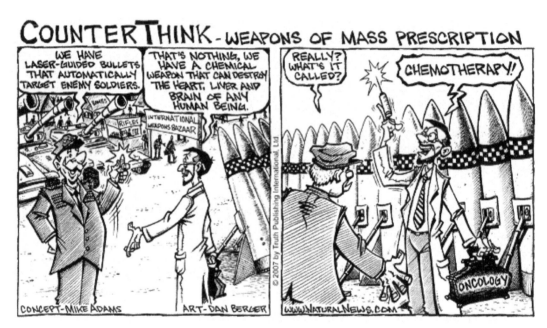

Thanks to Mike Adams and *www.NaturalNews.com* for the cartoon above.

❑ "Thirteen of the doctors who called me were eager to know how they could get access to treatments such as those devised by Gaston Naessens for themselves, their wives, or their relatives to treat grave cases of cancer with which they had become afflicted. In each case I asked them: 'Doctor, how come you're not advising yourself (or those close to you) to go the same prescription route you've been recommending for so long to your patients?' And each time, the answer came back: 'Because we know it doesn't work!'" – Christopher Bird, *The Persecution and Trial of Gaston Naessens*

❑ "Success of most chemotherapies is appalling... There is **no scientific evidence** for its ability to extend in any appreciable way the lives of patients suffering from the most common organic cancer... Chemotherapy for malignancies too advanced for surgery, which accounts for 80% of all cancers, is a scientific wasteland." – Dr. Ulrich Abel, The Lancet medical journal, 1991

❏ "Ironically, virtually all of the chemotherapeutic anti-cancer agents now approved by the Food and Drug Administration for use or testing in human cancer patients are (1) highly or variously **toxic** at applied dosages; (2) markedly **immuno-suppressive,** that is, destructive of the patient's native resistance to a variety of diseases, including cancer; and (3) usually **highly carcinogenic**... These now well established facts have been reported in numerous publications from the National Cancer Institute itself, as well as from throughout the United States and, indeed, the world." – Dr. Dean Burk, condemning the National Cancer Institute's policy of endorsing chemotherapy drugs when everyone knew that they caused cancer.

❏ "We have a multi-billion-dollar industry that is killing people, right and left, just for financial gain. Their idea of research is to see whether two doses of poison is better than three doses of that poison. [...] Sadly, some people will spend six figures a year poisoning their bodies because their 'doctor told them to do it.'" – Dr. Glenn Warner, one of the most highly qualified cancer specialists in the United States.

❏ "The thing that bugs me is that the people think the FDA is protecting them. It isn't. What the FDA is doing and what the public thinks it is doing are as different as night and day. [...] One case involved a professor who had tested almost 100 drugs for 28 different drug companies. Patients who died, left the hospital, or dropped out of the study were replaced by other patients in the tests without notification in the records. Forty-one patients reported as participating in studies were dead or not in the hospital during the studies." – Former FDA commissioner, Dr. Herbert Ley (U.S. Senate, Competitive Problems in the Pharmaceutical Industry, 1969), describing several cases of deliberate dishonesty in drug testing.

❏ "**Computed Tomography (CT) scans cause at least 29,000 cases of cancer and 14,500 deaths in the USA every year**. People may be exposed to four times as much radiation as estimated by earlier studies. Based on those measurements, a patient could get as much radiation from one CT scan as 74 mammograms or 442 chest X-rays." – Archives of Internal Medicine (2009)

❏ "Danish epidemiologists used cancer-registry data from the 1940s through the 1980s to first report a significantly increased risk of leukaemia among oncology nurses and physicians. Another Danish study of more than 92,000 nurses found an elevated risk for breast, thyroid, nervous-system and brain cancers. A just-completed study from the U.S. Center for Disease Control – 10 years in the making and the largest to date – confirms that chemo continues to contaminate the work spaces where it's used." – July 10, 2010 edition of The Seattle Times

❑ "Dr. Scott Reuben, a member of Pfizer's speakers' bureau, agreed to plead guilty to faking dozens of research studies that were published in medical journals. Reuben accepted a $75,000 grant from Pfizer to study Cerebrex and published his "research" in a medical journal. No patients were ever enrolled in the study! He faked the entire study and got it published anyways. According to the Wall Street Journal, <u>Reuben also faked study data on Vioxx, a drug which the FDA admits has caused over 50,000 deaths</u>! Reuben totally falsified 10 "scientific" papers and 21 articles published in medical journals. It turns out that Reuben had been faking research data for over 13 years." – Ty Bollinger, *Cancer: Step Outside The Box*

❑ "Why haven't you heard these things a thousand times on television or radio or in the major magazines? Because if they told you these things, the pharmaceutical industry would pull all of their advertising money and give that advertising money to a competing station or magazine. <u>The TV stations and other media don't dare broadcast anything which may hurt one of their biggest advertisers</u>... Also, to a large degree the same people who make huge profits supplying and working with orthodox medicine also own the large television and radio networks. For example, General Electric, which makes huge profits from supplying hospitals with expensive equipment, and by selling prescription drugs, etc. owns the NBC network and at least 30 major NBC affiliates. General Electric is a member of the Cancer Industry and they own NBC! What you know about cancer has been carefully designed and crafted by the pharmaceutical industry propaganda artists to keep you in the dark about the vast superiority of Mother Nature at treating cancer." – Ty Bollinger

False Diagnoses of Cancer Is Killing Millions

Many people are being told that their tissue lesions are "cancer" even though they would not lead to any real harm in the body even if left untreated. The National Cancer Institute themselves now admit that millions of people have been diagnosed with "cancer" by crooked doctors and oncologists in order to profit from highly profitable chemotherapy treatments, despite never having any sort of life-threatening condition to begin with. **These treatments destroy the patient's immune system and in the majority of cases lead to death.**

A panel of experts commissioned by the National Cancer Institute recently publicly admitted that **tens of millions of "cancer cases" aren't cancer at all**. In fact, two cancers have recently been struck off the list of 'cancers'.

According to Dr. H. Gilbert Welch, author of *Less Medicine More Health*, "Cancer screening is mostly a psychological terror campaign waged against women to enrich cancer treatment clinics."

The legendary Dutch football player Johan Cruyff recently died after being diagnosed with lung cancer. He stated *"I have an excellent team of doctors around me"* and described chemotherapy as a "friend" that the doctors had put inside his body to beat the cancer. Unfortunately, those "excellent" doctors and "friendly" chemo sent him to his grave. They destroyed his immune system and killed him in four months flat. But the media do not mention this. They talk instead of *a valiant battle with cancer.* It wasn't cancer he was battling. It was the medical establishment and their search for profits.

Study: Only 34% of Americans Trust Their Doctor

Is it any surprise that only 34% of Americans polled have confidence in the leaders of the medical profession? This number has fallen dramatically from 76% in 1966. They are responsible for nearly 800,000 deaths a year and prescription drugs injure over two million Americans each and every year.

CHAPTER 9

The Truth About Breast Cancer

Each year over 225,000 women are diagnosed with breast cancer, with a 25% mortality rate (mainly due to conventional treatments). Breast cancer is the leading cause of death among American women between the ages of 44 and 55. What *actually* causes Breast Cancer may surprise you.

Cause #1: Shaving & Antiperspirants

One of the causes of breast cancer is the use of antiperspirants. Most of these contain highly toxic substances such as aluminium chlorohydrate (aluminium is a known neuro-toxin, it causes a number of "autoimmune" disorders, and destroys the brain). This substance is also dangerous in antiperspirants because it blocks your skin from eliminating toxins. Aside from normal excretion of toxins via urine and faeces, the human body has a number of areas that it uses to purge toxins from the body through *sweat*. These includes the area behind the ears, behind the knees, the groin area, and the underarms. That is why most people have terrible body odour and need to perfume themselves – their bodies are highly toxic, and these waste products smell bad.

Antiperspirants work by *blocking* your pores from perspiring, thus inhibiting your body from purging toxins. Since it cannot sweat them out, the body deposits these toxins in the lymph nodes below the armpits, where they accumulate, day after day... This high concentration of toxicity leads to cancer. Clinical studies over the past 50 years have shown that nearly all breast cancers occur in the upper outer quadrant of the breast, precisely where these lymph nodes are located.

Dr. Kris McGrath published a study in 2004 showing a connection between antiperspirants, underarm shaving, and cancer. He found that women who performed these underarm habits more aggressively had a diagnosis of breast cancer 22 years earlier than the non-users. He theorized that substances found in deodorants were entering the lymphatic system through nicks in the skin caused by shaving.

Cause #2: Wearing A Bra

Medical anthropologist Sidney Singer discovered that the Fiji women who never wore bras experienced practically no breast cancer whatsoever, while those who wore bras had the same rate of breast cancer as American women. Specifically, he found:

- Women wearing a bra 24 hours a day had a 3 in 4 chance of developing breast cancer (75%).

- Women wearing a bra more than 12 hours a day, but not to bed, had a 1 in 7 chance of developing breast cancer (14%).

- Women wearing bras less than 12 hours a day had a 1 in 152 chance of developing breast cancer (0.65%), while women who rarely or never wore bras had a 1 in 168 chance of developing breast cancer (0.59%). Take off your bra when you get home!

According to Dr. David Williams, "Wearing a bra at least 14 hours a day tends to increase the hormone prolactin, which decreases circulation in the breast tissue. Decreasing circulation can impede your body's natural removal of carcinogenic fluids that become trapped in the breast's sac-like glands (lymph nodes). These glands make up the largest mass of lymph nodes in the upper part of your body's lymphatic system." Incredibly, the correlation between bras and breast cancer is four times greater than smoking is to lung cancer. Push-up bras are said to be the worst.

Cause #3: Mammograms – The $10 Billion Scam

At a cost of $150 each, mammograms are a $10 billion dollar a year industry in the US alone. They are prescribed to all 70 million American women over 40. In France, women over a certain age are *forced* to have an annual mammogram or else their health benefits are cut off. This will come as a shock to most people: **Mammograms actually *cause* breast cancer.** Furthermore, they DO NOT work well at detecting tumours – resulting in many false positives. A mammogram is simply an x-ray picture of your breast, and like all x-rays, mammograms use doses of ionizing radiation to create this image. This exposes breast tissue to cancer-causing radiation over and over again. In an article from the July 2006 issue of the *Journal of Clinical Oncology*, researchers showed that the radiation from mammograms actually *causes* breast cancer. According to Dr. Russell L. Blaylock, annual radiological breast exams increase the risk of breast cancer by 2% a year. So over ten years the risk will have increased 20%.

In his book *The Politics of Cancer*, Dr. Samuel Epstein states, "Regular mammography of younger women increases their cancer risks." And Dr. Charles Simone asserts: "Mammograms **increase** the risk for developing breast cancer and raise the risk of spreading or metastasizing an existing growth."

In a study of 1600 European women, **researchers found that women who had at least one mammogram were <u>54% more likely to develop breast cancer</u>** than those who never had one.

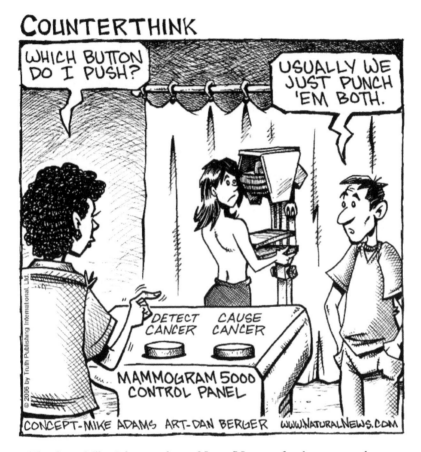

Thanks to Mike Adams and *www.NaturalNews.com* for the cartoon above.

Health advocate Mike Adams states: *"If you were an evil genius who wanted to design a* ***cancer-causing machine,*** *it would be difficult to beat the present-day mammography machine. It exposes human tissue to high-powered radiation that, if repeated often enough, practically guarantees cancer will eventually develop. [...] If you're an oncologist, the best way to ensure you'll have a cancer patient to treat at age 55 is to start exposing them to radiation at age 40 or earlier."*

Many physicians across the world have come to the same conclusion: mammography is not an effective tool for detecting tumours. In a Swedish study of 60,000 women, **<u>70% of the tumours detected by mammograms turned out to be false positives</u>**, but a quarter of these women *will* die regardless, because of the so-called "treatment" – deadly radiation and chemotherapy drugs.

Well-funded PR campaigns are in place to encourage women to have annual mammograms to "prevent" breast cancer by "early detection". We've all seen the pink ribbons. You may have even heard of Breast Cancer Awareness Month, purportedly launched to help women *avoid* breast cancer. But did you know the primary sponsor of these campaigns is AstraZeneca, the manufacturer of the controversial breast cancer drug Tamoxifen? They masterminded the initial event in 1985, to brainwash women into having annual cancer-causing mammograms. Why? Because more mammograms lead to more false positives, which lead to more sales for AstraZeneca.93% of "early detection" has no benefit to the patient according to a groundbreaking new study published in the *New England Journal of Medicine. "We found that the introduction of screening has been associated with about 1.5 million additional women receiving a diagnosis of early stage breast cancer,"* writes study co-author Dr. Gilbert Welch. The team of scientists discovered that there is virtually no reduction in late-stage breast cancer from all this "early" diagnosis, meaning that most women who were told they had breast cancer after a mammogram were being lied to. 93% of the "early detection" cancer cases studied were false positives. And yet more than a million women were told they had early stage cancer, most of whom underwent health-destroying chemotherapy.

Doctors are now even trained to tell patients: *"You have stage zero breast cancer".* What the heck does *that* mean? In some cases, they are even treated with radiation and chemotherapy, and are subjected to five years of hormone therapy! *They never had cancer in the first place!* Or in the case of colonoscopies: *"You have pre-cancerous lesions."* Does this mean you *actually* have cancer? *No it does not!* These types of statements strike fear in the patient and are used by doctors as *a sales tactic to sell more chemotherapy!*

Despite all of this data, governments continue to push mammograms onto the unsuspecting population. According to Dr. James Howenstine, *"This industry supports radiologists, x-ray technicians, surgeons, nurses, manufacturers of x-ray equipment, hospitals, etc. and will not be allowed to disappear by curing and preventing breast cancer."*

Cause #4: Monsanto's rBGH Bovine Growth Hormone in Milk

In his book *Milk: The Deadly Poison,* Robert Cohen states *"The single most disturbing aspect of rBGH from a human safety standpoint, concerns Insulin-like Growth Factor (IGF), which is linked to breast cancer."* According to Dr. Samuel Epstein, *"IGF is not destroyed by pasteurization, survives the digestive process, is absorbed into the blood and produces potent growth promoting effects."* Epstein says <u>it is highly likely that IGF helps transform normal breast tissue to cancerous cells,</u> and enables malignant human breast cancer cells to invade and spread to distant organs (more on milk later).

114

Cause #5: AstraZeneca's Tamoxifen Drug

Imagine this scenario. Your mammogram falsely reveals a "tumour", and your doctor tells you, *"You have breast cancer."* Devastated and fearful, you are ready to do whatever your doctor recommends. You do not stop to think about whether this diagnosis is correct, nor do you explore alternative ways of getting healthy. He prescribes Tamoxifen. Of course, you do not question him. But what if the treatment your doctor has just prescribed *actually causes breast cancer?*

The journal Science published a study from Duke University Medical Center in 1999 showing that after two to five years, Tamoxifen actually **initiated** the growth of breast cancer!

According to Dr. L.R. Wiseman of the Royal Victoria Infirmary, *"Tamoxifen stimulates cell proliferation by sensitizing cells to proliferative effects of IGF."* In his book *Indicted: Cancer Research*, Dr. Tibor J. Hegedus writes: *"Tamoxifen is given to women with breast cancer to block the entrance of estradiol into the tumour cells dependent upon this hormone to stimulate growth. When the hormones are blocked from reaching their primary targets, they are forced to travel to other organs."* This, in turn, stimulates proliferation of cells in the lining of the womb and in can even cause endometrial cancer!

In her article "Tamoxifen, Tears, and Terror," Betty Martini writes: "IGF is a hormone designed to make things grow up; it also stimulates and accelerates cancer in sensitized women, those taking Tamoxifen. One of the reasons for the uproar in Monsanto marketing the bovine growth hormone is the outrageous increase in IGF which will yield a firestorm of cancer from the milk. A chemical company is selling us a gasoline named Tamoxifen to put out the fire." […] "Tamoxifen has been tested and retested for more than 15 years. The testers admitted fraud, many contraindications were just ignored, test results were limited in duration and after-effects not tallied, though women sickened and died from them. Healthy women [are] buying the poison for a disease they don't have, but the drug will give it to them!".

In April 1996, the World Health Organization declared Tamoxifen to be a carcinogen, but AstraZeneca continues to market this toxic drug.

Cause #6: Pesticides and Xenoestrogens

AstraZeneca also makes herbicides and fungicides, including the organochlorine pesticide Acetochlor which has been implicated as a causal factor in breast cancer. Only 3% of the 80,000 chemicals in use have been tested for safety. These toxic health-destroyers are found in our water, air, and soil. Dr. Robert Rowen, MD states: *"We are so awash in a sea of poisons that even unborn babies are marinating in up to 200 different man-made toxic chemicals."* Some of these toxins come from plastics, and are called *xenoestrogens*. These xenoestrogens mimic oestrogen in the body, wreak havoc with women's hormonal system, and have been linked with an increased risk of breast cancer. Most women today have too much oestrogen and not enough progesterone in their body. This can be identified by strong PMS and menopausal symptoms.

Cause #7: Oral Contraceptives

Another drug that wreaks havoc with women's hormonal system is the contraceptive pill. According to international research, young women who take oral contraceptive pills before they become pregnant with their first child run a significantly higher risk of developing pre-menopausal breast cancer. The researchers, led by Dr. Chris Kahlenborn, found that those young women experienced a 44% increased risk of developing pre-menopausal breast cancer, while <u>women who took the pill for four years or longer prior to their first pregnancy ran an increased risk of 52%.</u>

Breast Cancer Emanates From Suppressed Anger, Sorrow, and Sadness

Breasts are the physical metaphor for *nurturing*. Breast cancer is related to women's need to be self-nurtured. Women give and give, but must learn to nurture themselves as well. Richard Moat's research points to the fact that breast issues and breast cancer commonly emanate from – or begin with – the behaviour of suppressing anger, being involved in and affected by inter-family feuding, experiencing significant separation from a loved one, having low self-worth, tending to put others first, long-standing shame, and conflicted inner feelings. Such patterns, as Richard's extensive work with clients has confirmed, lead to the creation of a toxic inner terrain that makes it possible for dis-ease to take hold (*see Chapter 16, 'Disease Starts In The Mind'*). Clear such patterns using the tools of love, forgiveness, and understanding… and you don't need to express that outcome anymore.

Actions You Can Take

So what should you do if you feel a lump in your breast? First of all, don't be alarmed, since it is highly likely it is benign. Secondly, you can use a thermography scan or an ultrasound to get it checked (rather than a mammogram). Thirdly, there are more than 300 ways to cure cancer naturally – start by detoxifying your body and changing your lifestyle. This includes removing your bra, using a natural deodorant (such as PitRok™), exercising, rebounding every day, drinking plenty of water, eating organic fruit and vegetables while cutting out toxic food, taking high quality nutritional supplements, and following the health advice outlined in this book.

The Angelina Jolie Effect?

Do you remember the massive, global media campaign about Angelina Jolie having a double mastectomy? Some people are questioning whether this was <u>a Big Pharma PR campaign</u> and whether she got *paid* to say to the media, *"My doctors estimated that I had an*

87% risk of breast cancer... My chances of developing breast cancer have dropped from 87% to under 5%." This statement to the media resulted in shares of diagnostic test maker Myriad Genetics Inc. to rise to a three-year high, and women all over the world getting their breasts chopped off for spurious reasons (double mastectomies rose by over 150% due to the "Angelina Effect"). At no point was diet, bras, antiperspirants, xenoestrogens, pesticides, drugs nor contraceptive pills mentioned in the media.

The Truth About Prostate Cancer – The Billion Dollar Scam

Similarly to the "breast cancer scam" described above, so-called "Prostate Cancer" is also coming under scrutiny. American men have a 16% lifetime chance of receiving a diagnosis of prostate cancer, but only a 3% chance of dying from it because the majority of prostate cancers grow **slowly** (again, they mostly die from the deadly medical *treatment*, not from "cancer").

The PSA test is what is used routinely for detecting prostate cancer. But does a high PSA score equal prostate cancer? According to articles in the New York Times and Washington Post, the PSA test is essentially worthless. The PSA test simply reveals *how much of the prostate antigen a man has in his blood*, which is a marker of inflammation. However, infections, benign swelling of the prostate and over-the-counter drugs (like Ibuprofen) can all elevate a man's PSA level, but **none** of them signal cancer. A high PSA score leads most men straight to biopsies, then to surgery. Removing the prostate leads men straight to incontinence and impotence.

The PSA test is the male equivalent of mammograms, since **it results in so many false positives and actually <u>causes more cancer than it prevents</u>**. Conventional prostate cancer treatment is the "billion-dollar scam", according to Dr. David Williams.

To proactively prevent prostate cancer you should be physically active and walk or rebound every day, since the movement of the muscles and organs in the pelvic area increases circulation to the prostate gland, and you should also follow the health advice outlined in this book (*lay off the meats, dairy, and alcohol, drink plenty of water, eat organic fruit and vegetables, cut out toxic food, take high quality nutritional supplements, etc.*) In any case, if ever diagnosed with 'cancer', you should get a second and third opinion, since over-diagnosis and false diagnoses of cancer is now very common.

Is Cancer Being Used To Lower The Population?

In 1931, Cornelius Rhoads, a pathologist from the Rockefeller Institute for Medical Research, infected human test subjects in Puerto Rico with cancer cells *on purpose*, and thirteen of them died. Despite stating that *all Puerto Ricans should be killed*, he was later named to the U.S. Atomic Energy Commission, where he began a series of radiation exposure experiments on American soldiers and civilian hospital patients! In 1952,

Chester Southam injected Ohio State Prison inmates with live cancer cells. In 1963 he performed the same procedure on 22 senile, African-American female patients at the Brooklyn Jewish Chronic Disease Hospital in order to watch their immunological response. He later became president of the American Association for Cancer Research!

Please note that the above are not merely isolated occurrences. There are hundreds more similar stories over the past century. It seems that the powers that be wanted to test *how to spread cancer more effectively*. The doctors that went along with it were rewarded with high positions and salaries. Read the sordid history of human medical experimentation at www.naturalnews.com/019187.html.

In a 1969 address to paediatricians in Pittsburgh USA, Dr. Richard Day – *an executive of Planned Parenthood (the rebranded name for the Eugenics movement) and a big Rockefeller 'insider'* – explained how the future would unfold, to a stunned crowd:

- Limiting access to affordable medical care will make eliminating the elderly easier.

- There will be an increase in infectious man-made diseases.

- Suppressing cancer cures is used **as a means of population control**.

- A cure to cancer exists in the Rockefeller Institute but is kept secret *for purposes of* **depopulation.**

It is interesting to note that fertility rates have plummeted while cancer rates have *skyrocketed* in the past few decades. Is it in the interest of the global 'Elite' to reduce the human population?

Governments are advised that lowering the global population will lead to higher standards of living for everyone, and that they will save on pension plans that indebted countries can no longer afford.

In 1969, White House National Security Advisor, Henry Kissinger, ordered the creation of bioweapons that could wipe out the immune system of specific populations, government documents have shown. Kissinger was a staunch advocate of African depopulation. He wrote: ***"Depopulation should be the highest priority of U.S. foreign policy towards the Third World"*, because these growing numbers of poor people would be competing for resources needed by Americans**. More and more people in these poor regions of the world would mean less and less resources for Americans and US companies. This was deemed a major threat to US power and continued pre-eminence.

Perhaps now you are starting to see why do **our healthcare and educational systems fail to educate the public** on how to prevent and cure diseases with nutrition, why immune-system-and-fertility-destroying vaccinations are so important to the ruling class, and why affordable healthcare is becoming more scarce. Their agenda calls for *fewer* people on our planet, not more.

Recap – The Truth About Cancer:

- ❑ Your body consists of trillions of cells. Your bloodstream brings oxygen and nutrients to every cell of your body. When cells do not get enough oxygen and nutrients they weaken and die.

- ❑ In a toxic environment, your cells mutate in order to survive this low-oxygen environment.

- ❑ Cells return to being healthy once they are placed in a clean, alkaline environment.

- ❑ Cancer is not a disease – it is a survival mechanism. The tumour is *not* the cancer.

- ❑ Typically, tumours are neither health endangering nor life threatening.

- ❑ The majority of people who "die from cancer" actually die from conventional treatments.

- ❑ Radiation and chemotherapy *cause* cancer, while surgery spreads the cancer *"like an explosion through the entire body"*. Biopsies are often responsible for cancer spreading.

- ❑ Surgery, chemotherapy, and radiation do not prevent the spread of cancer. They accelerate it.

- ❑ Chemotherapy is toxic, carcinogenic, destroys red blood cells, devastates the immune system, and kills vital organs. 91% of oncologists surveyed would not take chemotherapy themselves.

- ❑ Cancer is a $200+ billion a year industry. There is every financial incentive to "keep it going".

- ❑ <u>The medical profession has a cancer cure rate of only 2%</u>. Alternative treatments have a cure rate of 50% to 90%. There are over 300 known cancer cures that have virtually no side effects.

- ❑ Cancer is happening in your body – on a cellular level – because you are too toxic.

- ❑ Cancer-curing treatments are routinely being suppressed by the medical establishment.

- ❑ Human cancer is primarily attributable to chemical pollutants, bad eating habits, and unhealthy lifestyles, *not* genetics.

❑ Most cancer research by pharmaceutical companies is largely a fraud.

❑ Scientists and pharmaceutical companies routinely fake lab results to get FDA approval.

❑ The survival time of cancer patients today is no greater than it was 50 years ago because the medical establishment is treating the wrong thing. *26 times more people have cancer now!*

❑ Western medicine simply does not work. It is an outmoded system of medicine dominated by the financial interests of pharmaceutical companies.

❑ Cancer cells cannot thrive in an oxygenated environment.

❑ Cancer occurs when cells are denied 60% of their oxygen requirements.

❑ 94% of the information contained in promotional literature sent to doctors by Big Pharma is false and unsubstantiated (they are essentially *marketing lies*).

❑ Dr. Kanematsu Sugiura shrunk tumours in mice with a natural substance (Vitamin B17)

❑ Cancer patients who undergo radiation therapy are more likely to have their cancer metastasize to other sites in their bodies. When chemotherapy and radiation are given together, secondary tumours are 25 times more likely to occur than the normal rate.

❑ Patients who undergo chemotherapy are 14 times more likely to develop leukaemia and 6 times more likely to develop cancers of the bones, joints, and soft tissues.

❑ Children who are "successfully treated" by conventional medicine for Hodgkin's disease are 18 times more likely later to develop secondary malignant tumours (a 1,800% increase), and girls are 75 times more likely to develop breast cancer (7,500% more).

❑ The heads of US cancer clinics send their own parents to alternative cancer clinics abroad.

❑ Oncology nurses and physicians have an elevated risk for cancer, due to radiation and chemotherapy contamination of their workplace.

❑ The major media conglomerates are owned by the same financial interests that control the Pharmaceutical Industry.

CHAPTER 10

The Psychological and Emotional Root Causes of Colon Cancer

Now that we have explored the truth about *what really causes Cancer*, let's address Colon Cancer specifically.

Richard Moat states that Cancer begins with a mind pattern of **unexpressed anger; self-deprecation; deep hurt; long-standing resentment; lacking self-love; and being unforgiving**.

Richard describes the mindset that can lead to Cancer, as:

You are likely to be a loving person who has repressed or withheld their (unacknowledged) feelings of bitterness and/or resentment; most often, these feelings are towards one particular parent; Most cancers are underpinned by unresolved, unexpressed anger. [...] You may be a described as a 'rock' who handles and carries the problems of others (most often family), never complains and puts on a brave, unemotional face. If so, the version of you that you have been presenting to the world is unlikely to be the real you - it is more likely to be the you you think you should be." (find out more at www.RichardMoat.com)

For further clues as to the source of your Cancer, Richard advises you look up the part of body in question. For example, his research indicates:

- ❑ Breast cancer = Anger; Inter-family feuding; Low self-worth; Conflicted feelings.
- ❑ Kidney cancer = Feeling out of your depth, like an outcast, alone and/or abandoned;
- ❑ Larynx cancer = A fear of being stifled or choked from living fully and freely.
- ❑ Liver cancer = Fear of survival; Anger; Feeling as if 'territory' is under threat; Injustice, jealousy and envy are likely under-currents
- ❑ Lung cancer = Fear of dying, for self or someone else; Feeling threatened in a way that gives rise to fear and terror.
- ❑ Pancreatic cancer = Resignation from abuse of trust and good nature; Feel the sweetness has gone out of life; A perceived threat to territory and concern of being unable to fulfill your expected role fully.

❑ Prostate cancer = Intimate sexual conflict, often of an 'ugly' nature; Fear of loss of territory or valued person; threat to manhood, masculinity or role as husband/father

❑ Cervical cancer = Feeling inadequate and a failure; Angry at plans spoilt by others; Frustrated. no choice but to accept your lot; Feeling tied; Conflict of a sexual nature.

❑ **Colon cancer = Closed minded and rigid in thinking; Won't let go; Always battling something; A conflict arising from a vile, base, unspeakable and/or base act.**

Certain negative mindsets create energetic weaknesses in your body – *in a specific part of your body* – which is taken advantage of by toxicities that settle in the weakest parts of your body. According to British researcher and psychoneuroimmunology expert Richard Moat, the mind pattern that manifests itself as 'Irritable Bowel Syndrome' is one of *"Trying to hold on; fear of the unknown; general insecurities; deep-rooted irritation; feeling you shouldn't be angry."* Similarly, the mindset that manifests itself as 'Colitis' is: *"feeling irritated or frustrated with your situation; feeling anger around power/control issues; having difficulty letting something go."*

An English friend of mine, who suffered from colitis for a very long time and who wasn't aware of Richard's work, told me that he cured himself of his painful condition when he stopped his habitual mind pattern of *replaying in his mind over and over again* the things that annoyed him or hurt him, *and never 'letting them go'*.

Richard goes on to describe the psychological and emotional patterns of a person who will develop Irritable Bowel Syndrome, in more detail:

> *"There is conflict and confusion over control of certain aspects of your being; in fact there has been for some time now. When confronting unknown situations, you can experience extreme fears, lack of confidence and nervousness. Are there are issues around intimacy? Do you feel uncomfortable being too close to someone? Is there someone you are keen to eliminate from your life because you see them in some way as a threat to your security? Part of you is getting twisted as a result of holding onto something so determinedly that it becomes distorted and damaged. You need to release something. What are you desperately trying to hold on to that is not healthy for you - a relationship or situation for example? There is a huge, long-standing irritation which won't go away. Do you run and re-run in your mind this irritating and annoying scenario over which you have yet to get closure? Do you blame yourself to some degree for allowing it to happen? The anger that you hold toward yourself is eating away at you and in need of release but you fear expressing it because of the consequences."*

Do any of these emotional and psychological issues resonate for you? Which ones? *These* are the issues you need to address, on a psychological and emotional level, to stop your Colon Cancer in its tracks, heal it, and remove the possibility of it reoccuring.

Remember: you are *not* just a physical body. You are "Mind, Body, and Soul". If you just fix the "body" part of this equation but continue with the same mindset, your mind will just reproduce the same issues – or worse – in the body, until *you get the message*. All illnesses are a way for your body's innate intelligence to let you know the lesson you need to learn and *where you have not been loving*. Do some self-analysis and work on yourself. Get some healing. Change your mindset. Learn to let go, forgive, and find acceptance.

To find out more and get some help with these issues, go to www.RichardMoat.com and contact Richard or his team directly.

Stewart Swerdlow states: *"The mind-pattern of Irritable Bowel Syndrome involves rejection of what you learn in life. It is about needing to rapidly release the past and present and not hold on to anything of value. The mind-pattern of Crohn's disease is not being able to assimilate experiences in life and being angry at it."*

Louise Hay Healed Herself from "Incurable" Cervical Cancer

Echoing the work of Richard Moat, Louise Hay is the author of *"You Can Heal Your Life"*. In her book, she revealed that she was raped at the age of five, and how *decades* later, in 1977, she was diagnosed with "incurable" cervical cancer. She came to the conclusion that by holding on to her resentment for her childhood abuse and rape she had contributed to its onset. She refused conventional medical treatment, and began a regime of forgiveness, coupled with therapy, nutrition, reflexology and a thorough 'detox'. She successfully rid herself of the cancer.

Love, understanding, and compassion were the answer. And of course, getting great nutrition into the body to bring nutrients to your cells.

Anita Moorjani's Near-Death Experience

Anita Moorjani's is the author of *Dying To Be Me*. In 2002 she was diagnosed with cancer, and, after four years of struggling with the disease—having developed large tumours throughout her body—her organs began to fail. She slipped into a coma, doctors gave her just hours to live.

As her body laid there dying, Anita had an out-of-body-experience. In this state, Anita experienced profound peace and love. She also learned about the laws of life, including how she had caused her own cancer. She was then given the choice of remaining in the spirit world, or return to Earth. She was told that her body would heal itself if she returned. Anita awoke from her coma and within *days* her body was fully healed. Her doctors were at a loss to explain this miracle.

She writes of her near-death experience:

> "I felt free, liberated, and magnificent! Every pain, ache, sadness, and sorrow was gone. …I then had a sense of being encompassed by something that I can only describe as pure, unconditional love, but even the word *love* doesn't do it justice … I felt completely bathed and renewed in this energy, and it made me feel as though I *belonged*… I had finally come home … the combination of a sense of joy mixed with a generous sprinkling of jubilation and happiness. … It didn't feel as though I'd *physically* gone somewhere else—it was more as though I'd *awakened*. … My soul was finally realizing its true magnificence! […] I suddenly *knew* things that weren't physically possible, such as the conversations between medical staff and my family that were taking place far away from my hospital bed. […] To my amazement, I became aware of the presence of my father, who'd died ten years earlier, and it brought me an unbelievable level of comfort to sense him with me. …I was also aware of other beings around me. I didn't recognize them, but I knew they loved me very much and were protecting me."

She had not been close to her father, while he was alive, but in this moment, she only felt unconditional love emanating from him. And he reminded her of this important spiritual truth:

> *"Dad, it feels like I've come home! I'm so glad to be here. Life is so painful!* I told him. *But you're always home, darling,* he impressed upon me. *You always were, and you always will be. I want you to remember that."*

The souls of her father and her recently-deceased friend Soni urged her to return to her body, with this message: "*Now that you know the truth of who you really are, go back and live your life* _fearlessly!_"

When she awoke in her body, she astounded her doctors and her loved ones by recounting their conversations in other parts of the hospital, and even more so by becoming cancer-free *within days*. She explains that her miraculous recovery was due to no longer feeling fear, having replaced it by a sense of unconditional love *for herself*:

> "The question I get asked most frequently when sharing my story is: *So, what caused your cancer? I* can sum up the answer in one word: *fear*. What was I afraid of? Just about everything, including failing, being disliked, letting people down, and not being good enough. I was a people pleaser and feared disapproval, regardless of the source. I bent over backward to avoid people thinking ill of me; and over the years, I lost myself in the process. I was completely disconnected from who I was or what I wanted, because everything I did was designed to win approval. […] I understood that the cancer wasn't a punishment or anything like that. It was just my own energy, manifesting as cancer because my fears weren't allowing me to express myself as the magnificent force I was meant to be.

[...] Why, oh why, have I always been so harsh with myself? Why was always beating myself up? Why was I always forsaking myself? Why did I never stand up for myself and show the world the beauty of my own soul? Why was I always suppressing my own intelligence and creativity to please others? I betrayed myself every time I said yes when I meant no! Why have I violated myself by always needing to seek approval from others just to be myself? Why haven't I followed my own beautiful heart and spoken my own truth? How come I never knew that we're not supposed to be so tough on ourselves?

[...] There was nobody punishing me. I finally understood that it was *me* I hadn't forgiven, not other people. *I* was the one who was judging me, whom I'd forsaken, and whom I didn't love enough. [...] I saw myself as a beautiful child of the universe. Just the fact that I existed made deserving of unconditional love. I realized that I didn't need to *do* anything to deserve this. ...I'm loved unconditionally, for no other reason than simply because I exist ... I saw that I'd never loved myself, valued myself, or seen the beauty of my own soul. ...*we already are what we spend our lives trying to attain,* but we just don't realize it!

[...] I understood that my body is only a reflection of my internal state. If my inner self were aware of its greatness and connection with All-that-is, my body would soon reflect that and heal rapidly."

This experience had a profound impact on Anita's life, as one can imagine. After leaving the hospital, her outlook on life had transformed. She states:

"I danced and drank champagne gleefully. <u>I knew more than ever that life was to be lived with joy and abandon</u>. ... I saw divinity in everything—every animal and insect. I developed a much greater interest in the natural world than I had before. ... Every day was a fresh adventure. I wanted to walk, drive, explore, sit on the hills and the sand, and just take in this life! ... I was awed by it all. The deliciousness of each day made me feel as though I'd just been born. [...] I feel that people had lost the ability to see the magic of life. They didn't share my wonder or enthusiasm for my surroundings—and just being alive. They seemed caught up in routine, and their minds were on the next thing they had to do. ...they've forgotten how to just be in the moment."

Is it any surprise so many people feel anxious, depressed, and lost, when they are disconnected from such truth and beauty?

Anita then adds:

"I understood that I owed it to myself, to everyone I met, and to life itself to always be an expression of my own unique essence. Trying to be anything or anyone else didn't make me better—it just deprived me of my true self! It kept others from experiencing me for who I am, and it deprived me of interacting authentically with them. Being inauthentic also deprives the universe of who I came here to be and what I came here to express. [...] I danced and drank champagne gleefully. I knew more than ever that life was to be lived with joy and abandon. I knew that the purpose of my life was to expand my tapestry and allow more and greater experiences into my life."

Anita Moorjani stated that her cancer was due to her not being true to herself. The moment she realized her own magnificence, and replaced all her fears with a deep feeling of *love*, she was healed. She writes: *"I'm at my most powerful when I allow myself to be who life intended me to be."*

She adds: *"It's one of the best-kept secrets of our time: the importance of self-love. I can't stress enough how important it is to cultivate a deep love affair with yourself. I don't recall ever being encouraged to cherish myself. ... my* NDE *allowed me to realize that this was the key to my healing. ...True joy and happiness could only be found by loving myself, going inward, following my heart, and doing what brought me joy."*

Exercise: Grab your journal and a pen. Identify in your own life where you have not been loving, towards others and towards yourself. Then, write down why you are worthy of love, what you are proud of. Also, write down what you are committed to creating in your life.

CHAPTER 11

Is Colon Cancer Due To The Over-Acidification and Over-Toxification Of Your Inner Terrain?

It is important to understand that 'Cancer' is a scary-sounding label that the Medical Establishment puts on what is essentially *your body healing itself*. What *you* need to do is *assist* your body in this process, by detoxifying and changing to a healthier lifestyle.

While our 'toxic emotions' can set the stage for weakening our energetic body, that is just the beginning. Cancer is due in great part to the over-acidification of the body, where the acid accumulates and breaks down your cells day after day—in the areas of your body that are too weak to eliminate them properly—causing toxicity buildup, inflammation, mutation, and eventually cellular death.

Eliminating Cancer from your life is therefore not just a one-off thing you do – it requires a change in your mindset, as well as a change in your lifestyle habits for it to go away and not come back.

It is vital to understand that **cells mutate in a toxic environment!** If your bloodstream is polluted and sludge-like, oxygen and nutrients are not going to reach your cells. Your cells mutate in order to *survive* this anaerobic and toxic environment.

Once you understand cancer as a condition of the environment the cells are in, rather than a disease of the cells themselves, you begin to realise how much control you have over your condition, and how you can reverse it naturally. So the big question is: *"How can I provide the right environment for my cells? What do my cells need?"*

Dr. Robert O. Young writes, in his bestselling book *Sick and Tired*:

> *"Simply cutting out a cancerous tumour **does not cure the symptoms,** because the acid pH conditions responsible for the cancer's development still exist, allowing for a recurrence of the cancer at the same or another site in the body. This theory of how an acid pH plays the major role in all symptoms presents a new paradigm in medicine, which to date has been centred primarily on seeking out and destroying germs with little or no regard for the apparent "soil" in which symptoms are expressed."*

"Without acidosis (an over-abundance of acid in the body) there can be no sickness or disease and there can be NO CANCER!"

"One of the first things to do to get rid of any so-called disease is to get rid of all the acid. For it is this state of the blood and tissues that makes disease possible. Infection, drugs and food poisoning may kill but if they do not, they will be short-lived in a subject free from enervation and acid. Conversely, the poisoning will linger in the system until the acid is overcome".

"So there is only one sickness, one disease, and NOW one treatment. *The one sickness and disease is the over-acidification of the blood and tissues due to an inverted way of living, eating, and thinking. These acids are systemic and they localize at the weakest part of the body like in diabetes or pancreatic cancer."*

"Now, if you were to ask an allopathic doctor to explain cancer in a few words what would he say? He might mention cell mutation or a missing gene, or maybe a so-called virus, but after all these years of research, the medical profession still has no answer as to why. Let me help you understand cancer in a new light. It is my conclusion, based on years of research and study, that cancer is nothing more or less than a cellular disturbance of the electromagnetic balance, disorganization of the cellular microzymas, their morbid evolution to bacteria, yeast, fungus and mould, and their ensuing production of exotoxins and mycotoxins. Cancer, therefore, is a four-letter word —acid, especially lactic acid, a waste product of yeast and fungus".

"Yeast, fungus and mould can aggressively plunge into the cells of the body, even penetrating the nucleus. The fungus can now damage the genetic structure by feeding on (fermenting) it. Eventually, the cell may be converted entirely from normal fermentative metabolism (metabolism in the presence of oxygen — referred to as oxidative metabolism in traditional biology) to abnormal fermentative metabolism (metabolism in the deficiency or absence of oxygen) — CANCER."

In other words, allowing your body to become acidic results in it gradually being taken over by yeast, fungus and mould that develop from inside your own cells. These organisms then feed on the body, weaken it, take over and cause cancer.

At the end of the day, what matters is *results*. Here are just a few testimonials from Dr. Young's patients who started cleansing and alkalizing (source: www.phmiracleliving.com):

"I am a 67 year old male. I was healthy up to 1984 when I had a heart attack. I had by-pass surgery in 1995. One year later the Doctor, found cancer in my right kidney. They had to remove my kidney. One year later they found cancer in my bladder. They removed the tumors, I was on Chemo for a year. The cancer cleared up for about three months. Then the cancer came back in my bladder, so they did surgery again. In three months after surgery, the Doctors called me into the office to tell me that they found tumor in my right lung. A few months later they did surgery on my lung. They couldn't get all the cancer, because it was to close to an artery. Doctors want me to have radium therapy, but I have emphysema bad, if they did the therapy it may kill me. So I decided not to do it. I didn't have long to live.

I started SuperGreens, Ph, and vegetables diet. I have been in this program for nine months. Three weeks ago I had an IVP done, **Doctors didn't see any tumor in my left kidney or my bladder anymore.** *Two weeks ago I had a CT on my lung, the Doctor said,* **the tumor was shrinking in my lung,** *no lesions from the tumor and it was the size of a pea. Doctor told me that I was looking real good, and whatever I was doing 'just keep it up'. I have lost weight from 198 to 160. I can walk and work without getting out breath. I feel great and I am going to lick this with my SuperGreens, PH and Alkaline diet. Also* **I was a diabetic and had high cholesterol and treglyceride. They are all normal now.** *God Bless Dr. Young"* – S.L. Slane

"I was told over 10 years ago that I have a condition called HPV (Human Papilloma Virus). For years I have been diagnosed as HIGH RISK HPV for pre-cancer of the cervix. In June of 2003, I started using Super Greens. On March 4th, 2004 I was re-tested again. My Doctor told me **I had been high risk... now I was low risk!** *I was stunned! They also started seeing some weight loss, and toned muscles, which they made positive comments on."* – **Carmen Bennett – Ziegler,** Apple Valley Minnesota

"Last June it was recommended that I have a lumpectomy and do chemotherapy, radiation and drugs. After serious thought, I decided to do a different approach: your complete program of alkalizing and energizing my body.

This past Friday, my doctor called to tell me the results of my AMAS test (Anti-Malignin Antibody Screen for all types of cancer). His words: **'Great news, you have NO cancer cells'.** *I was ecstatic!!! I've never felt healthier, and that is because of changing my "inner terrain" on a cellular level, regenerating my cells, and bringing my body back into balance. Alkalizing my body made complete sense to me. Thus, I was able to embrace the "cancer" with love from the very beginning."* – Dorothy Torrey

"Who needs stage 4 liver cancer or even a liver transplant when you can have a brand new liver every six weeks? That's right. Your liver recycles itself every six weeks. So why not a healthy new liver, cancer free in six weeks?

I wanted to share about a patient of mine. Stage 4 liver cancer, 48 year-old male.
U of I medical center and several other doctors have given up on him. Since he had tried traditional medicine and they gave up on him, I knew I couldn't. Thank God for Dr. Young. **With these products, in 3 weeks we have witnessed a change in his liver enzymes and body function.** *I already knew which particular nutrients to go after, but these products are outstanding."* – Dr. Larry Hopkins *(my great great uncle is John Hopkins of the famous Johns-Hopkins Medical School)*

Alkalizing and detoxifying the body *works*. It requires, as I said, a different mindset and a different lifestyle.

The Power Of Alkalinity

" I just got a text message from Patty Webb on the results from her doctor regarding the 403-point drop in her cal25# reading (cancer measurement; below 35 is considered normal). Her count had a 19-point drop when she started back on the water at 8.5ph (alkaline) and a drastic drop of 403pts in a two-week period when she started on the 9.5ph water!!! Her doctor said that it was not normal for that to happen and he was very surprised and she thanked me for as she said "taking a chance on me." She is almost in the safe zone now with her cancer count at 69, safe zone being 0-35. We will see what the next test shows and hopefully her body will have the support it needs to get rid of this ovarian cancer that she has been told is terminal and there is no cure for. Our bodies have such an amazing ability to heal themselves if we support that healing process. I am so excited about the news that I had to tell all of you about it. " – Donna

Source: http://www.healthywaterlife.com/cgi-bin/d.cgi/kangenwaterclinic/ge/testimonials.html

The Impressionable Colon

The colon is a very changeable and susceptible part of the body. An injury, surgery or other stress such as emotional upset or negative thinking can alter the flora (no one needs to be told how negative emotions affects the stomach, for example). Usually written off as a minor disturbance, incomplete digestion from emotional upheaval will quickly set the stage for intestinal imbalance, and the colon can become a putrid, toxic mass of unwanted material. Birth control pills, broad-spectrum antibiotics like penicillin and tetracycline, antifungal drugs and other chemicals, such as the chlorine in water, will all cause the pleomorphosis of healthy flora to symptogenic forms. This can result in mycelized fungus almost immediately. Therefore, it is not unreasonable to say that the use/abuse of many so-called wonder drugs of modern medicine has been instrumental in bringing cancer and AIDS down on our heads, among a few other problems! In a matter of days after antibiotic treatment, a growth of fungal cells can occur. This can linger for life if ignored, especially when one regularly consumes poultry, eggs, meat, and milk, since these foods also contain antibiotic (and hormone) residues, not to mention fungus itself.

It is usually a combination of factors that makes a person ill. For example, cancer-causing (carcinogenic) substances called *nitrosamines* can form by the interaction of *nitrates* and *nitrites* (chemicals in processed deli meats, for example) with certain other chemicals in your body. These certain other chemicals are mycotoxins! Nitrosamines are therefore secondary mycotoxins from fungus, which needs our help to feed it raw material. Nitrosamines cause cancer by creating severe electrochemical imbalance, thus disturbing the central balance of the microzymas. Morbid evolution to the mold stage then follows. It is important to understand that the friendly bacteria help prevent this. They neutralize toxins, thus preventing their absorption (no –you can't take some acidophilus pills and eat a salami sandwich!).

CHAPTER 12

To Get Rid of Cancer You Must Cleanse & Purify Your Body!

In order for cells to be healthy and vibrant, they need oxygen, nutrients, and *the ability to eliminate their own waste*. At its basic essence, the process of life revolves around *'Consuming and Eliminating'*. Both need to happen smoothly in order for your cells to be healthy.

What happens if the cell is living in an environment (i.e. the bloodstream) that is polluted? Pretty soon the cell starts to run out of energy. If day after day we consume more things than can be assimilated by the body – junk food, processed foods, 'dead' foods, alcohol, etc. – the body accumulates and stores excess waste, instead of eliminating it through faeces, urine, or *through the skin*. This is rather like never throwing out the trash – your house would soon become disgusting!

It is not long before the bloodstream starts to accumulate waste and toxins. In this toxic environment, oxygen and nutrients do not reach your cells as effectively. As your cells become weaker, the functional efficiency of your system begins to drop. They don't produce as much energy. The real health challenge most people have is <u>not that some 'bug' is attacking them, but that their inner environment has been compromised</u>. Their lifestyle has weakened their body and has caused their inner environment to become polluted, resulting in their body getting *out of balance*. The first step on your way to breaking this cycle and getting *back in balance,* is: **YOU MUST CLEANSE!**

David Wolfe states in his book *Longevity Now*: **"Detoxification is the process of the body cleansing itself of wastes and poisons.** These toxins can include metabolic waste heavy metals, pathogenic organisms, volatile organic compounds, distressed emotions, spiritually stuck energy and other energies. Though every tissue and organ is able to go through its own detoxification, it is the liver, kidneys, lymph fluid, skin, brain, gastrointestinal tract, along with the entire immune system, that are the key facilitators of this process. By decreasing the pathogen, viral, and nanobacteria load in our bodies, we improve our physical and mental energy and acuity. Raw plant foods, superfood, medicinal herbs, fresh spring water, laughter, bliss, joy, positive thoughts,hope, and unconditional love all exist in the same frequency range. Tuning into this frequency range raises the overall vibration of your energy field, causing anything that is vibrating at a lower frequency, such as fear, pain, doubt, cancer, ugliness, depression, toxins, parasites, bad calcium, and so on, to eventually percolate out and be ejected from the body. This process is known as detoxification."

After attending my first ever health seminar in the summer of 2003, I rushed home and threw out all the processed foods in my fridge and cupboards, I threw out the meats, cheeses, milk, cereal boxes, sugary snacks, chips, etc. and went out to buy lots of fresh fruit, fresh vegetables, brown rice, quinoa, and a juicer. I spent the next 30 days doing a detox. While the first 4-5 days were quite tough, by the end of the week I was feeling *amazing*. My energy levels were tremendous, I only needed 6 hours of sleep (instead of ten hours previously), my skin cleared up, I had incredible clarity of thought, my gum ulcers didn't flare up anymore, and my mood remained constant and positive.

My Detoxification Routine

I now regularly do a 10-day detox at home, where I cut out all meat, dairy, and starch. I have cut out sugar from my life (I still have a piece of chocolate from time to time). I start my day with an alkalizing glass of water, **lemon juice**, aloe vera juice, MSM powder and chlorella (to help remove heavy metals from my system), or freshly made wheatgrass juice that I grow myself. I have a **sauna** once a week, as well as play squash and basketball on the weekends, to sweat the toxicity out. I **walk** my dog twice a day and I use my **rebounder** for 10 minutes a day and this stimulates my lymphatic system further. I have a bath with Epsom salts twice a month. I have removed 90% of all the plastic and chemical products we used routinely. I got my **mercury fillings** removed by a biological dentist. And once every couple of years, my wife and I go do a *thorough* **mucoid plaque cleanse**.

Colon Cleansing – Death Begins At The Colon

Your colon – or 'large intestine' – is a major way for your body to eliminate waste and toxins. The fastest it eliminates that toxic waste out of your system, the better. Your stomach and intestines use billions of germs to break down your food, so that you can digest what is digestible and eliminate the rest. Imagine if all that resulting waste and billions of germ kind of stick around, multiply, and fester for a while… Imagine having a whole container of dangerous, highly toxic chemicals stored in your basement, leaking out and contaminating your entire house. You would want to get rid of that container pretty quickly, right? Unfortunately, most people don't use their colon very effectively, and consequently it gets clogged up. Whenever you ingest something that your body can't use right away (live foods), it 'clogs' up the system. The modern diet is incredibly clogging, because it consists of mostly *dead foods*. The average American has 15 pounds of faecal matter lodged in their system! It's been there for years! When your colon remains so clogged up and toxic, all these toxins back up into your bloodstream (this is known as toxaemia), compromising the integrity of your inner terrain. *You are literally poisoning yourself.*

After reading Richard Anderson's book ***Cleanse & Purify Thyself*** in 2006, where he recommended doing a mucoid plaque cleanse, I flew to Thailand to spend a couple of weeks at The Sanctuary on the island of Koh Pang Yang. Their cleansing protocol involved fasting for ten days, doing colonics every day, taking specific herbs recommended in Anderson's book (designed to loosen the mucoid plaque from your intestinal walls), and drinking a specific clay with psyllium husk and watermelon juice (this is to absorb toxins and scrape away the mucoid plaque from your intestinal walls). We had a thin vegetable broth for dinner, and we could drink coconut water during the day as well. <u>Mucoid plaque slows down intestinal action, waste excretion and nutrient absorption</u>. It can harbour pathogens such as bacteria and parasites.

What surprised me initially, was that despite not having eaten in five days, my body was still excreting, um… a lot of 'waste'. We truly have a lot of backed up waste lodged into our digestive system! But the biggest surprise occurred on day six, when after a colonic I saw that I had excreted green, red, and brown rubbery pieces into the toilet! You could rinse away the rest of the waste (it was collected in a mesh basket placed in the toilet bowl), but these bizarre pieces of rubbery mucoid plaque remained. You could even pick them up with a plastic glove to examine them. They literally felt like rubber. It made me wonder whether all the plastics and chemicals in our environment – things that our body simply cannot break down naturally – remain lodged in our intestinal walls for our entire lives.

I had been a very health-conscious vegetarian for two years at that point, and I was drinking my alkalizing "Green Juice" smoothie every morning for *three* years. Other people were excreting entire one-meter-long "tubes" of mucoid plaque! (See picture above).

I believe that it is extremely doubtful that people can maintain any degree of good health past a certain age, if they are walking around with 10 to 25 pounds of lodged faecal matter in their colon. You will never have vibrant health if you don't **clean out your personal "sewer pipes."**

Doing a thorough detox should be a matter of priority. *Please* go on a cleanse and get yourself a colonic irrigation – you will be amazed at the difference it makes to your health and levels of energy.

By the way, bad breath is often due to the rotting, putrefying food in your stomach and intestines… It could be due to what you ate *a year ago!* Also, why does body odour increase with age? And why do people use underarm deodorants and perfumes? Because they are *spoiled rotten* from the inside. All that toxicity is escaping through your mouth, skin, armpits, and *backside*, and *makes you stink!*

Dr. Richard Schulze states that 80% of all maladies, whether arthritis, acne, chemical sensitivity, or cancer were cleared up within two weeks of cleaning the bowel. And according to Dr. Darrell Wolfe, "There is one major cause of disease and this is acidosis (low pH). Do you know that **its major cause is putrefaction of faecal waste reabsorbed into your system**? This causes toxaemia, which means dirty blood. Let me pose a question to you. Do you believe that you could have systemic candida, chronic fatigue, headaches, sore throat, skin disorders, heart disease, gout, arthritis, sinus problems, even cancer – without your blood being dirty and toxic? The only way for your blood to become toxic is by reabsorbing your own toxic faecal waste from the large intestine."

Check out Dr. Schulze's Intestinal Corrective Formula at www.herbdoc.com.

The MMS (Miracle Mineral Solution) Cleanse

MMS is good for clearing Allergies, Arthritis, Cancer, Cardiovascular Problems, Cirrhosis, Chronic Infections, Chronic Inflammations, Heavy Metal Toxicity, Kidney Disease, Lyme disease, Liver Disease, Malaria, Sinusitis and sinus problems, Thyroid issues, and many more ailments still.

I am keen to try out the MMS cleansing protocol, for removing any remaining parasites and viruses from my system, considering the number of vaccination I was subjected to as a child in the 1980s.

Many people have posted videos on YouTube describing their results with using MMS. It is quite a harsh cleansing protocol, but the results are there for all to see. Recently, field trials conducted with a team of Red Cross humanitarian workers in Uganda found that **100% of malaria victims treated with a simple MMS solution mixed in water were healed within 24 to 48 hours**, without any side-effects! This has the potential to improve the quality of life for millions of people living in Africa and elsewhere, and prevent millions of deaths. And despite this entire field test having been filmed and released to the public, the Red Cross is now claiming the trial never even happened... This is yet another cover-up by the Medical Establishment, protecting its vaccination and pharmaceutical cartel.

Stewart Swerdlow's Recommendations for Detoxifying Your Body

❑ Start your day with a glass of water with some **lemon juice** to alkalize it.

❑ Get **Rife treatments**/ foot baths frequently.

❑ Detoxify your body from **heavy metals** such as mercury.

❑ Take **sea salt baths** frequently (I use Epsom Salts in my bath and swim in the sea frequently)

❑ Take far infrared saunas as often as possible.

❑ Do a **colon cleanse** twice per year.

❑ Consider taking a course of **MMS** to kill viruses and bacteria.

❑ **Fast for 24 hours once a month**, and for three days every 6 months.

David Wolfe lists the following detoxification 'tools' in *Longevity Now*:

❑ **Detox products** that remove artificial environmental toxins: fulvic acid, MSM, zeolites, shilajit, EDTA, clay, and Patrick Flanagan's Crystal Energy

❑ Dissolve and **remove parasites** and their waste products, and remove **bad calcium**.

❑ **Herbal detox** systems such as *Triple Herbal Treasures* and herbal cleansing systems – these are designed to remove hardened **mucoid plaque** from the small intestines

❑ **Fasting**: Juice fasting (usually enters on alkaline green vegetables and beet juice); blended fasting (no solid food, this fast usually enters on detox lemonades and raw green soups); water fasting (should be done with spring water); dry fasting (alternate days of dry and water fasting have been shown in Russian research to reduce dangerous deuterium or heavy hydrogen levels in the body, thus increasing longevity)

❑ A thinned-down **raw detox diet** (with low-fat, low sugar, and high fiber/alkalinity): this type of diet should be done temporarily and not as a maintenance diet

❑ **Sauna**: this can include traditional Water Cure, Russian *banya* therapies, Finnish saunas, variations of Ayurvedic panchakarma, etc. The idea behind these therapies is that heat expands your tissues and cold contracts them; in the dynamic between heat and cold, the body is purified and detoxified like the squeezing of a sponge.

❑ A lymphatic activating exercise program (inversion-oriented yoga, **rebounding**, etc.)

❑ Enemas and **colonics** (it is important to pull the plug and let all wastes drain out regularly)

❑ Deep-tissue **bodywork** (Romi Romi, Rolfing, etc.)

❑ *Grounding* and ***Zapper* technology**: Zappers draw toxins right through the skin to the negatively charged electrode on the zapper. Being grounded by touching the Earth directly or via grounding technology alters the exchange of gases excreted when we breathe.

David Wolfe also gives the following "common-sense" warning when embarking on a detox: "All detoxification strategies should be adopted with common sense. **Too sudden a shift can "shock" the body**. Everything comes as it should, in its own time. The Universe rewards the virtues of discipline and perseverance."

This passage from his book will be of extreme interest to women, in particular: "Women with high levels of toxicity (pesticides, chemicals, solvents, petroleum byproducts, xenoestrogens, heavy metals, etc.) tend to experience **more challenging PMS symptoms, as well as a more extreme menopause experience**. Detoxification tools can assist one in normalising extremes of hormonal imbalance."

Ty Bollinger lists in his book *Cancer: Step Outside The Box* the following toxicities that need to be address when doing a cleanse:

- ❑ **Heavy metals** such as mercury, lead, antimony, nickel, cadmium tin, arsenic, uranium, as well as a host of others. In addition to causing significant oxidative damage, heavy metals are doubly dangerous because they have the ability to displace many of the essential minerals your body needs to function properly. Adding insult to injury, heavy metals and mercury in particular wreak additional havoc on the endocrine system, which regulates hormonal levels.

  There are 358 studies linking mercury with heart disease, 643 linking mercury with cancer, and 1445 studies linking mercury to neurodegenerative disease (such as autism, Alzheimer's, etc.). And mercury is just *one* of the many heavy metals known to have serious health issues.

- ❑ **Persistent Organic Pollutants** – These POPs exist in pesticides, insecticides, varnishes, cleaning solutions and virtually every product in an aerosol can, a bottle underneath your kitchen sink or in your garage right now. The placental cord blood of newborn babies was tested for 413 different industrial chemicals and found to be positive for 287 of these substances, which included PCBs, mercury, DDT, dioxin, fluorinated hydrocarbons, organophosphates, and many other categories of POPs!

- ❑ **EMF frequencies** – Energetic toxicity includes all the high-powered energy waves that pass through our bodies every day. In modern society, our bodies are bombarded by energetic toxicity from things we can't see, including electromagnetic radiation (from power lines and microwaves) and ambient radiation (from cell phones, military radar systems, TVs and computer screens). And this toxicity is increasing at a stunningly rapid exponential rate.

- ❑ **Negative emotions** are one of the most toxic forms of oxidative stress because it's insidious and often suppressed. Dr. Rashid A. Buttar writes: *"Every patient suffering with cancer I have seen did not begin to recover until they had addressed their emotional issues. Only those who were able to successfully come to terms with and*

138

release their anger, to forgive and choose to love unconditionally have a chance of winning the battle."

❑ **Toxic family members** – some people act as energetic 'vampires' and can drain you of energy.

❑ **Toxic Food** – Completely avoid GMO produce and irradiated produce.

❑ **Bacteria, viruses, parasites, fungi, yeast and a host of other critters** – All the other toxicities suppress the immune system and render the body vulnerable to opportunistic pathogens…

Ty also recommends doing the following cleanses in *Cancer: Step Outside The Box* (reproduced with kind permission of Ty Bollinger):

❑ **A Parasite Cleanse** – Scientists have identified **over 300 types of parasites thriving in the USA today,** including pinworms, tapeworms, hookworms, ringworms, whipworms, roundworms, and heartworms. The USDA tells us that the average cubic inch of beef contains up to 1,200 larvae. It is estimated that over 90% of Americans suffer from parasites and don't even know it. When symptoms appear, these parasites have probably been in your system for over a decade, growing fat on sugar, processed food, and excessive carbohydrate consumption…

Dr. Hulda Clark was the leading expert on parasites, up to her death in 2009. She developed a device called "The Zapper", which kills pathogens in the body. She also claimed that three herbs can rid you of over one hundred types of parasites: Black Walnut Hulls, Wormwood (from the Artemisia shrub), and Common Cloves (from the clove tree). These three herbs must be used together. According to Dr. Hazel Parcells, *"Make no mistake about it, worms are the most toxic agents in the human body. They are one of the primary underlying causes of disease and are the most basic cause of a compromised immune system."*

Check out the TV series "Monsters Inside Me", where they show a patient have their skull cracked open for the doctors to remove parasitic worms *with tweezers…*

When professors Henry Lai and Narendra Singh, researchers at the University of Washington, tested the combination of Artemisin with transferrin (an iron-enhancing molecule), they saw a 98% reduction in breast cancer cells within 16 hours! Other studies have shown that <u>100% of Leukaemia cells are destroyed with this combination in only eight hours</u>.

Dr. Clark's parasite cleanse can be purchased at www.drclark.com.

❑ **A Kidney Cleanse** – Every day, your kidneys process the blood and help to sift out waste products (like mercury, lead, arsenic, copper, and other toxins) and extra water. The waste and extra water become urine. The urine then flows to your bladder through the ureters. Crystals form in urine from various salts that build up on the inner surfaces of the kidney. Eventually these crystals become large enough to form kidney stones. A kidney cleanse is a procedure which is used to dissolve deposits inside the kidneys that can lead to kidney stones. We now know that hard minerals (mainly from tap water) cannot be assimilated by our bodies; thus, they begin to build up in our kidneys and other organs, contributing toward many diseases, including cancer. According to Dr. Charles Mayo, "'Water hardness' is the underlying cause of many, if not all, of the diseases resulting from poisons in the intestinal tract. These hard minerals pass from the intestinal walls and get into the lymphatic system, which delivers all of its products to the blood, which in turn, distributes to all parts of the body. This is the cause of much human disease."

One popular way to cleanse kidneys is to do a watermelon cleanse. Just purchase a few huge watermelons and eat them all throughout the day. Another popular kidney cleanse is celery seed tea. Just pour boiling spring water over a tablespoon of freshly ground celery seeds and allow it to steep. Celery seed tea is very potent in case of kidney stones and chronic kidney diseases. Celery seeds have a direct action on the kidneys, speeding up the clearance of accumulated toxins from the joints. Celery seed tea is oftentimes combined with dandelion root to increase the efficiency of elimination by both the kidneys and the liver. However, if you are pregnant, do not drink celery seed tea since it is a uterine stimulant! Also, check out Dr. Hulda Clark's kidney cleanse: www.curezone.com/clark/kidney.asp.

❑ **A Liver & Gall Bladder Cleanse** – The liver performs over 1,000 tasks daily and filters every drop of blood that flows through it. 80% of the liver can be damaged without producing any symptoms! Plus, the liver regenerates itself every 6 weeks! Dr Leo Roy stated in 1994: "No disease, especially degenerative diseases including cancer and AIDS, could survive longer than a few weeks in the presence of a healthy liver." Dr. Kasper Blond of Vienna, Austria, in his book The Liver and Cancer, refers to the liver as the "gateway to disease." [...] The best liver flush I have seen is the five-day liver and gallbladder flush from Jon Barron. You can find it at www.jonbarron.org. Another good liver flush is from Dr. Schulze at www.herbdoc.com. Drink a quart of organic, unprocessed, apple juice every day for three days. You don't have to fast during this period, but it is recommended that you do fast. On the evening of the third day, drink eight ounces of organic, cold pressed, extra virgin olive oil. Stir it up (along with the juice of one lemon) and drink it down quickly. Then grab a small trashcan and lie in a foetal position, curled up on your right side of half an hour. Keep the trashcan by your face just in case you vomit. The next norming, you should find a few small green or black objects in your stool. These are gallstones. Apple juice is high in malic acid, which acts as a solvent to weaken adhesions between solid globules. The organic olive oil stimulates the gallbladder and bile duct to contract and expel its contents. Dr. Schulze claims our diets are just too sweet, that we must get some bitter herbs and greens to stimulate the bile flow. He recommends eating some parsley or kale (or any bitter herb/green) just prior a meal to get the bile flowing. Beet juice, alfalfa juice, wheat grass juices are a delight for the liver. And I've already mentioned, coffee enemas also stimulate the flow of bile.

When the blood becomes overburdened by these deadly toxins and poisons, the liver has to pick up the overload. Your liver already does over 500 different functions for the body and intestines. The liver works overtime until it becomes chronically fatigued, and then the body starts experiencing an array of negative side effects.

❑ **Cleanse Your Blood** – Your bloodstream is your "river of life". Blood-cleansing herbs include red clover, burdock root, chaparral, poke root, and sheep sorrel. These are the herbs you will find in the famous blood cleansing formulas such as Hoxsey tea, Essiac tea, and Dr. Schulze's formula. They literally drive tumours out of the body.

CHAPTER 13

17 Natural Cancer Remedies "They" Don't Want You To Know About

There are hundreds of effective, safe, natural remedies for eliminating cancer. The reason you rarely hear about them is that the pharmaceutical industry and Medical Establishment fight tooth and nail to suppress this information, as it threatens their $300-billion-dollar-a-year "Cancer Industry". A lot of jobs, and a lot of profit is at stake.

It is important to understand, first and foremost, that **Cancer Is Not A Disease**, even though we have been brainwashed to believe it is. Cancer is actually *a symptom* that occurs when the human body is too acidic and toxic and your cells don't get enough oxygen to survive – or when our 'toxic emotions' wreak havoc with our biochemistry.

Dr. Otto Warburg, a cancer biochemist and the 1931 Nobel Laureate in Medicine, discovered that **cancer occurs whenever any cell is denied 60% of its oxygen requirements**. His thesis was that cancer is a fermentative disease caused by cells which have *mutated from aerobic respiration to anaerobic respiration*, resulting in glucose fermentation and uncontrolled cellular growth.

Tumours are nothing more than <u>walled-off toxic waste dumps</u> inside the body sustained by fermenting sugar. *Remove the source of toxic waste, and your body will break down and eliminate the "tumour" naturally.*

According to Warburg, most, if not all degenerative diseases, are a result of lack of oxygen at the cellular level. **Cells mutate when they don't get enough oxygen.** It stands to reason that cleansing the body and doing things that bring oxygen to the cells helps patients regain their health.

"The cause of cancer is clear: poor diet, lifestyle and poor mental attitude result in toxic build-up which overloads the self-cleansing mechanism. Cancer is manifestation of long term nutritional and environmental irritation, resulting in cellular oxygen starvation, leading to uncontrolled cell replication."

Dr. Saul Pressman

"Cancer cells cannot thrive in an oxygenated environment. Exercising daily, and deep breathing help to get more oxygen down to the cellular level. Oxygen therapy is another means employed to destroy cancer cells."

Johns Hopkins hospital

Your cells *mutate and expand*, in an all-out attempt at surviving your body's toxic, low-oxygen wasteland. As we saw in Chapter 6 and Chapter 11, Dr. Robert O. Young explains that blood cells mutate and expand in order to survive, when the bloodstream surrounding them is too polluted and toxic. If your blood becomes *sludge*, nutrients and oxygen can't reach your cells, and they weaken and die. But first, they mutate in order to adapt to this toxic oxygen-less environment! **Cancer is not a disease – it is a survival mechanism!**

Conventional Treatments Are DEADLY and Have a Measly 2.1% Cancer Cure Rate

Cancer is not a disease. It is a survival mechanism. Even more surprising, is that cancer does not kill – *conventional treatments do.*

According to a 2004 report by Morgan, Ward, and Barton: *"The contribution of cytotoxic chemotherapy to 5-year survival in adult malignancies... survival in adults was estimated to be 2.3% in Australia and 2.1% in the USA."*

Despite the fact that oncologists are successfully able to shrink tumours, the cancer patient still dies in the majority of cases. Why? The reason is the tumour size has nothing to do with curing cancer, and furthermore, patients are dying from the toxic chemotherapy treatments.

"Most people think that cancer is caused by DNA damage and that orthodox medicine is frantically searching for a cure for cancer. Both beliefs are complete nonsense and come from the propaganda and deceptions of television. Cancer is not caused by DNA damage. The definition of a cancer cell is a cell with low ATP energy. [...] Yet the media glorifies all of the "cancer researchers" who are diligently trying to "fix" the DNA damage of cancer cells. It is all a scam to make sure that cures for cancer are never found!

The 5-year cure rate of orthodox medicine (e.g. oncologists) is 2.1%. In other words, in 97.9% of the cases, their cancer patients are dead within 5 years of diagnosis."

"A true cure rate of 90% or more can easily be achieved by cancer patients who avoid orthodox medicine, go with alternative medicine first, and do their homework."

Webster Kehr

"Orthodox medicine, with its focus on the highly profitable tumour, has **brainwashed the public into thinking that the tumour is the cancer**" says cancer expert Webster Kehr. The tumour is not the cancer. The tumour is your body's way of telling you that you are really *toxic*, and it doesn't have enough *energy* to break down and eliminate all that excess waste.

Your body has to maintain enough energy to run your heart, your brain, your nervous system, your digestive system, your liver, your lymphatic system, etc. AND deal with the *poisons* you ingest numerous times a day in the form of coffee, sugar, alcohol, pesticides, pollution, pharmaceutical drugs, chemicals in household cleaning products, chemicals in toiletries, perfumes, and skincare products. Your body can heal itself. *But not if it is under constant assault and not provided with the nutrients and minerals it needs to survive!*

Cancer is happening in your body – on a cellular level – because you are too *toxic*. But doctors don't label this as such, and they don't recommend what we now know cures cancer naturally: cleansing and alkalizing your bloodstream, exercise, rest, and healthy nutrition. Instead, they label it 'Cancer' and they recommend the most toxic chemical cocktail possible, that destroys your immune system! And then for good measure they cut your body open, creating even more stress on the body.

145

As a result, many people who "die from cancer" *actually* die from the conventional treatments long before they would have actually died from the cancer itself.

Dr. Leonard Coldwell states that <u>radiation and chemotherapy *cause* cancer, while surgery spreads the cancer *"like an explosion through the entire body."*</u>

Alternative cancer treatments focus on detoxifying the body and returning the body to a state of *health and strength*. Some of these treatments can be combined, for maximum treatment, but ultimately it is a change of *lifestyle and mindset* that is required to maintain one's health.

Note: make sure you get a formal test before, during, and after you commence one of these treatments. Ty Bollinger, author of *Cancer: Step Outside The Box*, recommends the AMAS test (www.oncolabinc.com).

> "Orthodox Medicine is a racket, and the orthodox cancer treatment industry is the biggest racket of them all. Wake up now or wake up later after you've lost your loved ones to the cancer industry. It's completely up to you. You can cure yourself of any form of cancer, at home, for next to nothing if you simply educate yourself about the therapies that actually work versus the high priced, phony baloney, half baked, 'hopeful' assurances that you'll get from the oncologist poison-peddlers of the cancer industry."
>
> Ken Adachi, Canadian writer and literary critic

Natural Anti-Cancer Solution #1 – Raw Food, Alkalizing and Detoxifying

Removing *weakened, diseased, mutated, "cancerous"* cells from the body requires *giving your cells what they actually need: oxygen and nutrition.*

This involves, as a first step, cleansing and alkalizing your "inner terrain" (your bloodstream). Start by cutting out alcohol, cigarettes, coffee, sugar, sweets, chocolate, milk, ice cream, cheese (all dairy products), GMO foods, meat, eggs, fluoride and chlorine from tap water, toxic personal care products, pesticides in produce (go organic), processed food, aspartame, MSG, and food additives, to name a few.

Instead, adopt a raw food or vegan diet – at least while you are recovering – that includes 80% fresh greens, vegetables, and fruit. Juicing can be an excellent way to make this transition. Some excellent **alkaline-forming foods** are: lemon juice, most raw vegetables, wheatgrass, barley grass, Aloe Vera, lima beans, olive oil, green tea,

most   herbs,   sprouted   grains,   and   sprouts   (see   full   list   here:
www.rense.com/1.mpicons/acidalka.htm)

The American author Anthony Robbins begins his "Living Health" seminars by sharing the story of how, many years ago, his friend came to him in tears, because her mother had been diagnosed with Cancer. She had tumours the size of a *baseball* on her shoulders and in her female organs. The doctor gave her 9 weeks to live.

Robbins said to his friend: *"Look, hundreds of thousands of people have had cancer and beaten it. I know you don't hear much about it, but it's a fact. All we've got to do is find people who got cancer and beat it, find out exactly what they did and what they had in common, and model that. If we model what most people do, we'll get what most people get."*

He gave this woman a couple of books to read (including Dr. Kelley's classic *One Answer To Cancer*), and within a few days she started detoxifying her body – essentially, getting rid of the poisons that were in her body, without cutting the body open.

Waste and toxins started streaming out of her system. Within 4 weeks she lost 28 pounds. After just 8 weeks, she was feeling amazing, she is in the best fitness of her life, the best *health* of her life, and she doesn't feel any sense of 'dis-ease' in her body.

The doctors still insisted on performing an exploratory operation. So they opened her up, and found... nothing. No tumours. In her whole body. In 9 weeks. The doctors couldn't understand how that was possible. They said: *"It's a miracle!"* She tried to explain to them what she did, but they just repeated: *"No! It's a miracle!"*

You can find *thousands* of stories online of people who cured themselves naturally of practically every disease imaginable, including Cancer, when they turned to a more natural, "raw food", healthy diet that includes much more "greens". One such story is the case of Natasha Grindley, a 37-year-old nursery teacher and mom from Liverpool, England, who was diagnosed with "terminal" cancer. Doctors told her she only had two weeks to live.

With two young children to take care of, Liam, 5, and 6-year-old daughter Gabriella, she refused to accept their death sentence, and instead proceeded to *educate herself* about_Cancer. After coming across the author known as Deliciously Ella, she transformed her diet: she started juicing and getting a lot more proper nutrition into her body. This involved cutting out all the "bad" stuff, and increasing dramatically her intake of organic vegetables, particularly carrots.

She would later tell journalists, *"I noticed that every time I made a change to my diet, I saw a positive difference in how I felt."*

It has been two years, and Natasha is healthier than she has ever been! She is now sharing her message with more people through her talks and social media.

Source: *Mother Beats Cancer With JUICING After Told She Only Had Two Weeks To Live*
     http://www.naturalnews.com/053006_juicing_beating_cancer_plant_medicine.html

Natural Anti-Cancer Solution #2 – Sodium Bicarbonate (Baking Soda)

Sodium Bicarbonate (baking soda) is extremely alkaline, and –under proper medical supervision– can be used to alkalize one's bloodstream extremely rapidly.

Dr. Robert O. Young started curing Stage IV Cancer patients by administering Sodium Bicarbonate intravenously – combined with his full protocol of juicing green vegetables, detoxifying the body, and using his "Supergreens" powder which includes wheatgrass, barley, broccoli, etc. The idea is that **cancer cells revert to healthy** cells (and healthy cells don't mutate into cancerous ones) when the bloodstream is cleansed and alkaline. Furthermore, oxygen is delivered much better to the cells in such an environment (a clean, alkaline bloodstream).

His amazing results put him directly in the crosshairs of the FDA and their agenda of protecting the financial interest of the Cancer Industry. He is currently on trial, as they attempt to block his work from reaching a wider audience.

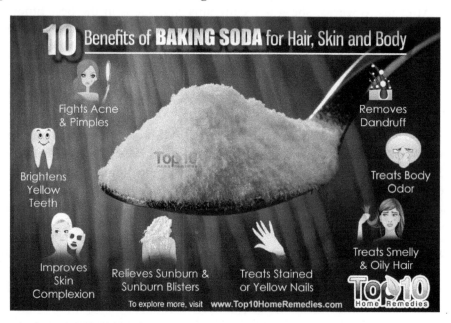

Dr. Tullio Simoncini is an Italian doctor who also uses sodium bicarbonate Perhaps the success is due to the fact that baking soda floods the cancer cells with alkalinity and oxygen, thus reversing the low oxygen levels usually present in cancerous tissue.

According to Dr. Simoncini, *"My methods have cured people for 20 years. Many of my patients recovered completely from cancer, even in cases where official oncology had given up. [...] If the fungi are sensitive the sodium bicarbonate solutions and the tumour size is below 3cm, the [cure rate] will be around 90%, in terminal cases where the patient is in reasonably good condition it is 50%."* Dr. Simoncini can be reached at t.simoncini@alice.it and www.cancerfungus.com.

Check out on YouTube the short video of Vernon Johnson explaining **how he cured himself of cancer with sodium bicarbonate** by raising his urinary pH to over eight: https://www.youtube.com/watch?v=Yl8Y8I_TsjI

The original diagnosis from his doctors was: *"You've got prostate cancer Stage IV, that has metastasized to the bones (Bone Cancer)".*

His website is http://www.phKillsCancer.com.

Mark A. Sircus in his book **Rich Man's Poor Man's Cancer Treatment** says that sodium bicarbonate is a "nothing-to-lose-everything-to-gain" treatment for cancer as well as the general acid conditions behind a host of modern diseases.

It is of also of great help to patients receiving radiation treatments as it protects the kidneys and other tissues of the body from radiation damage.

Note: Baking soda should not be considered a standalone cancer treatment, and should be used in conjunction with a full protocol.

Source: http://www.naturalnews.com/033385_cancer_ph_levels.html

Baking Soda and Lemon Juice Eradicates Cancer Cells 10,000 Times Better Than Chemotherapy

"More than 20 studies dating as far back as 1970 have showed that lemon and lemon extracts are able to destroy at least 12 different varieties of cancer cells, and also prevent cancer from metastasizing. At least one study showed that lemon extract was 10,000 times stronger than mainstream chemotherapy drugs such as Adriamycin. To prepare a pH-boosting drink, mix a teaspoon of baking soda with about 7 ounces (just under a cup) of lemon juice. The beverage can be diluted with distilled water, as long as you drink the whole thing. For best benefit, it should be taken on an empty stomach, first thing in the morning."

Source: http://www.naturalnews.com/054329_lemon_juice_baking_soda_cancer_prevention.html

You won't hear about cheap Baking Soda as a simple cure for Cancer from your doctor or oncologist, because there simply is no money in it for The Medical Establishment (and they might even lose their job – or *be* out of a job).

Natural Anti-Cancer Solution #3 – The "Garlic, Ginger, Broccoli, Lemon Juice, Turmeric, and Dandelion Root" Concoction

Recent studies on garlic have shown that it contains over 200 biologically active components, it is powerfully antibacterial, antifungal, and antioxidant, and in fact kills parasites, bad bacteria (Candida), and fungi in the body.

It can also help eliminate tumours, lower blood sugar levels, lower blood sugar levels, lower harmful fats in the blood, and prevent clogging of the arteries.

There are cases on record where cancer was beaten with a good detox program and garlic alone.

Ty Bollinger writes: "**Here's a powerful anti-cancer concoction: blend up some ginger, onions, raw broccoli, and garlic juice.** *If you can stand the taste, it's one of the most potent cancer-fighting concoctions available.*"

According to www.NaturalNews.com, garlic's healing properties are so intense that <u>it is 100 times more effective than antibiotic treatments</u>. But make sure you don't cook it, as cooking kills garlic's cancer-fighting properties.

Other awesome natural antibiotics to survive infections include: Oregano and oil of oregano, Raw apple cider vinegar, Honey, Turmeric, Grapefruit seed extract, Echinacea, Extra virgin coconut oil, Fermented foods, and Colloidal silver.

Together with the Raw Garlic, Ginger, Onions, Broccoli blend, I recommend adding Lemon Juice, Ginger, Turmeric, Soursop, and Dandelion Root to this "anti-cancer concoction". Here are five articles from www.NaturalNews.com explaining why:

"Ginger Eliminates 10,000 Times More Cancer Cells Than Chemotherapy"

Georgia State University succeeded in eliminating 10,000 times more cancer cells in mice than chemotherapy was able to. The mice experienced a reduction in the size of prostate tumours by as much as 56% when taking 6-shoagoal, a compound in ginger. By comparison to the treatment of control subjects, ginger proved to be a staggering 10,000 times stronger. Besides slowing down cancer, ginger was proven to be effective for over 100 other ailments, including diabetes, and osteoarthritis. Unlike chemotherapy, ginger acts as a remedy, with virtually no side-effects. It is worth noting that Chinese medicine has been using ginger for over 2,000 years.

Source: http://www.naturalnews.com/053177_ginger_chemotherapy_cancer_cells.html

"Lemon Eliminates 10,000 Times More Cancer Cells Than Chemotherapy"

After more than 20 laboratory tests since 1970, lemon has been shown to destroy the malignant cells in 12 cancers, including colon, breast, prostate, lung and pancreas. The compounds of the lemon tree were 10,000 times more effective than the chemotherapy drug Adriamycin (also known as "Red Death"). It is worth noting that lemons are extremely alkalizing and cleansing, which is why I start my day with a glass of water with lemon juice. Cancer cells cannot thrive in an alkaline environment.

Source: http://www.naturalnews.com/054329_lemon_juice_baking_soda_cancer_prevention.html

"Turmeric Is Able to 'Smart Kill' Cancer Cells"

A study published in the journal *Anticancer Research* reveals that the primary polyphenol in the spice turmeric (also known as 'curcumin') has the ability to selectively target cancer stem cells, which are at the root of cancer malignancy, while having little to no toxicity on normal stem cells, which are essential for tissue regeneration and longevity. Titled *"Curcumin and Cancer Stem Cells,"* the study describes curcumin's powerful properties that inhibit the spread of cancer at a cellular level. It inhibits a particular cancer-promoting enzyme (COX-2), impedes blood supply to cancer cells, induces tumour-suppressing genes, stops metastasis (the spread of cancer throughout the body's organs), kills lymphoma cells and prevents the regrowth of cancer stem cells. (source: www.GreenMedInfo.com)

It is best to find a source of organic Turmeric, as most Turmeric sold in the US contains high levels of lead and microbes.

"Dandelion Root Destroys Cancer Cells in 48 Hours"

"Recent research from the University of Windsor in Canada, has found that dandelion root may be especially effective in treating and defeating cancer, and much more so than immune system-destroying chemotherapy. The dandelion root formula in use in the Pandey lab is about five times more concentrated than the extract that can be purchased over the counter and has been proven to kill leukemia, melanoma and pancreatic cancer cells in lab mice. [...] The website Healthy Solutions reported last month that the trials found that cancer cells were destroyed within 48 hours. The dandelion greens contain extremely important vitamins and minerals such as vitamin B6, thiamine, riboflavin, vitamin C, iron, calcium, potassium, folate, magnesium and manganese. They may contribute up to 535% of the suggested daily intake of vitamin K, not to mention over 110% of the recommended daily intake of vitamin A. It is believed that some of its flavonoids such as zeaxanthin and cryptoxanthin have specific healing properties".

Source: http://www.naturalnews.com/053880_dandelion_root_cancer_cell_suicide_chemotherapy.html

"Tropical Fruit Proves 10,000 Times More Effective At Treating Cancer Than Chemo"

The compounds found in the Soursop fruit (a.k.a. 'Guanabana', 'Graviola', or 'prickly custard apple') – especially its seeds – attack and destroy malignant cancer cells, and are 10,000 times more effective than chemotherapy at treating cancer.

Source: www.naturalnews.com/042768_graviola_cancer_treatment_chemotherapy.htm

Natural Anti-Cancer Solution #4 – Vitamin B17 (Laetrile)

Jason Vale cured himself of cancer by eating the seeds from apples and apricots (which contain vitamin B17, also known as *laetrile*). The FDA then threatened him with jail time if he revealed this to anyone…

Dr. Ernst Krebs theorized in the 1940s that cancer was caused by the lack of an essential food compound in modern-man's diet, identified as part of the nitriloside family which is found in over 1200 edible plants.

Dr. Krebs learned of the kingdom of Hunza in the Himalayan Mountains of Northern Pakistan, who were said to be "cancer-free." They ate huge quantities of apricots, but they did not believe that the fruit contained any cancer fighting substances.

It turns out that the Hunzakuts also eat the *pits* of the apricot seeds, which are one of the richest sources of nitrilosides! Nitrilosides are especially prevalent in the seeds of apricots, peaches, apples, millet, bean sprouts, buckwheat, and other fruits and nuts, including bitter almonds. The substance they contain received the name "Vitamin B17".

Why haven't you heard of Vitamin B17? The Cancer Industry has suppressed this information and has even made it illegal to sell B17. Big Pharma has mounted highly successful "scare" campaigns based on the fact that vitamin B17 contains an amount of cyanide. Studies show that vitamin B17 is harmless to healthy tissue.

In truth, the hydrogen cyanide becomes utterly devastating to the cancer cells since the benzaldehyde unit unlocks at the same time. The result is a poison 100 times more deadly to cancer cells than either in isolation. **The cancer cells are literally obliterated.**

Another enzyme, rhodanese, always present in far larger quantities than the unlocking enzyme beta-glucosidase in healthy tissues, has the ability to completely break down both cyanide and benzaldehyde into a thiocyanate (a harmless substance) and salicylate (which is a pain killer similar to aspirin).

Why is Big Pharma so intent on eliminating this "competition"? Apricot seeds are very, very cheap… not nearly as expensive as the latest chemotherapy drug cocktail.

The most effective method of B17 treatment has been six grams, intravenous once a day, usually given for three weeks. You should also add **zinc,** since it is the transportation mechanism for B17 in the body.

Biochemists and researchers have found that you can give massive doses of B17 to a patient, but if the patient was deficient in zinc, none of the B17 would get into the tissues of the body. Also important with B17 therapy are **pancreatic enzymes,** which form the first layer of defence the body has against cancer. If you have a low supply of these digestive enzymes then it will be difficult for B17 to work. Also, emulsified vitamin A is usually used as an additional supplement to B17 therapy. And laetrile therapy is best used in conjunction with a very strict nutritional regimen, oftentimes one with a raw food diet.

Ty Bollinger writes: *"It is recommended that you eat the apricot seeds rather than taking the pill form of the vitamin. According to Dr. Ernst Krebs, cancer patients should start with a few apricot seeds a day and build up to around thirty apricot seeds per day, preferably eaten on an empty stomach and spread throughout the day between meals, taking around ten seeds between breakfast and lunch, then ten more between lunch and dinner, then ten more at bedtime."*

Source: *Cancer: Step Outside The Box*, by Ty Bollinger. Visit http://www.CancerTruth.net

Editor's Note: Bitter almonds are the most easily accessible source of vitamin B17 . Interestingly, the FDA banned them in the US and they are now illegal in that country. The bitter almond tree had already been banned from the US in 1995.

Stewart Swerdlow has stated: *"If you eat 3 raw (bitter) almonds daily, you will prevent cancer cells from growing."*

Dr. Philip Binzel, MD had **an 81% cure rate using liquid laetrile from apricot seeds**.

Personally I buy apricot seeds online and I add 3-4 a day in my "Green Juice" avocado smoothie, as a source of nutrition and as a cancer "preventative measure".

Natural Anti-Cancer Solution #5 – Wheatgrass Juice

Wheatgrass juice is *incredibly* healing. It contains all the minerals needed by your body (including calcium, phosphorus, magnesium, sodium and potassium in a balanced ratio), as well as vitamins A, B-complex, C, E, and K. Two ounces of wheatgrass juice has the nutritional equivalent of five pounds of the best raw organic vegetables.

Wheatgrass is a complete source of protein, supplying all of the essential amino acids. Wheatgrass juice is one of the best sources of living chlorophyll available (to get the full benefit, it is best to juice the living plant). It floods the body with therapeutic dosages of vitamins, minerals, antioxidants, enzymes, and phytonutrients. It is also a powerful detoxifier, especially of the liver and blood, and cleanses your body of heavy metals, pollutants and other toxins.

According to Webster Kehr, ***"The number of ways Wheatgrass deals with cancer is incredible.*** *It contains chlorophyll, which increases haemoglobin production, meaning more oxygen gets to the cancer.* **Selenium and laetrile are also in wheatgrass**, *and both are anticancer. Chlorophyll and selenium also help build the immunity system. In addition, wheatgrass is one of the most alkaline foods known to mankind. And the list goes on."*

At the Hippocrates alternative health center in the US, their cancer healing protocol includes drinking two ounces of wheatgrass juice twice a day. They recommend consuming it fresh, within fifteen minutes of juicing, undiluted and on an empty stomach, so that the nutrients are absorbed more efficiently. Studies have shown that wheatgrass powders and supplements are only 2% as effective as freshly juiced wheatgrass.

They state on their website: *"When it is consumed fresh it is a living food and has bio-electricity. This high vibration energy is literally the life force within the living juice. This resource of life-force energy can potentially unleash powerful renewing vibrations and greater connectivity to one's inner being. These powerful nutrients can also prevent DNA destruction and help protect us from the ongoing effects of pre-mature aging and cellular breakdown.*

Recent research shows that only living foods and juices can restore the electrical charge between the capillaries and the cell walls which boosts the immune system. When it is fresh, wheatgrass juice is the king of living juices. Wheatgrass cleanses and builds the blood due to its high content of chlorophyll. The high content of oxygen in chlorophyll helps deliver more oxygen to the blood. Chlorophyll is the first product of light and therefore contains more healing properties than any other element. All life on this planet comes from the sun. Only green plants can transform the sun's energy into chlorophyll, via photosynthesis. Chlorophyll is known as the 'life-blood' of the plants. This important phytonutrient is what your cells need to heal and to thrive. Drinking wheatgrass juice is like drinking liquid sunshine."

You can buy wheatgrass-growing kits online, which includes organic compost, seeds, growing trays, a wheatgrass juicer, and a set of instructions. It's super-healthy and fun for the whole family! It is part of my daily routine.

Dr. Robert O. Young's "Supergreens" powder, made up of over 40 grasses and herbs, is extremely alkaline and is a very good alternative in you do not wish to grow your own wheatgrass. His Prime pH is a stabilized oxygen product, and I highly recommend it. Take one drop per two ounces of water.

Natural Anti-Cancer Solution #6 – Aloe Vera and Glyconutrients

Aloe Vera contains over 200 active components including vitamins, minerals, amino acids, enzymes, polysaccharides, and fatty acids. Aloe Vera has been used therapeutically for over 5000 years. It contains many vitamins including A, C, E, folic acid, choline, B1, B2, B3 (niacin), B6, and even the rare vitamin B12.

Some of the 20 minerals found in Aloe vera include: calcium, magnesium, zinc, chromium, selenium, sodium, iron, potassium, copper, and manganese. Aloe Vera is also full of Amino Acids & Fatty Acids (the building blocks of protein). There are about 22 amino acids that are necessary for the human body and it is said that 8 of these are essential.

Aloe Vera contains at least 18 of these amino acids, including all 9 essential amino acids. Aloe vera also includes quite an impressive range of fatty acids, such as campesterol, and B-sitosterol, linoleic, linolenic, myristic, caprylic, oleic, palmitic, and stearic.

Researchers have identified eight essential "glyconutrients" which are crucial to the proper structure and function of the 60 trillion cells in the human body. Unfortunately, six of those are missing from our modern diet. This is why it is important to supplement your diet with a product that contains all eight. Aloe Vera contains all eight glyconutrients.

It is thought that Aloe Vera is a powerful adaptogen, which balances the body's system, stimulating the defense and adaptive mechanisms of the body. This allows you an increased ability to cope with stress and resist illness. Aloe also helps with digestion, it promotes weight loss, and it soothes and cleanses the digestive tract. It has been a great remedy for people with problems such as irritable bowel syndrome as well as acid reflux. Aloe also helps to decrease the amount of unfriendly bacteria in our gut keeping your healthy intestinal flora in balance. Aloe is also a vermifuge, which means it helps to rid the body of intestinal worms.

Aloe Vera also helps detoxify and alkalize your body, as well as boost your immune system. The polysaccharides in aloe vera juice stimulate macrophages, which are the white blood cells of your immune system that fight against viruses. Aloe is also an immune enhancer because of its high level of anti-oxidants.

Aloe Vera also great for the skin, known to help heal wounds, burns, abrasions, and psoriasis. It also helps reduce inflammation, as well as being a Disinfectant, Germicidal, Anti-bacterial, Anti-septic, Anti-fungal & Anti-viral! Next to wheatgrass, this is the best single plant to have around your home.

Dr. Robert Siegel **cured himself of three different cancers** (prostate, colon, and kidney) using the *Aloe Immune* available at www.aloeimmune.com. Precautions: This is an incredibly potent plant and should be used with a level of respect for its potency. Avoid taking Aloe internally during pregnancy, menstruation, if you have hemorrhoids or degeneration of the liver and gall bladder.

I recommend the MPS GOLD glyconutrients or the Mannatech glyconutrient product range. I have seen hundreds of testimonials from people who have cured themselves thanks to supplementing their diet with glyconutrients.

Ty Bollinger recommens using Aloe Arborescens as a supplemental Cancer treatment. It involves creating a mixture from half a kilogram of pure honey, 350 grams of Aloe Arborescens leaves (3-4 leaves), 40 to 50 ml of a distillate such as whisky, cognac, or other pure alcohol (this represents just 1% of the mixture, and is used to preserve the product and to dilate the blood vessels).

It is recommended to take one tablespoon three times a day, 20 minutes before a meal, on an empty stomach. Shake the bottle very well just before pouring, never have it in come into direct contact with sunlight, and keep it stored in a cool, dark place.

Apparently, Aloe Vera contains 300 phytotherapeutic biochemical and nutrient constituents that enhance the immune system and protect against diseases, and its "cousin" species of Aloe Arborescens contains 200% more medicinal substances than Aloe Vera and almost 100% more anti-cancer properties.

You can purchase Aloe Arborescens at www.aloeproductscenter.com.

Natural Anti-Cancer Solution #7 – Essiac Tea

In 1922 A Canadian nurse named Rene Caisse found a woman who had cured herself from breast cancer thanks to a herbal tea recommended by an old Indian medicine man. She would later heal thousands of terminal cancer victims with Essiac Tea in her clinic between the mid-1920s and the late 1930s. She saw up to 600 patients a week at one point.

In 1937 she was introduced to Dr. John Wolfer, then Director of the Cancer Clinic at Northwestern University Medical School. Wolfer arranged for Caisse to treat 30 terminal cancer patients under the direction of five doctors.

She commuted from Canada across the border to Chicago, carrying her bottles of freshly prepared herbal brew. After supervising 18 months of Essiac therapy, the Chicago doctors concluded that the herbal mixture *"prolonged life, shrank tumours, and relieved pain."*

Because her discovery threatened the Medical Establishment and pharmaceutical companies' profits, Caisse was heavily persecuted and continually threatened with arrest. She closed the clinic in 1942 and went into seclusion.

You can find the formula for Essiac Tea at www.octagonalhouse.com (click on the 'Essiac' hotlink). It includes 6 ½ cups cut up Burdock Root, 1 pound powdered Sheep Sorrel, ¼ cup powdered Slippery Elm Bark, and 1 ounce powdered Turkish Rhubarb Root. These herbs are known for helping cleanse the blood!

Source: *Cancer: Step Outside The Box*, by Ty Bollinger. Visit http://www.CancerTruth.net

This story is reminiscent of what happened with The Hoxsey Treatment, in the 1920s. Harry Hoxsey was the son of a rural Illinois veterinarian who used a herbal tonic on animals. The formula, long used by Native American healers, was very successful on humans with cancer. It consists of Red Clover blossom, Licorice root, Buckthorn bark, Burdock root, Stillingia root, Poke root, Barberry root, Oregon Grape root, Cascara Sagrada bark, Prickly Ash bark, Wild Indigo root and Sea Kelp, all of which possess anti-cancer properties.

A supplement of potassium iodide was included along with the tonic, and a diet that excluded pork, bleached white flour products, alcohol, sugar, soft drinks, and excess salt was advised.

Journalist James Burke was sent by Esquire magazine in 1939 to expose Hoxsey as a fraud. After witnessing Hoxsey's generosity and how dozens of his patients were recovering from cancer, he submitted an article in favour of his treatment. Esquire never published it.

After he refused to sell his formula to the head of the American Medical Association, Harry Hoxsey was harassed and persecuted by the AMA for 40 years, until they shut down his clinic in the US in 1960. His work continued at the Bio-Medical Center in Tijuana, Mexico.

Source: http://www.naturalnews.com/027020_cancer_AMA_treatment.html

Natural Anti-Cancer Solution #8 – Bio-Oxidative Therapies

Ty Bollinger writes in his outstanding "Bible" of alternative cancer therapies, *Cancer: Step Outside The* Box:

"Dr. Otto Warburg pointed out that any substance that deprived a cell of oxygen was a carcinogen. In 1966, he stated that it was useless to look for new carcinogens, because the end result of each one was the same: cellular deprivation of oxygen. The incessant search for new carcinogens was counter-productive because it obscured the prime cause, lack of oxygen, and therefore prevented appropriate treatment.

Dr. Charles H. Farr was nominated for the Nobel Prize in Medicine in 1993 for his work. He was the foremost researcher of bio-oxidative therapies, that use **hydrogen peroxide** *(H_2O_2) and* **ozone** *(O_3). If the oxygen system of the body is weak or deficient (due to lack of exercise, poor diet, environmental pollution, smoking, or improper breathing), therapies are used to provide the body with active forms of oxygen (orally, intravenously, or through the skin) in order to eliminate toxins and fight disease.*

Ozone *is an activated form of oxygen with three atoms (Oxygen is* **O_2** *and ozone is* **O_3***). Ozone therapy accelerates the metabolism of oxygen and stimulates the release of oxygen atoms from the bloodstream. It has been shown that ozone can "blast" holes through the membranes of viruses (HIV), fungi, yeasts, bacteria, and abnormal tissue cells (cancer cells) before killing them, without harming normal tissues. In Germany, it was successfully used to treat patients suffering from inflammatory bowel disorders.*

How do you get the ozone into the body? One excellent method is via ozone IV (injecting a fluid saturated with ozone into the blood). Another effective method is autohemotherapy (via infusion bottle) where 10-15 mL of Blood is removed from the body, saturated with ozone, and then put back into the body. Perhaps the most effective ozone therapy of all is the ozone sauna, with the dual application of ozone and hyperthermia.

Ozone has been used for human health since 1860, and is presently employed in over 16 countries. Its widest use is in Germany, where over 7,000 doctors have treated more than 12,000,000 people since World War II. However, as you might expect, the FDA has not allowed testing of ozone, and has actively persecuted physicians who use it. According to Dr. Hans Nieper, who used ozone in Hanover, Germany, "You wouldn't believe how many FDA officials come to see me as patients in Hanover. You wouldn't believe this, or directors of the AMA, or ACA, or the presidents of orthodox cancer institutes. That's the fact." President Ronald Reagan, John Wayne, and Princess Caroline of Monaco have gone as well.

Hydrogen peroxide *is involved in all of life's vital processes and must be present for the immune system to function properly. Colostrum, found in the mother's milk, contains tremendously high concentrations of H_2O_2. The cells in the body that fight infection produce H_2O_2 naturally as a first line of defence against invading organisms (i.e. parasites, viruses, bacteria, and yeast. Dr. Charles Farr has shown that H_2O_2 stimulates oxidative enzyme systems throughout the body, which triggers an increase in the metabolic rate, causes small arteries to dilate and increase blood flow, clears out toxins, raises body temperature, and enhances the body's distribution and consumption of oxygen. H_2O_2 also stimulates the production of white blood cells, which are necessary to fight infection.*

In the 1950s, Dr. Reginald Holman conducted experiments involving the use of H_2O_2 added to the drinking water of rats that had cancerous tumours. <u>The tumours completely disappeared within fifteen to sixty days</u>.

In the 1960s, European physicians began prescribing H_2O_2 to their patients. Before long, the use of H_2O_2 became an accepted part of the medical mainstream in Germany and Russia, as well as Cuba. Dr. Kurt Donsback wrote: "One ounce of 35% hydrogen peroxide (per gallon of water) in a vaporizer every night in an emphysemic's bedroom, and they will breathe freer than they have breathed in years! I do this for my lung cancer patients."

Treatments are usually given about once a week in chronic illness, but can be given daily in patients with illnesses such as HIV and cancer. Tens of thousands of patients have received H_2O_2 treatment without serious side effects.

Bathing in hydrogen peroxide is the best way to get it into the body and is an inexpensive treatment. The recommended rate is 8 ounces of 35% grade hydrogen peroxide in a tub of non-chlorinated water, soaking 30 minutes. If you feel like you're getting sick, try dropping a few drops of H_2O_2 into each ear. The H_2O_2 begins working in minutes killing the cold or flu. It will probably bubble, which is a sign that it's killing the "bad guys". Hydrogen Peroxide is one of the few "miracle substances" still available to the general public. And best of all, it is safe and dirt cheap!

*I want to emphasize very strongly that, for internal purposes, you should not use any type of hydrogen peroxide unless it is "35% food grade." The hydrogen peroxide you buy at the grocery store is only 3% and contains toxic chemicals. It is for **external use only.** Cancer patients should stay away from this form of H_2O_2.*

Also, cancer patients who use H_2O_2 internally should also use a quality proteolytic enzyme (such as Vitälzym) which will cut through the protein coating on the cancer cells and will enable the H_2O_2 to penetrate the cell wall.

Almost 200 years ago, people in India found that H_2O_2 added in small amounts to drinking water cured a variety of sickness, including colds, flu, cholera, and malaria. This knowledge threatened the "British Big Pharma" drug sales, so Britain sent an "undercover" agent who masqueraded as a doctor and claimed that taking H_2O_2 causes viral brain damage. The fabricated story was accepted as "Truth", and the Indian people bought the British drugs.

A large portion of the medical community continues to overlook or purposely ignore these incredibly simple and inexpensive treatments. One clinic that uses bio-oxidative therapies is Dr. Frank Shallenberger's Nevada Center for Alternative and Anti-Aging Medicine."

Source: *Cancer: Step Outside The Box*, by Ty Bollinger. Visit http://www.CancerTruth.net

Natural Anti-Cancer Solution #9 – Intravenous Vitamin C

Dr Linus Pauling and Dr. Ewan Cameron in 1976 reported that patients treated with high doses of Vitamin C had <u>survived three to four times longer than similar patients who did not receive vitamin C supplements</u>.

Studies show that Vitamin C kills cancer cells while leaving normal cells alone. Intravenous Vitamin C is the best protocol. Of course, you will need to be under the supervision of a doctor. The key is to be consistent with large quantities of vitamin C. It needs to be taken several times every day.

Check out the Riordan Clinic in Wichita, Kansas. And Dr. Cameron's entire protocol is available at www.doctoryourself.com/cameron.html.

Dr. Leonard Coldwell states:

> *"Cancer can be gone in 2 to 16 weeks. Sometimes in just days. 100cc's a day of vitamin C, intravenous injections, three times a week. Very often <u>the tumours and cancerous growth are gone in a couple of days</u>. Beware, though. They are now producing ARTIFICIAL Vitamin E and Vitamin C, with chemicals. And what a surprise, it doesn't work."*

159

Natural Anti-Cancer Solution #10 – The Bob Beck Protocol

Dr. Bob Beck writes: *"I read an article in Science News that [...] stated that Steven Kaali, M.D., from Albert Einstein College of Medicine, had found a way of inhibiting AIDS in blood, but that years of testing would be required before the virus-electrocuting device was ready for use. [...] The U.S. Government Patent Office described the entire process. You can obtain patent #5188738 in which the same Dr. Kaali describes a process, which will attenuate any bacteria or virus (including AIDS/HIV), parasites, and all fungi contained in the blood, rendering them ineffective from infecting a normally healthy human cell. [...] We found a patent, #4665898. That cured all cancer, dated May 19, 1987. Why has this been suppressed? Why hasn't your doctor told you about an absolutely proven, established cure for cancer? The answer is that doctors get $375,000 per patient for surgery, chemotherapy, x-ray, hospital stays, doctors and anaesthesiologists. Unfortunately, the medical patient cured is a customer lost."*

Dr. Beck's early research had to be done outside the USA. His first electromedicine machine is called the Blood Purifier or Blood Electrifier. [...] He then developed his second electromedicine machine (the Magnetic Pulser) to disable those microbes which were not circulating in the blood. <u>Dr. Beck's protocol also included colloidal silver and ozonated water</u>. Since this protocol could potentially destroy the "friendly" bacteria in the digestive tract, you should consider adding some potent probiotics to your diet to help replenish them.

Important: no other alternative treatment can be used with the Bob Beck Protocol. The Bob Beck Protocol must be used by itself (no prescription drugs, no herbs, etc.)

Please visit http://www.cancertutor.com/bobbeck-bp if you decide to use the Bob Beck protocol. Study the list of "forbidden substances" and make sure you read the entire article.

Source: *Cancer: Step Outside The Box*, by Ty Bollinger. Visit http://www.CancerTruth.net

Natural Anti-Cancer Solution #11 – Cesium Chloride / DMSO / MSM

Cesium Chloride is one of the most popular alternative cancer treatment for patients who have been *"sent home to die"*. It is often combined with other treatments, such as DMSO, hydrogen peroxide (H_2O_2), ozone (O_3), etc.

Unfortunately, conventional treatments such as toxic chemotherapy, radiation, and surgery have often wiped out the patient's immune system and critically damaged one of more of their vital organs by that stage... And yet, Cesium Chloride manages to achieve an astonishing 50% survival rate on patients who were given "just weeks to live."

The protocol described here is considered to be "High pH therapy for cancer", just as Baking soda with lemon juice aims to achieve. Cesium Chloride is **an extremely**

alkaline mineral. This treatment can help *all* cancer patients, but has proven particularly effective for Sarcoma, Carcinoma with bone metastasis, and Colon Cancer (a 97% improvement).

When Cesium is transported into the cell, it is able to radically increase the intracellular pH of the cell (it does not make the *blood* alkaline, but only the inside of the cancer cells), it limits the cancer cell's intake of glucose and stops the fermentation process (cancer cells survive anaerobic environments by fermenting sugar), and it neutralizes lactic acid.

In one study, approximately 50% of patients on Cesium Chloride with breast, colon, prostate, pancreatic, and lung cancer survived for at least three years, despite the fact that conventional doctors gave them only a few weeks to live.

Thirteen patients died in the first two weeks of therapy – but keep in mind what conventional medicine had done to their immune system and organs. Autopsy results in each of these thirteen disclosed reduced tumour size from the Cesium therapy, within only two weeks. Amazingly, pain disappeared in all the patients within one to three days after initiation of Cesium therapy.

On the other hand, those who use cesium chloride FIRST, instead of orthodox medicine first, and do not lose any time to orthodox treatments, **have a very high chance of survival, most likely around 95%** if they do their homework and keep to their strict cancer diet.

Dr. Keith Brewer determined that Cesium could raise the pH of cancer cells, and that a number of vitamins and minerals (including DMSO and vitamin B17) greatly enhanced the *absorption* of these elements by the cancerous cells. By administering these substances in conjunction with the Cesium, the level of the Cesium absorbed was sufficient to kill the cancer cells. The Cesium proceeded to alkalize the cancer cells, thus causing them to re-establish aerobic metabolism. It also caused normal apoptosis to occur within a few days.

In 1981, tests were performed on 30 patients with cancer, and in all 30 patients, the cancerous tumours disappeared and the pain ceased within a couple of days. This protocol became the basis for what is no commonly referred to as "High pH Therapy".

According to Dr. Robert R. Barefoot in his book *The Calcium Factor*, *"Cesium Chloride is a natural salt, and where it is found, cancer does not exist. This is because Cesium is the most caustic mineral that exists and when it enters the body, it seeks out all of the acidic cancer hotspots, dousing the fire of cancer, thereby terminating the cancer within days. Also, when dimethyl sulfoxide (DMSO) is rubbed near a painful cancer, the pain is removed, and* **the DMSO causes the Cesium to penetrate the cancer tumour much faster.**"

However, since this can also cause excessive swelling, in some cases it is better not to rub the DMSO directly above the tumour. Any level of swelling or inflammation can be dangerous, so Cesium Chloride *with* DMSO is not recommended for everyone.

It is interesting to note that the Hunzakuts of Northern Pakistan have water high in Cesium and **never** develop cancer unless they move away from their homeland. The Hunzakuts also eat apricot kernels (which contain vitamin B17) on a regular basis.

Webster Kehr writes: *"When it comes to treating advanced cancers, fast growing cancers, cancers that have spread significantly, high fatality cancers, cancers which have spread to the bones, etc., the cesium chloride protocol is one of the most proven cancer treatments in existence. This treatment can be used on patients with all stages of cancer, from Stage I to Stage IV, even if they are being fed by feeding tubes or I.V. The only downside to this treatment is the potential for swelling and inflammation caused by the immune system attacking cancer cells which are in the process of dying. The good news is that experts in this protocol know how to adjust doses and add other products to keep the swelling and inflammation at safe levels. It is actually a very safe and easy to use treatment."*

He recommends working with the team at Essense of Life who can provide high-quality and safe Cesium Chloride and give appropriate advice and support over the phone. They have worked with several thousand cancer patients over the years: http://www.essense-of-life.com

Dimethyl sulfoxide (DMSO) is an organosulfur compound with the formula $(CH_3)_2SO$. Methylsulfonylmethane (MSM) is an organosulfur compound with the formula $(CH_3)_2SO_2$. It is also known by several other names including $DMSO_2$. DMSO and MSM can work in synergy with other treatments, such as Cesium Chloride. DMSO grabs the Cesium Chloride and drives it through the skin and into the cancer cells. **For brain cancer patients, it blasts past the blood-brain barrier** like it wasn't even there.

Kehr gives a word of caution, though: *"While DMSO is very non-toxic, it can be mildly dangerous to handle, so it is absolutely critical to read this article which covers the safety warnings about using DMSO (e.g. it should NOT be used by pregnant women or women who might be pregnant, it should not touch cloth or gloves, etc.)".*

Kehr also recommends the following "anti-cancer diet" supplements containing extremely high concentrations of nutrients, while following this protocol: Fucoidan (16 ounces a day if possible) from Limu Juice; Juiced red, black or purple grape (with seeds if possible); Juiced blueberry juice; Youngevity Multi-Vitamin Mineral Complex; Xango Mangosteen Juice; Tahitian Noni Juice; One of the wolfberry juices (or goji berries juice).

Sources: http://www.cancertutor.com/alkaline and *Cancer: Step Outside The Box*, by Ty Bollinger.

Natural Anti-Cancer Solution #12 – Vitamin D

Vitamin D slashes Cancer risk by an astonishing 77%. Exciting new research conducted at the Creighton University School of Medicine in Nebraska has revealed that supplementing with vitamin D and calcium can reduce your risk of cancer by an astonishing 77 percent.

This includes breast cancer, colon cancer, skin cancer and other forms of cancer.

And yet, the American Cancer Society – *that continues to have strong financial ties to pharmaceutical companies* – opposes vitamin D.

Source: http://www.naturalnews.com/021892_vitamin_D_American_Cancer_Society.html

Many people are reporting healing from Arthritis, Crohn's disease, fatigue, and a host of other conditions **by taking extremely high doses** of Vitamin D3 (from 5,000 to 30,000 IU per day or more).

In Jeff Bowles' book *"The Miraculous Results Of Extremely High Doses Of The Sunshine Hormone Vitamin D3 – My Experiment With Huge Doses Of D3 From 25,000 To 50,000 To 100,000 IU A Day"*, he states that:

> *"Appropriate vitamin D supplementation makes most conventional drugs and treatments obsolete (e.g. osteoporosis, fibromyalgia, cancer, schizophrenia, psoriasis, or arthritis).* **Sufficient vitamin D prevents all kinds of cancer and even depression.** *Vitamin D is antiestrogenic, anticortisol, and it promotes an adrogenic metabolism of healthy hormones."*

New studies show that over 87% of all newborns and over 67% of all mothers had severe vitamin D deficiencies. Sufficient vitamin D levels can reduce your risk of having a premature delivery. It can also help protect your newborn baby from other health problems:

❑ Mothers who took 4,000 IU's of vitamin D a day during pregnancy had their risk of premature birth reduced by 50%.

❑ Women taking high doses of vitamin D had a 25% reduction in infections, particularly respiratory infections such as colds, and fewer infections of the vagina and gums.

❑ The "co-morbidities of pregnancy" were reduced by 30% in the women who took high doses of vitamin D (Including diabetes, high blood pressure, and pre-eclampsia).

❑ Babies getting the highest amounts of vitamin D after birth had fewer colds and less eczema. In addition, numerous other studies have found that <u>Vitamin D may protect against a number of birth defects and autism</u>.

Natural Anti-Cancer Solution #13 – The Kelley Metabolic Protocol

Dr. William Donald Kelley is the author of *Cancer: Curing the Incurable Without Surgery, Chemotherapy or Radiation*. He achieved an astonishing cure rate of 93% in patients who did not have chemotherapy, radiation or surgery. He worked with more than 30,000 cancer patients. This protocol is not necessarily fast-acting, so it might not be suited for patients who went through conventional treatments and were *"sent home to die…"*.

His treatment protocol includes:

❑ <u>Eliminating pasteurized milk, peanuts, white flour and sugar, chlorinated water, and all</u> **processed foods**

❑ Restricted proteins

❑ A diet that is **70% to 80% raw**, <u>and emphasizes whole grains, fruits, vegetables, raw juices, spouts, and pancreatic enzymes.</u> He recommended high dose juicing of specific vegetable combinations, and he worked to rebuild the glandular function of the body with glandular supplements.

❑ **Coffee enemas** to help the body detoxify and to eliminate toxins secreted by tumours as they dissolve; His protocol included an aggressive detox program, done in sequence, very carefully.

❑ **Pancreatic enzymes** (*they help your digestive system and strengthen your immune system; they also strip the protein coating off of cancer cells so the immune system can identify and kill the cancer cells*); Dr. Kelley talked of the importance of the pancreas in eliminating Cancer, as it works with the liver to regulate hormones and produces over 30 different enzymes. Dr. Kelley saw a close correlation between diabetes and cancer.

One study followed 22 pancreatic cancer patients who had been treated by Dr. Kelley between 1974 and 1982. Interestingly, the five patients who followed the protocol completely achieved long-term remission. Those that never went on the protocol all died.

Webster Kehs recommends combining this protocol with a major cancer treatment, such as the Cellect-Budwig protocol. He also recommends Life Clinic (Kelley Protocol) in Hong Kong, a clinic specializing in this protocol.

Sources: http://www.cancertutor.com/metabolic and *Cancer: Step Outside The Box*, by Ty Bollinger.

Natural Anti-Cancer Solution #14 – MMS

Chlorine Dioxide (ClO_2) is a substance that releases oxygen in the body, helping oxygenate cells and eliminate yeast and fungus at the same time. MMS stands for *"Miracle Mineral Supplement"*. It can be made at home by combining drops of Sodium Chlorite with lemon juice or 50% citric acid (best choice) to produce chlorine dioxide.

The creator of MMS, Jim Humble, wrote in his newsletter:

*"**They Don't Want You to Know How MMS Kills Cancer**... Over the past 100 years there have been more than 100 successful cures for cancer. Royal Rife and William F. Koch [...] had records of well over one hundred thousand successfully treated cases of cancer.*

Let me tell you how MMS cures, because MMS is one of the few cancer cures now available to the public worldwide, free of charge. Basically, MMS is a highly diluted solution of chlorine dioxide and water. Solutions 1,250 to 10,000 times stronger than MMS are used in industry as industrial bleaches. [...] Chlorine dioxide is approved by the FDA for food contact use, and home bleaches cannot be used for that purpose. [...] Last year, 2011, more than 7 million cancer patients worldwide died while under the care of a medical doctor, yet if one single cancer patient dies under the care of an alternative doctor using herbal medicine, the public is up in arms and the alternative doctor is usually prosecuted. [...] Isn't it getting obvious that medical doctors are the wrong place to seek help for cancer? They had 7 million failures last year. Check it out. It isn't something they can hide. [...]

MMS destroys cancers of all kinds. The reason is that chlorine dioxide with the formula of ClO_2 is an oxidizer with very unique characteristics. One important point is that the chlorine dioxide in MMS is a 1000 times more diluted than the weakest bleach. It runs through the body never touching the body but killing the pathogens. It is simply too diluted to harm the body in any way. [...] MMS kills the pleomorphic organism in the cancerous cell. The cell then reverts back to a normal body cell or it dies and is carried off by the blood in a normal body action. The pleomorphic organism is destroyed using oxidation, as MMS has no other chemical reaction. [...] There have been quite a few hundred testimonials of MMS cancer cures on the internet. [...] If you get a lethal cancer and you begin the MMS cancer protocols, you will have, in my opinion about a 90 percent chance of a cure. If, however, you have had radiation, chemo, or surgery treatments, your chances of a cure using MMS protocols drop to about a 50 percent chance of living through the experience. The more radiation, chemo, and surgery treatments you have had, the worse your chances are for recovery. If you continue medically, according to AMA reports of several years ago, your chances drop to less than 3 percent for survival. There has been no improvement or change in the medical treatment for cancer for a 100 years. I make no money from the sales of MMS directly, or indirectly. My goal and the goal of this church is a world without disease. [...] Normally the pain is reduced in hours and all pain is usually gone in less than a week. The cancer usually heals in a few weeks but may take months."

Source: http://educate-yourself.org/cn/humblemmsandcancer07jan12.shtml & http://jimhumble.biz

Natural Anti-Cancer Solution #15 – The Brandt/Kehr Grape Cure

Johanna Brandt of South Africa shared in the 1920s how she cured her stomach cancer with *'The Grape Cure'*, eating lots of grapes, including their skins and seeds.

Grapes —especially purple Concord grapes— contain several nutrients that are known to kill cancer cells, such as **resveratrol, ellagic acid, lycopene, oligomeric proanthocyanidins (OPCs), selenium, catechin, quercetin, gallic acid, and vitamin B17**. A powerful combination!

This treatment typically involves:

❑ Twelve hours of fasting;

❑ Followed by twelve hours of grape consumption (grapes, grape mush, and fresh grape juice, consumed slowly over the twelve-hour period. Use organic purple Concord grapes, as most store-bought grapes are full of dangerous pesticides.

❑ Drink at least a gallon of pure spring water or artesian well water, spread over both twelve hour periods, and taken with the grape mush during the consumption period.

Webster Kehr writes: *"This is a very potent cancer treatment. However, not all people can live on red, purple or black grapes for several weeks. Also, the grapes must be virtually free of pesticides because the patient will eat so many grapes. There are several options described in this article which will supercharge this protocol. [...] I do NOT recommend this treatment for fast-growing cancers, such as pancreatic cancer. I also do not recommend this treatment for any type of brain cancer. [...] If you have bone cancer, this is not the best treatment. [...] For those who cannot obtain the proper grapes, a vegetable juice containing carrot juice and some beet juice can be substituted for the grape juice. [...] The water fasting is used to "trick" the cancer cells into consuming the first thing that comes along. The water fast is absolutely critical to this treatment, and should not be taken lightly."*

He adds that this "Grape Cure" should not be mixed with other cancer treatments (Cesium Chloride blocks glucose from getting into the cancer cells). He *does* recommend, however:

❑ Colloidal Silver (ASAP Plus or Angstrom Silver)

❑ Cellect powder (*contains Calcium, Magnesium, Vitamin A, Vitamin C, Vitamin D3, Natural Vitamin E, Chromium Polynicotinate, Zinc, Iron, Iodine, Shark Cartilage, Colostrum, Selenium, L-Glycine USP, AlgaeCal™, Milk Thistle, and 74 Trace Minerals*).

❑ Fucoidan, present in Limu juice (16 ounces a day)

❑ Transfer Point Beta-1, 3D Glucan

❑ Glyconutrients from Aloe Immune (from the Aloe Vera plant)

❑ Exercise – *"Exercise is critical for cancer patients. It pumps the lymph system and is critical to getting the toxins out of the body."*

Source: http://www.cancertutor.com/grapecure and *Cancer: Step Outside The Box* by Ty Bollinger.

166

Natural Anti-Cancer Solution #16 – The Cellect-Budwig Diet

German biochemist Dr. Johanna Budwig found that the blood of seriously ill cancer patients was deficient in certain important essential ingredients, including phosphatides and lipoproteins (Omega 3 and 6 fats), whereas the blood of a healthy person always contained sufficient quantities of these ingredients (personally, this is why I use Udos Oil every day).

The theory behind the Budwig Diet is: **the use of oxygen in the organism can be stimulated by lipoproteins** (sulphur-rich proteins and linoleic acid). Electron-rich fats interact with sulphur-rich proteins to bind oxygen and promote aerobic metabolism in the cells.

Bill Henderson (author of *Beating Cancer Gently*) has worked with over a thousand "terminal" cancer patients. The keystone to his treatment protocol is the Budwig Diet.

This treatment uses Cellect, a multi-mineral, multi-amino acid, multivitamin supplement, with some anti-cancer products added. The biochemist Fred Eichhorn had "terminal" pancreatic cancer in 1976. He is still alive today thanks to this protocol.

Webster Kehr states that Cellect-Budwig is *"one of the crown jewels of alternative medicine. It is the strongest and fastest-acting alternative cancer treatment which does not have any restrictions placed on its use. It does not cause any inflammation or swelling. It frequently shrinks tumors and reduces pain within a couple of weeks. It can be used by any advanced cancer patient dealing with any type of cancer."*

Mike Vrentas of the Independent Cancer Research Foundation has added the Budwig Diet, Vitamin B17 and juicing to *Cellect*, making it a very potent treatment:

1 – **Cellect Powder** *(can be purchased at www.cellect.org; choose 'maxi-blend' powder)*

2 – **The Budwig Diet** *(but do not take the Cellect with it within 1.5 hours of each other)*

3 – **Vitamin B17**

4 – **Organic Vegetable Juicing** *(vegetables are typically very high in cancer-fighting nutrients and phytochemicals. Also, by filling up on fresh, organic vegetable juice you won't have as much room left for the toxic food that most folks love to eat; It is recommended that you drink the juice in several smaller amounts spread over the entire day, rather than drinking the entire juice in one sitting).*

5 – **Sunshine** *(Vitamin D; get thirty minutes of sunshine a day).*

Sources: *Cancer: Step Outside The Box*, by Ty Bollinger. Visit http://www.CancerTruth.net

Natural Anti-Cancer Solution #17 – The Unlimited Power Protocol

The "Unlimited Power Protocol" was created by Webster Kehr. It includes more than 30 **inexpensive but highly potent natural remedies** for returning cancer cells to normal, healthy cells. Many of these treatments are known for curing cancer in and of themselves. Combining them can be very powerful, according to Kehr. This treatment protocol includes:

- ❑ Protandim – **required**
  This product consists of Milk Thistle seed extract, Bacopa extract (Brahmi), Ashwagandha root, Green Tea leaf extract, and Turmeric rhizome extract. It is claimed that this formula is 18 times more powerful when combined in the proportions available in this product. Protandim is scientifically proven to be **a million times more effective at getting rid of free radicals than anti-oxidants**. It activates the Superoxide Dismutase enzyme in the body, a scavenger of free radicals, and apparently, a single Superoxide Dismutase enzyme can neutralize up to one million free radicals every second, *for two weeks*. Protandim is designed to get inside of cancer cells, and has been shown **to shrink tumors**.
- ❑ MSM/LIPH or MSM/Vitamin C – **required**
- ❑ Beta Glucan (by "Transfer Point") – **required**
  According to Webster Kehr, *"Transfer Point's Beta Glucan is by far the best product to build the immune system".*
- ❑ Several "liver flushes" each day for two or three weeks – **required**
  (High RF Frequency Generator with Plasma Amplifier, Photon Genie, etc.)
- ❑ Vitamin D3 – *"Vitamin D3 is critical for many biochemical reactions in the body. For cancer, D3 should be combined with MSM because it also kills microbes and the MSM will help the D3 get inside the cancer cells."*
- ❑ Cellect powder (Cellect-Budwig cancer protocol)
- ❑ Natural, organic purple Grape Juice (contains 12 different cancer-killing compounds)
- ❑ Fucoidan (present in Limu juice, made from an algae from Hawaii) – scientific studies show it targets and safely kills cancer cells. A highly potent cancer treatment in itself.
- ❑ Moringa Juice (Moringa Oleifera)
- ❑ Carrot Juice with beetroot juice (many have cured themselves with this alone)
- ❑ Oxalic Acid (present in spinach, for example)
- ❑ Extra-Virgin Olive Oil (oleocanthal in extra virgin olive oil kills cancer cells)
- ❑ Salvestrol or Silvestrol (also kills cancer cells)
- ❑ Kelley Metabolic diet (with pancreatic enzymes)
- ❑ DCA (Sodium Dichloroacetate) (stimulates apoptosis in cancer cells)
- ❑ Mangosteen juice
- ❑ Tahitian Noni Juice
- ❑ NingXia Red Wolfberry Juice
- ❑ Goji Juice (www.gojijuiceandvitamins.com)
- ❑ Blueberry Juice
- ❑ Sea Cucumber

- ❑ Oleander
- ❑ Coconut water
- ❑ Cancer Cell Treatment (protocol)
- ❑ 3-bromopyruvate (3BP) (only available at clinics)
- ❑ Asparagus (very alkaline and detoxifying, known to cure cancer in and of itself)
- ❑ Fresh broccoli sprouts
- ❑ Six Lemons a Day, frozen and grated (two at a time, three times a day)
- ❑ Essiac Tea
- ❑ Laetrile / Vitamin B17 (present in apricot seeds, apple seeds, bitter almonds)
- ❑ Wheatgrass
- ❑ Vitamineral Green (by *HealthForce*)
- ❑ Oceans Alive 2.0 (marine phytoplankton)
- ❑ PolyMVA (I.V. drip used frequently at cancer clinics)
- ❑ Black Cumin (Nigella Sativa seeds)
- ❑ Bitter Melon
- ❑ Vitamin K
- ❑ DMSO Potentiation Therapy (DPT)
- ❑ Soursop fruit (a.k.a. Guanabana, Graviola, or prickly custard apple)
- ❑ Paw Paw fruit
- ❑ Protocel (causes cancer cells to fall apart) – cannot be used with DMSO, MSM, or electromedicine devices.
- ❑ Cantron (causes cancer cells to fall apart)
- ❑ Modified Citrus Pectin (also chelates heavy metals)
- ❑ Escozine (derived from Caribbean Blue Scorpion venom)
- ❑ Colloidal silver
- ❑ Hemp oil
- ❑ Dandelion root (Dandelion Tea)
- ❑ Ozonated Water
- ❑ Ionized alkaline water (Kangen, or Jupiter Water Ionizers)
- ❑ Anti-cancer herbs (see list below)

List of anti-cancer herbs:

- ▪ Cayenne Pepper
- ▪ Habanero Pepper
- ▪ Sheep Sorrel (in Essiac Tea)
- ▪ Burdock Root (in Essiac Tea)
- ▪ Slippery Elm (in Essiac Tea)
- ▪ Indian Rhubarb (in Essiac Tea)
- ▪ Chaparral
- ▪ Wormwood
- ▪ Red Clover
- ▪ Poke Root
- ▪ Echinacea
- ▪ Barberry

- Garlic
- Turmeric (Curcumin) (mixed with honey)
- Ginger (mixed with honey)
- Cinnamon (mixed with honey)
- Aloe Vera plant (mixed with honey)
- Aloe Arborescens plant (mixed with honey)
- Green Tea leaf extract (Camellia Sinensis)
- Bacopa (Brahmi, or waterhyssop)
- Ginkgo Biloba
- Eucalyptus plant
- Black Currant
- Ashwagandha root
- Blushwood
- Dong Ling Cao
- Yi Yi Ren (Semen Coicis)
- Tu Fu Ling
- Ling Zhi
- Ren Shen

You will notice that the items listed help **alkalize** and cleanse the blood, bring much more **nutrients** to your cells, or increase *oxygenation* levels in your body. Why does this cure cancer? Because your cells need oxygen, nutrients, and a clean inner terrain **to survive!**

Rules of The Unlimited Power Protocol

According to Kehr, there are two very important rules when following this protocol. First, <u>at least 14 items from the list above must be used every single day</u>. You can use up to 30 different items from the list, every day. Secondly, <u>only ONE highly alkaline protocol per day should be used</u> (e.g. **baking soda**, or a cup of **asparagus**, or **wheatgrass**, or **Cesium Chloride**…). You can alternate, on different days, but only one can be used on any given day.

And of course, it goes without saying that you need to be on an anti-cancer diet. This means not giving your body things that *feed* the cancer, such as sugar, glucose, dairy, processed meats, junk food, fried food, processed foods, soft drinks, etc.

Alcohol, smoking, and drugs are big no-no's, of course.

Read more: https://www.cancertutor.com/unlimited_power_protocol

How Much Cancer Do You Have? (How To Measure Your Progress)

Kehr also recommends you use cancer tests regularly to determine how your treatment is going. Tests include "The CA Profile" (a blood and urine test that measures a combination of 6 different biomarkers); The Navarro Urine Test (not as accurate as blood tests, but very useful because it is so inexpensive – www.navarromedicalclinic.com); Infrared thermographs (can tell you exactly where the cancer or tumours are located).

If the amount of cancer has stayed the same or gone up, then switch to a different protocol, or use more elements from the Unlimited Power Protocol.

Read More http://www.cancertutor.com/reference

Check out, also, Webster Keh's "Perfect Storm" cancer protocol that combines DMSO and Chlorine Dioxide (the 'MMS' solution mentioned earlier). *"This is rated one of the top cancer treatments on the planet earth, including natural medicine cancer clinics"*, writes Kehr. Find out more at https://www.cancertutor.com/perfect_storm

CHAPTER 14

Healing From Colon Cancer By Using
The Power Of Your Mind

Do you have a strong 'will to live'? It might surprise you to realize how many people out there feel resigned and even *welcome death*. Many more experience 'secondary gains' (subconsciously) when being diagnosed with Cancer, such as gaining attention and sympathy from others, escaping an unfulfilling life, making loved ones feel guilty, having an in-built excuse for not going after their dreams, etc.

Exercise: What 'Secondary Gains', if any, do you experience from your condition?

Webster Kehr highlights the importance of having an unshakable and powerful "Will To Live", as you embark on your journey back to health. **You must be DETERMINED AND ABSOLUTELY 100% COMMITTED AND FOCUSED to overcome cancer.** There is no room for negativity or doubt, from yourself or from within your environment (family, partners, friends, spouse, co-workers).

Those who do not believe in natural medicine should stay away or keep their opinions to themselves. **Do not spend time with negative people that focus on disease, bad news, and "problems" rather than focusing on solutions and getting healthy.**

Having *no will to live*, or *a weak will to live*, well… no amount of nutrition, healing, detoxing or alkalizing. will help. This journey starts with adopting a positive mindset and being upbeat and determined!

Exercise: Write down 100 Reasons Why You MUST Regain Your Health!

This exercise will give you tremendous motivation to get well again! Do it!

The Limiting Beliefs of Cancer Patients

According to Jen Caruso ("Holistic Jen"), the limiting beliefs of cancer patients include:

"It is common and natural that many people have cancer..."

"Sickness is normal..."

"I will need chemo..."

"I'm going to have a hard time getting better..."

"It's going to take a really long time to get better..."

"I'm probably going to die..."

"I only have a short time left..."

"I better start making arrangements for my death..."

"It's all my fault..."

"It's all HIS/HER fault...!"

"I don't have the finances to get better..."

"Since I can't quit smoking, I expect things to continue badly..."

"I know I'll have to change my lifestyle and diet, and I don't think I can..."

"All the doctors say I only have 6 months to live..."

"My doctor won't be supportive of my ideas..."

"It's really hard doing through cancer..."

"I don't want to be sick..."

"I don't want to live in pain..."

"I don't want to be a burden to my family..."

"I'm unable to care for my family with this..."

Unless each and every of these beliefs are eliminated, and replaced by new, EMPOWERING beliefs, it is doubtful a patient can overcome their condition and return to a state of health, regardless of their diet, supplements, or treatment.

Exercise:

1) Do some self-analysis to identify your own limiting beliefs and negative beliefs.
2) Write down 10 reasons why each limiting belief is WRONG.
3) Write the OPPOSITE, new, empowering belief for each one, and write down 10 reasons why *this* new belief is TRUE!

Reprogramming Your Subconscious Mind

Note that your subconscious mind does not process negatives. If you say to yourself *"I don't want to be sick..."* your subconscious simply hears, repeatedly, *"I want to be sick"*.

Instead, here are some positive beliefs about health and healing, taken from the Prosperity Power™ subliminal message software, that helps people reprogram their mind:

Vibrant Health

- ❏ *I am healthy and strong*
- ❏ *Every day in every way I am healthier and stronger*
- ❏ *My body is my temple*
- ❏ *I am calm and I am happy*
- ❏ *I am healthy, healed and whole*
- ❏ *Every cell in my body vibrates with energy and health*
- ❏ *I choose health*
- ❏ *I naturally make choices that are good for me*
- ❏ *I take loving care of my body*
- ❏ *My body heals quickly and easily*
- ❏ *I have boundless energy*
- ❏ *My cells enjoy the benefits of maximum nutrition*
- ❏ *I hydrate my body regularly with pure water*

Youth & Feeling Younger

- ❏ *Every day in every way I am healthier and stronger*
- ❏ *I am youthful and vibrant every day of my life*
- ❏ *I am positive, energetic and enthusiastic*
- ❏ *I live my life with passion*
- ❏ *I look amazing*
- ❏ *Every day in every way I feel younger and stronger*
- ❏ *Every day in every way my body rejuvenates itself*
- ❏ *I am full of radiant health and youthful energy*
- ❏ *I live powerfully in the present moment*
- ❏ *Today I bless my being with infinite youth*
- ❏ *People constantly remark on how young I look*
- ❏ *I look 20 years younger than my age*
- ❏ *I am healthy, healed and whole*
- ❏ *My body looks and feels younger every day*
- ❏ *My skin glows with youthful radiance*
- ❏ *I look younger and healthier every day*
- ❏ *I take loving care of my body*
- ❏ *I look and feel forever young, strong, and vibrant.*
- ❏ *I love looking 20 years younger than my age*
- ❏ *Every cell in my body vibrates with energy and health*

Increased Energy

- ❑ *I am healthy and vital*
- ❑ *I have boundless energy*
- ❑ *I feel vital and alive*
- ❑ *I enjoy maximum vitality and energy*
- ❑ *I am energetic*
- ❑ *Every day in every way I am healthier and stronger*
- ❑ *Every day in every way I am more powerful and energetic*
- ❑ *Every day in every way my energy increases*
- ❑ *I enjoy my abundance of energy and wonderful feelings*
- ❑ *I love my life and I have lots of FUN*
- ❑ *I am excited about my life's purpose and my vision*

Healing (following surgery or medical treatment)

- ❑ *My body heals quickly and easily*
- ❑ *Every day in every way I am healthier and stronger*
- ❑ *I know that my healing is already in process*
- ❑ *Every hand that touches me is a healing hand*
- ❑ *I now receive the treatment I need in the perfect time, place and way for me*
- ❑ *I am healthy and strong*
- ❑ *My body is my temple*
- ❑ *I am calm and I am happy*
- ❑ *I am healthy, healed and whole*
- ❑ *Every cell in my body vibrates with energy and health*
- ❑ *I take loving care of my body*
- ❑ *I am grateful for my amazing body*

The Power of Visualization and Affirmations

If you focus on your disease, you will only experience *more* disease. Instead, you should focus on –and visualize yourself—being healthy and vibrant. **Visualize and focus on a mental picture of yourself being healthy, vibrant, and happy**. Visualize yourself as HEALTHY, VIBRANT, STRONG, HAPPY, SMILING, ENJOYING LIFE.

Use **affirmations** daily, such as *"Every day in every way I am healthier and stronger"*, *"Every day in every way my bones are healing and getting stronger"*.

CHAPTER 15

Healing From Colon Cancer Naturally – The Stories

My sources 'in the field' have sent me many stories of people healing themselves naturally from cancer, over the years. In this chapter I share a few of these wonderful stories. May these stories provide you with hope and inspiration.

How Jim Unknowningly Cured Himself of Prostate Cancer with One Simple Treatment

"Jim did not know anything about alterative medicine. He had extensive chemotherapy and radiation for his colon cancer. **He was sent home to die. He quit his job and sat at home waiting to die.**

Because Jim was in pain due to oxidation, a friend of his gave him a couple of bottles of Protandim. Jim took 2 Protandim pills every day to deal with oxidation. In fact, he took these two pills solely because of the side-effects of large doses of chemotherapy and radiation. Neither Jim, nor anyone else, suspected that Protandim might be a cancer treatment.

Protandim almost immediately helped with his symptoms of pain, energy and sleeping, but more importantly it dealt with his cancer as well."

Source: http://www.healitself.com/protandim

How Jerry Went Against His Doctor's Advice and Treated His Colon Cancer Naturally

"I am a 77 year old gentleman who never smoked in his life time and drank alcohol very moderately. I have had comparatively good health all my life up until November 8th, 2001 at which time I went to the emergency room. I was diagnosed with Atrial Fibrillation which will continue for the rest of my life.

On April 20th, 2004 I was operated on for malignant colon cancer and had a colostomy. *Dr. S. Midwell, my surgeon said he removed 95% of the cancer and only 5% remained. That was left due to my not being physically able to endure 2 major surgeries at one time.*

177

I chose not to undertake radiation/chemotherapy treatment advised by my surgeon. *I decided to go to the Hoxey Clinic (alternative medicine therapy) in Mexico. They put me on a strict vegetarian diet with a special herbal tonic and I improved rapidly. During all this time I had no pain.*

A couple weeks prior to November 8th, 04 I began to have pain in my lower rectum area. I returned to my surgeon and he found another tumor the size of a walnut. ***Reluctantly, I then began a 7 week radiation program under the strong advice of my surgeon.***

The radiation made me sick and nauseated. I should mention that during the month of October everyone, including myself, thought my life was ending. I began to lose weight, and was in pain when I would go to my house of worship for services. I had to lay on a lounge chair I was too weak and in too much pain to sit.

Through the concern of a dear friend in December 2004, I reluctantly started Mangosteen Juice. ***I thought to myself, "another gimmick.***

At that time I was on 10 prescription drugs.

I then started taking a Mangosteen juice regimen on December 4th, 2004.

I was on many medications prior to taking Mangosteen Juice. ***Freedom from so many prescribed drugs in 30 days made me feel 10 years younger.***

It was during the last three weeks of my radiation therapy, that I informed my radiation doctor that I was on the Mangosteen Juice. ***He advised me to discontinue it, which I chose not to follow through with.*** *I continued taking my 2 oz's of juice daily with meals along with the radiation.*

My radiation treatments then ended December 20th, 2004; at which time ***my doctor was unable to physically find any trace of cancer.***

I personally feel very positive it is all gone. Only time will tell. From the day I started taking Mangosteen I immediately started feeling better.

Today I feel like I could run a 10 mile marathon. *I can truthfully say I feel as strong and youthful as I was 10-15 years ago. I can only speak for myself.*

Yvonne, my wife started taking Mangosteen about 3-1/2 wks ago. She has much more energy now, and also has no more arthritis pain in her hands and fingers. The eczema she has had since childhood has completely cleared up.

Every M.D. I have seen this past month cannot believe the changes in me. *They say, "Jerry, we don't know what you're doing but keep it up!"*

Source: http://www.mangosteen-juice-online.com/mangosteen-testimonials-colon-cancer.html

How Mangosteen Juice Cured Marshall
of Terminal Colon Cancer

"On July 18, 2004, we left Brooke Army Medical Center in despair. Marshall (73) had just been released after undergoing colon cancer surgery. He had cancer in his intestines, his stomach cavity lining, and his colon. He had also undergone treatments for prostate cancer.

The Doctors at BAMC told him he only had 4 months to live, and maybe 5 months, if he took chemotherapy. *He said to his doctor that he didn't want to take the chemo, and he didn't.*

*We told our good friend Jim about this and he said he knew of something which might possibly help. At that point, Marshall could barely walk, was very weak, had no energy, was ashen gray, and **literally looked like "a walking corpse."** It was like he had one foot in the grave and the other on a banana peel. Marshall was also very depressed, and so was I.*

Jim took us to see his friend, Ed, and they told us all about the scientific research reports they had read about the "Garcinone E Xanthone" in the pericarp of the Mangosteen fruit, and had learned at a recent medical seminar.

*They spoke with a doctor who said there were no guarantees, or any claims that could be made, but he said that if he had these conditions, he would follow the doctor's advice, and also **take a 25oz bottle of mangosteen extract a day for 21 days,** along with a gallon of distilled water every day, and then go on 6oz a day of mangosteen and be re-tested.*

Marshall did just that. After the first 21 days, Marshall went to drinking 6oz a day (3oz in the am and 3oz in the pm), of the mangosteen juice, with lots of water.

*On November 29, 2004, over four months after his diagnosis, Marshall had blood work done, and on December 9, 2004 a cat scan was done at Brook Army Medical Center. A few days later, the doctor met with Marshall and me, and said **"it really looks good." That "there are just a few small spots left, with nothing life threatening."***

*Marshall is now feeling and looking really good. He has his strength and his life back. We walk a mile a day and dance every Friday night. **We are so thankful to God, and for Jim and Ed for introducing us to the Mangosteen Juice!"***

Source: http://www.mangosteen-juice-online.com/mangosteen-testimonials-colon-cancer.html

179

How Changing to a Healthy Lifestlye Cured
Allan Taylor of Colon Cancer

"When doctors told Allan Taylor he had incurable cancer, he decided he wasn't just going to give up and die. Instead the 78-year-old grandfather determinedly searched the internet for help.

And when he found what he was looking for, he began an intensive alternative diet to try to cure his sickness.

It included powdered grass, curry spices, apricot seeds and selenium tablets. Now, four months later, retired oil rig engineer Allan has had the "all-clear" from doctors.

"I got a letter on April 30 and I was told there was no point having any more chemotherapy, it wouldn't cure me and neither would an operation," he says.

"They said if they cut out the cancer it would just pop up somewhere else. But I was determined to stay positive and decided to find my own cure.

"On August 6 I got a letter from North Tees hospital to say a scan had shown my cancer had gone and **'the abnormality is no longer visible'. I'm all clear."**

Source: http://www.chrisbeatcancer.com/ann-cameron-cured-her-cancer-with-carrot-juice/

How Ann Cameron Shocked Doctors By Curing
Her Colon Cancer with this One Natural Remedy

"On June 6 I had surgery for a newly diagnosed Stage 3 colon cancer. I declined the recommended chemotherapy and felt better and better from that date. But six months later, on November 6, I had a CT scan followup that showed probable cancer in my lungs.

The oncologist said I had Stage 4 colon cancer metastasized to the lungs. Later I learned that the colon cancer surgeon believed the cancer in the lungs was unrelated to the colon cancer, an independent development. His reasoning was that colon cancer, even metastasized, grows very slowly, and the two lung tumors were growing fast.

The oncologist also said radiation wouldn't help me. She recommended chemotherapy to retard my demise, but said chemotherapy wouldn't cure the cancer. I asked the surgeon about my life expectancy. **He told me that without chemo I probably had only two to three years to live—and not much more with chemo.**

I was very distraught. I read everything I could find on the internet about alternatives to chemotherapy and radiation. I already had a list of twenty or so recommended substances that didn't work, that my husband had tried for six months before dying of lung cancer in 2005.

180

I hit upon a letter on the internet by a California man maned <u>Ralph Cole</u>, saying **that drinking the juice of five pounds of carrots daily had eliminated small squamous cell cancers on his neck,** *and that a few others had told him the juice had helped with a variety of cancers. Ralph was very detailed in describing his own experience, and wasn't selling anything or engaging in self-aggrandizement. On November 17, I started drinking the juice in the quantity Ralph recommended.*

I Juiced 5 lbs of carrots per day.

On November 27, a PET scan confirmed the findings of the CT scan: the presence of "spots," swollen lymph nodules, and two small tumors in enlarged lymph nodes between the lungs, each about an inch long by 1/4 inch diameter. According to the radiologist 's report, these tumors were "avid for sugar" and "rapidly growing."

Drinking carrot juice, unlike some supplements that oncologists prohibit during conventional treatment, is perfectly compatible with simultaneous radiation or chemo; but I didn't want the recommended chemo because I had researched and dreaded its side effects.

So I had no chemo, no radiation, no other treatments, and no dietary changes beyond the carrot consumption, *and continuing eating meat and ice cream and indulging in other dietary vices.*

On January 7, after eight weeks on the carrot juice (a quart to a quart and one third daily) I had my first follow-up CT scan. **It showed no growth of the cancer, some shrinkage of the tumors, and fewer swollen lymph nodes. In just eight weeks, the growth of the tumors had stopped.**

For the next six months, until the end of July, 2013, I continued drinking the juice faithfully every day, except when I was traveling. A CT scan at the end of March 2013 showed no growth of the cancer, no new cancer, no swollen lymph nodes, and further shrinkage of the tumors.

A CT scan on July 30, 2013 showed no evidence of cancer!

The swollen cancerous lymph nodes had returned to normal size and were stable. I told my oncologist for the first time about my carrot juice treatment, saying I hadn't told her because I thought she would be skeptical. **She said that she was sure that many natural substances are effective against cancer, but that she can't recommend them because of the lack of formal studies and statistical support.**

My understanding is that M.D.'s must rigidly conform to recommending chemotherapy or radiation, and nothing else, lest they fly in the face of proven published research and cause a patient's injury or death with unorthodox advice–which could get them a big medical negligence law suit. **So you can bring up carrots, or cabbage, or curcumin**

with your doctor, but even if they are interested, they are not free to to recommend these substances to you.

My oncologist recommended a new scan in six months, but in six months I'll likely be in Guatemala where a scan involves drinking a lot of a very nasty-tasting contrast medium. So I've decided to wait a year to have the next scan. In the meantime, I will keep on with occasional carrot juice, and aim for less meat and ice cream, and more salads."

Source: www.anncameronbooks.com

Incurable Colon Cancer CURED with the Budwig Protocol

"I am a 42 year old male and was diagnosed with colon cancer in May 2004. I went the surgery, chemo and radiation route and almost said goodbye to everybody. There was no hope left by September 2004, I was very fatigued, by then bleeding constantly - not to mention the excruciating pain I felt due to the cancer having spread to my bones. In fact, I was busy getting my affairs in order. My son was 9 and my daughter only 2.

Enter Dr. Johanna Budwig, Cheryl - and my determination to heal

Then a friend told me about Cheryl. I had realized by then that the allopathic doctors I had been dealing with knew nothing about the healing of cancer. Wasting no time indulging in self-pity, I phoned Cheryl and after talking with her realised that I would have to do this myself. Cheryl immediately got me started on the Budwig protocol.

At first I never thought I would be able to do this protocol... but by October I could feel life returning to my body. I was able to walk normally again, most of the pain was gone and **in November I went back to work**. *My oncologist reckons that I am a miracle - imagine that!! It was in fact simple work and dedication - I had to learn how to eat properly etc., but Cheryl trained my wife and myself and made it all easy and simple. We had to learn how to make sauerkraut, kefir, our own bread and sprout our own seeds, not to mention the juicing, correct foods and of course the flaxseed oil and cottage cheese mix and sunlight on a daily basis. I used the Eldi oil rubs we purchase from Germany as well as body brushing and a mini trampoline(rebounder) [to activate the lymphatic circulation] every day.*

I am healthy now - the Budwig protocol saved my life. *My advice to anyone in a similar situation would be that you need to believe that you can cure yourself and start immediately - life is too precious to wait.*

While Dr. Budwig did not address the subject of detoxification in any specific detail, she mentioned the importance of proper elimination of wastes and was in favour of all natural modalities that have been traditionally used to enhance and recover health such as bathing, massages and other therapeutic processes, and her diet and protocol with its abundance of fresh organic foods, fresh herbs such as dandelion as well as sunlight has, as she was aware, an intrinsically detoxifying effect. Personally I feel that when you have cancer, you must work intensely at getting the toxins out of your system. Drink plenty of water with lemon, maple syrup and cayenne pepper (also known as The Master Cleanser Formula). During the first days when I was too sick to even eat, Cheryl told me to drink lemon water throughout the day. It is apparently a good way to detoxify your body.

I had plenty of fever spells, but felt better after each one. In fact, while I still had the terrible pains in my bones, I used to take extremely hot baths with epsom salts, using 500g (a bit more than a pound) of epsom salts per bath. These baths made my temperature go right up, but were a good way to detoxify and get some magnesium into my aching bones. Afterwards, I regularly felt much better."

Source: http://www.healingcancernaturally.com/colon-cancer-cure-testimonials.html

How Tony Jackson Beat Colon Cancer – Against All Odds

"The dull ache in my groin and the appearance of a small amount of blood should have sent me rushing to the doctor. But it didn't. I hoped it would go away. The mind, that master of self-deception, invented an endless list of ridiculous possibilities. Diverticulitis, irritable bowel, ulcerative colitis, haemorrhoids, washing-up scourer. Anything but cancer. That happened to other people.

Eventually, cornered by unimaginable pain, I dragged myself to my GP who referred me for tests. Following a colonoscopy, I was informed that a tumour blocking my colon was so advanced it had prevented passage of the camera. My blood had also tested positive for hepatitis C. I was a mess. The doctors explained that an appointment had been made to arrange for urgent surgical intervention during which any further spread would be assessed.

'You mean that you want to take out half of my colon without knowing the full extent of my condition,' I gasped, **visions of colostomy bags filling my mind's eye.** *The pressure to conform was intense. I wanted six weeks to think about it, I told the doctors. 'You probably don't have that long to live,'* **they said. 'Immediate surgery, <u>chemotherapy</u>, radiotherapy is the only cure. Everything else is snake-oil quackery.'**

One in two people in the West will be afflicted with cancer at some point despite the trillions of dollars spent on decades of research. I wanted better odds than those. I took my six weeks. In fact, in the end, I took three months.

Returning home, I decided to take time to go deep into myself mentally in order to make what was probably the most crucial decision of my life. Sitting back, I took a breath and let go. When I'd left behind the chatter of a restless mind, something remarkable happened. I felt as though I was embraced by a vibrant stillness, a feeling that would stay with me for the next 20 months. In that very moment, I knew I had reached the heart of listening that lies at the core of the healing process and that whatever happened it was going to be OK.

A lifelong interest in holistic therapies meant that I could make informed choices. I'd read a book by a Dr. Max Gerson about his successful use of nutrition in the cure of chronic metabolic diseases and advanced cancers. He recommends the use of copious, freshly made organic vegetable juices, detoxing coffee enemas and intense supplementation designed to help regenerate a compromised metabolism.

Accordingly, **I put myself under the guidance of a holistic physician who favoured a modified model of the Gerson therapy** *that took into account the increased toxicity of contemporary life. He included cutting-edge, high-dose supplements and enzymes uniquely geared to fighting cancer, a sweeping detoxification programme and a total revision of diet and lifestyle. The key was to boost and nurture the immune system so that the conditions of cells are transformed, no longer providing a toxic ground for cancer to flourish.*

After three months of this therapy combined with a six-week fast, during which I sustained myself on organic vegetable juice, my immune system was boosted to help protect my cells against metastasis during surgery.

Sue Rose, my partner, and I were lucky enough to find a surgeon, who although she didn't profess to understand my methods, was sympathetic, agreeing to remove the minimum amount of malignant tissue, for I needed as much of my colon as possible for the enemas. Her major concern was that given the amount of time I had left it there was a real danger of the cancer having spread into the liver, in which case it would be inoperable. A CT scan showed that it hadn't. **For this I thank my regime.**

After surgery, the biopsy showed the cancer had spread into the lymph, hardly surprising given the amount of time I had been in denial. This didn't concern the holistic physician I was under, who was completely confident of being able to deal with it. Not wishing to have chemotherapy, I was discharged.

My day would begin around 6am when I drank the morning mid-stream of my own urine (urea helps to protect the liver), took my first juice, followed by the first of three daily coffee enemas. I grew my own wheatgrass, which formed part of a daily requirement of 10 freshly prepared juices. Three times a day I ate a porridge bowl full of pills and capsules, knocked back with a witch's brew of liquid supplements administered under the guidance of the physician, who understood the importance of not disturbing the balance of electrolytes when using high-dose supplements.

Every moment was taken up with preparing the next fresh juice, washing equipment, preparing and taking enemas, pills and potions along with daily saunas and hyperthermic baths which help the process of detoxification. Sacks of organic vegetables and fruit were organised in industrial quantities. A water purifier was installed. Supplements were ordered from around the world.

One of the demands of a diagnosis of cancer is that everything must change. All activities inessential to survival stopped. Some days, overwhelmed, I crawled around the floor sobbing. At the same time, my monthly blood tests showed a steady improvement, as my cancer markers dropped.

One night, nauseated by a blinding headache, the process reached a crisis. Becoming progressively weaker, I lay down like a dying animal. Gaunt and hollow-eyed, I lost muscle mass rapidly. Physical anguish penetrated deep into my bones with every attempted movement, preventing me from sleeping, even though I was exhausted.

For the first time, I acknowledged the possibility of death. Yet deep down, I understood this heavy torpor to be nature's way of imposing the long healing rest that was needed. In the end, I surrendered, trusting the process.

By December 2002, my legs had swollen and my belly grotesquely bloated with fluid pressed painfully up under my diaphragm, making it hard to breathe. My haemoglobin count had halved. Catching myself naked in the mirror I gasped in horror at the pestilential image that stared back, unrecognisable with its big belly, protruding ribs and skeletal limbs. Friends sat around, whispering in hushed tones.

Just when it seemed as if death had me checkmated, a miracle turned the tables and I began to recover. Before Christmas, I went to hospital, and a barrage of painful, scary, intrusive cameras, needles and probes explored every orifice. Then we waited for the results. **No gift could have been more wonderful than the morning of Christmas Eve when the doctors telephoned to tell me that there was not a sign of cancer anywhere.**

In January, the liver doctors diagnosed advanced cirrhosis due to long-term hepatitis C. Thinking of Muhammad Ali on the ropes during 'the rumble in the jungle', I continued with my regime.

There is no evidence to date of the return of cancer and my liver tests are normal. *Happier than I have been for years, I cycle around London while friends tell me I look 10 years younger than I did before all this started."*

Source: https://www.theguardian.com/society/2004/jan/04/health.medicineandhealth

The Incredible Story of How Robin Saved His Own Life

"16 years ago I was diagnosed with cancer (tumors in the sigmoid curve of the decending colon) and was told I could possibly live another 6 months if I took the chemo. Whether it was stage 1,2,3, or 4 (terminal) I do not know. I know only that the surgeon and the radiation and chemo oncologist present during the surgery all agreed that I would live maybe 6 months. That is if I took the chemo. NO-BRAINER at least for me. I wouldn't take the chemo no matter what they said. I saw too many friends go that route and I preferred not to die like that.

So, fortunately I had paid attention in my short life and knew from my past friends' experience that if ever confronted with this antagonist, I would take my chance with the cancer for there had to be a far better way to cross over to the other side of life than a dance with the chemo.

During surgery (simply because I did not know better at the time) they found tumors in some lymph nodes as well as others attached to the prostate and stomach. They were saying they thought other organs may be affected as well.

Biopsies showed malignant and of course they did not need to tell me when I came out of surgery because I could see it in their faces. They said I was in denial because I didn't cry or get mad. I was thinking of what I was going to do. One night the nurses were talking that they should call my family because they didn't think I would make it through the night, but I told them to let me die in peace. I didn't want people there crying and all emotional about a natural event. As I lay there I just couldn't see myself dying. **I knew I had to get out of the hospital or I would be carried out feet first.**

The next day I hung the bags, one for urine, one for drainage coming out the left side of my abdomen, the huge IV in my neck, I hung these on the IV tree and began walking up and down the halls a few times a day. **They were freaking on this, the hospital staff, but I was going to walk out on my own.** *After a week of begging the docs to let me go they finally sent me home.*

The oncologist that administers the chemo told me all the things he would do but I told him no way I was going out of this life like that. He was an arrogant SOB. **They called me at home for several weeks after, telling me that I was giving up and I was a coward.** *They could give me 6 more months, was I stupid? I had a follow-up appointment with the surgeon a few weeks later, the day after I began my self-healing, and he told me, "the stronger I got from the diet and exercise, the stronger the cancer would get." He was brilliant. I still laugh at that one.*

The day after I was out of the hospital my best friend and his dad came to visit. His dad had a book called "Back to Eden" by Jethro Kloss written in the 1920s. It lay on my coffee table for a couple of weeks before I opened it and read his words. **If I did the veggie diet and drank the violet leaf tea, it would cure the cancer.** *I began the next morning by boiling onions and carrots and drinking a large pot of this tea each day.*

The treatment I used changed as I was ready. I began the journey with Mr. Kloss's information. The violet leaf tea. Which I simply boiled in a big pot and then drank at least 6 quarts a day. A bit extreme but I liked it. Of course no sugar or sweetener. I ate only fresh fruit and vegetables for a few weeks, then began oatmeal in the morning. **No sugar or milk, no poison.** *I put a little honey in the water as it heated and then stirred in the oats.*

186

But I was very strict, I was wanting to live. I did not falter in the least. I gave up drinking everything but water and lots of it and the tea only. No fruit juice. No veggie juice. No vitamins or anything else.

I have talked with people about this for many years and the first thing I ask is if they smoke. If they say "do I have to stop smoking"? then I know they don't have the mettle to heal themselves. What are you prepared to do for good health? I didn't drink beer, booze, wine, nothing alcoholic. I guess I was willing to do whatever made logical sense

I also began walking 3 miles a day and visualization, a change in attitude towards life and living. The daily walking was important, as was the visualization and meditation. I went back in my life and would visualize the people that I thought I needed to forgive and that needed to forgive me, of course in my mind. I asked them for forgiveness and forgave them. **A clean mind is healing itself.**

I have learned there is only one type of cancer, it begins in the marrow where cells are produced and "cancer" as we call it is the body's way of dealing with abnormalities. The cells find the weakest link and the body isolates these cells in the form of a tumor to save our lives. **We need to work with the body's natural healing system to rid ourselves of these tumors.** *But it all starts in the marrow in the blood and by cleansing the blood we heal ourselves.* **Nature is very logical and very simple.** *We do not fight against nature but we bend to the wind and storms of life and we not only survive but we thrive.*

Originally I think my only thought was to die like a man. With my head up and a smile on my face. **But I can assure you the chemo or radiation is no way for a person to live or die.** *It is barbaric and not even the bloodletters of the early centuries could match the AMA. The modern time quacks. Hippocrates was a brilliant man and said it all, "let your food be your medicine and your medicine your food". They take a hypocritic oath today, not hippocratic.*

If you look at my healing from a medical standpoint you would say what many doctors have said since then. **"It is a miracle", "it was misdiagnosed", "I just got lucky".** *I believe in only one God and that is this precious Earth Mother that gave me life along with that spark of energy from Our Father Sun. I wish I was lucky and win the lottery. But perhaps those doctors as learned as they were did mis-diagnose my condition. It was not an easy thing to do, to disregard medical advice and fly by the seat of my pants with what was my life, my future. What, me put my life in the hands of another? No way! But as I said before, I am a rebel spirit and as I said then and now like Frank sang, "I did it my way".*

I am now 54 years old and enjoy good health *and travel each winter to South America. Last year I spent two months in Brazil hiking the amazon jungle and telling My Earth Mother how wonderful she is and how thankful I am for her and the beauty of life that surrounds me.*

If you have further questions or comments I would be happy to correspond. I would be very happy to help anyone that wishes, and by all means, you can use my name, I am not ashamed of my life nor the path I travel. Of course you can add my e-mail if someone wants to chat. I am often friendly. My life is an open book and I enjoy telling of experiences."

Source: http://asyouheal.com

How A Complete Lifestyle Change Cured Colon Cancer

"In January 2007 and at the age of 57, I was diagnosed with colon cancer which had spread to the liver. As a non-drinker, non-smoking fella who had exercised most of his life, this was a bit of a shock to put it mildly.

However, I am a person that gets stressed quite a bit and had recently experienced a very tragic bereavement, which I think was the tipping point for my immune system.

Surgery was necessary as the colon was almost blocked and I had 2 small tumours removed from the liver in a second operation 3 months later. **I knew enough about chemotherapy to avoid it completely.** *I refused all other follow up treatment that was offered, much to the disgust of the highly paid oncologist.*

When I told him about the alternative treatments that I would be using instead, all of which were non-toxic, he remarked arrogantly that none of these had any proven benefits. I did point out that neither has chemotherapy, which did not go down too well. I could see that there was no point in discussing this with him any further and so I took my leave. I have not been back to a hospital since that time.

My experience of some conventional medicine is that is saves many lives in emergency and acute medical situations and I applaud all doctors and nurses for their compassion and dedication to their patients. However on the dark side of this is the complete disregard for lives and human suffering by Big Pharma. **They continue to deceivie the public into thinking that they are actually trying to develop a cure for cancer when they have no intention of doing so.**

I knew what I had to do, which was to address the toxicity, deficiency and stress which all seem to be a factor in cancer. I bought a book by Dr. Sherry Rogers entitled Detoxify or Die and that book became my bible.

From it I learned why we get so toxic in our modern world and how these toxins lead to serious and degenerative illness. The book also explains how to go about getting the toxins out of the body. I used a variety of supplements and the famous Coffee Enemas, which is **the best thing I ever did.**

From my research I knew that cancer cannot survive in an oxygen-rich environment and one which is alkaline. So my next step was to make my body as inhospitable as possible for the cancer cells.

I started out gently at first using FlorEssence (Essiac) which is an herbal tea and has anti-cancer properties.

Once the cancer cells started dying off, I would need all the elimination channels working as effectively as possible, otherwise the liver gets overloaded.

I invested in an ozone generator from Ozone Guru Dr. Saul Pressman in Canada and self-administered Ozone Therapy. Having read about the benefits of Infrared Sauna treatment, for not only detoxing but also stressing cancer cells to destruction, I invested in a small one person unit.

I also combined the two therapies by heating up my body to a high level with the sauna and then funnelling Ozone, whilst still in the sauna (pores wide open) to the site of the removed tumour.

I juiced organic celery, carrots and a green apple every morning to which I added ground Bitter Apricot Kernels.

*I also followed the complete **B17 Protocol** which includes Pancreatic Enzymes, Zinc and several other supplements. There is lots of information about B17 on both Philip Day's site www.credence.org and also www.anticancerinfo.co.uk*

Every afternoon I made fresh fruit smoothies and tried to include pineapple and Papaya, because they contain some very potent anti-cancer enzymes, Papain and Bromelain. I also included some of the Brazilian Super Fruits, Acai and Acerola which I bought frozen from a juice bar supplier (you cannot buy these fresh) I cut out red meat and ate chicken and fish for protein.

*I supplemented with high doses of Vitamin C, Vitamin A, COq10, Selenium, Zinc, Magnesium, and several more. I got back into exercise as soon as I could because that brings so many benefits both physically and mentally. **That was 5 years ago and looking back, the whole journey has been a blessing.***

It is so important to take control and responsibility for your own health and educate yourself about the options available. Do not be bullied into going down the conventional route without checking out other options first and don't make the mistake of thinking that doctor's know everything about health matters, they don't!"

Source: www.mumsnothavingchemo.com

How Lindsay Cured Her Colon Cancer
With Cannabis Oil

"My name is Lindsey, and I live in Cape Town, South Africa. I was diagnosed with Colon Cancer – Sept 2012. On the 12th August 2011 my life changed forever. I had been to the doctor three times before about experiencing pain in my lower abdomen. He did the usual urine and blood test and announced it was a bladder infection. Weeks of antibiotics later, I was sicker than ever.

That morning I woke with the most excruciating pain I had ever experienced, I could barely walk. Deep inside me, I knew it was something terrible.

My now husband, Brett, took me to another doctor who remarked "yes, I can definitely feel something in there, you need to go for an ultrasound", which confirmed a ovarian cyst, about 9cm in diameter which had twisted on itself and was "causing chaos in my abdomen" -quoting the radiologist.

The gynaecologist, a sweet young woman, assures me everything will be okay, and I have surgery an hour later to remove the rogue ovary. Waking up from that operation and hearing the news confirmed my biggest fear.

Apparently, while in the process of removing my ovary and cyst, they noticed something wrong with my colon, but closed me up anyway. I really don't understand what happened here. **But after that operation, my colon and bladder had been punctured.**

What follows is just too horrible to talk about, but slowly my body was becoming septic…and then, they sent me home. I'm sure it had nothing to do with the fact that I was a private patient. My gynecologist, bless her, in her good conscience, used her contacts to get a surgeon to operate at another much cheaper hospital, and a day later, I am in the ward waiting.

On the 25th August 2011 I go into surgery for the repair of my bladder and colon, and the temporary fitting of a colostomy bag – **I found out later that the doctors were pleasantly surprised to see me alive the next morning….***the op was difficult, and they literally had to remove my insides and wash everything out with betadine!*

It's hard to describe how survival instinct kicks in…but it's there…and you can feel it…when you need it.

I surprised everyone with my quick recovery and the doctors were happy with my progress, just one final CT scan to make sure that I don't have any remaining infection, and then I can go home. It was the 7th September 2011. Brett had come to fetch me – we were waiting for a doctor to discharge me. I was already dressed when I watched his face and body movements as he walked towards me – I knew then! I was crying, maybe from relief, because I just knew there was something else.

I felt so sorry for the young doctor, he was very cute, and in the days I was there looking awful and puking up green stuff, he would always have a flirty chirp, like "you don't look old enough to be a mother with grown children" – that kind of makes your day.

He blurted it out, I could see his eyes turning off, like they must be trained to say this without emotion. He spoke a whole lot of words I didn't hear, and then it came, and he apologised before he said it too. Quote **"Sorry, you have cancer.** *You can go home and be with your family for the weekend (it was Friday), but you have to be back Monday. I'm giving you a weekend pass."*

That evening, my daughter Kerry, my son Warren, Brett and myself spend time together talking. Life takes on a new perspective; you're completely alert, aware of every moment, taking it in all in…taking in the value of the people in your life, and the precious memories you have. Then you realise that's actually all that counts.

I go back to hospital on Monday, they monitor me (I had some "mass" in my abdomen) they were worried about, two days later, they discharged me with an appointment to the oncology ward in a few weeks. **The diagnosis – Stage 3 Colon Cancer.** *They had cut out a tumour in my colon, but it was in my nodes, and there was spot on my liver.* **Only course of action, 6 months of chemotherapy, once a week, for 30 weeks, and we see what happens from there.**

Chemo started on 14th October 2011. Some people react okay to chemotherapy, but most feel the terrible side effects as it builds up in your body. I honestly can say that it sucked the life out of me…I could feel it slipping away. I found myself in limbo – trying to survive to the next week, to be strong enough for the chemo and the bouts of nausea and general luckiness that sap your energy and leave you feeling morbidly depressed.

Half way through my chemo (3rd February 2012 -15 weeks in), I go for my halfway ct scan. My spirits are soaring! I've been living on a virtually organic vegetarian diet, berry smoothies, brown rice, greens and salad are what I live for, I've been taking supplements every day for about 6 months now: Vitamin C, green powder, hemp powder, spirulina, milk thistle and bicarb. I have no red meat or caffeine in my diet! I had every reason to believe I am clear and healthy and then all I had to do was to convince them to reverse my op so that I can get rid of the colostomy bag.

It didn't work out that way.

*In the doctors words, "there are now 4 spots on your liver, one on your kidney and one on your gall bladder, but let's wait until we see the final report and I meet with the specialists to discuss." A week later I go back, well apparently, this is damage by the chemo….***the spot in my gall bladder is actually a 2.8cm stone caused by the chemo.***…the "spots" on my liver turn out to be lesions caused by the chemo…and kidney, turned out to be a cyst….again, caused by the chemo. Nothing more to say.*

The chemo was causing more harm than good.

191

That day I made life a changing decision (either way), I told the oncologist I want the chemo to stop and the remainder of my "treatment" to be an opportunity for me to heal myself holistically. She wasn't happy but gave me an appointment for the 23rd May 2012. Saying they will still follow protocol and treat me even if I don't take the chemo. I wondered whether she didn't worry too much because she probably believed I wouldn't be alive on the 23rd May.

Around that time I met some interesting people on facebook who had a lot to say about **cannabis oil** *curing cancer, I did all the research I could do and could only come up with positive things about the plant. The testimonials of people who have been cured were incredible. I can't mention names, but I wrote on the wall of one of the groups that are fighting to legalize cannabis, asking if anyone knew where I could get my hands on some cannabis oil. I already knew about the benefits while on chemo.*

A few days later the universe hooked me up with just the right person – and within days I was sorted.

I managed to connect with some people who are taking the legal issue to parliament. These people knew some people who were growing the herb to heal people with cancer.

Cannabis is very strong and the idea is to build up the daily dose over time. One dose is a drop on your finger about the size of "half a grain of rice". I took all 6 syringes, which totalled 18 grams, in 46 days. Most people take about 90 days.

Now, after doing more research, I plan to buy a <u>*Vaporizer*</u> *to get the oil (like Shona Banda) or will* <u>*juice raw cannabis*</u>*, which will work out MUCH cheaper.*

I feel strong, brave, invincible…and I'm so loved…that's worth staying for, I would say!

28th March 2012:

I'm at the hospital to see the oncologist and the surgeons who did my operation to ask for them to schedule my "reversal" Operation. I undergo a whole range of tests and scans and meet later in the afternoon with four doctors present.

There is no sign of any cancer in my body!!

If this story encourages someone in a similar situation to do the same, then my reason for writing this has been achieved! I've spent months researching every aspect of cancer and the holistic healing modalities to cure or at least put up a bigger fight, which is better than what chemo can do for you. If this story helps others to make the move, then none of my experience will be for nothing.

Lastly, I have to say that my cancer diagnosis was a true blessing …it facilitated a change within me on every level – emotionally, physically, mentally and spiritually…it formed an unbreakable bond of love and support with my husband. I've become brave and confident in my own power to heal myself…and this is truly the biggest blessing…and I really want to help inspire others to do the same…"

Source: http://www.chrisbeatcancer.com/lindsey-cures-colon-cancer-with-cannabis-in-48-days/

Colon and Rectal Cancer

Marty Gscheidmeier Story

Colon and Rectal Cancer – resolution of liver metastasis in 14 days

My colon/rectal cancer was discovered Sept. 2002. After radiation & chemotherapy, I had surgery in Jan, 2003 in which a section of my colon was removed & given a colostomy.

During surgery it was found that I had 5 lesions on my liver, where the cancer had metastasized. I was told that no further surgery could be done on the liver because of the number of lesions. I was further treated with 2 types of chemotherapy to stop the growth of the cancer. The doctor told me that I had 6 months to live if I did not take the chemo treatments and about 18 months to live if I used the chemo.

I proceeded with the chemotherapy and in August, 2003, I was introduced to Mangosteen Juice by a friend. I was told about the effectiveness of the Xanthones in Mangosteen Juice to fight cancer cells and I decided to try this alternative.

I began taking one bottle per day of Mangosteen Juice along with a gallon of distilled water. I did this for twenty-one days. I was previously scheduled for a CAT scan about 14 days into the program. The scan showed that four of the five lesions in my liver were no longer discernable in the scan. My doctor was surprised and asked that I have a more detailed scan, using the MRI. I had this scan and the results confirmed that there was only one lesion left.

At this point I had not told the doctor about the mangosteen juice, & still didn't at that point. The doctor reminded me how I would have only about 1 in a million chance of recovering from liver cancer. He said, "Marty, you may be that one!

The doctor then suggested a PET scan. This resulted in confirming the same results as the CT and MRI. There appeared to be just the one remaining lesion, which by then had been reduced to less than one centimeter in size.

Then I told the doctor about the mangosteen juice, & gave him some literature. I continued taking the Mangosteen Juice for the remainder of the 21 days & THEN I REPEATED the process for another 21 days.

I am still drinking Mangosteen Juice, however, have decreased the amount to 3 - 4 oz / day. I believe that the Xanthones in Mangosteen Juice (along with the power of prayer) were responsible for the disappearance of the cancerous lesions in my liver.

Source: Mangosteen Stories

Colon Cancer

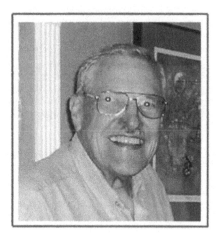

Tom Sarver's Story

I recently received some great news from my doctor....

My father had colon cancer and survived it.   My oldest sister had colon cancer and survived it.   Unfortunately, we lost my next oldest sister to colon cancer this past September.

Given my family history, I thought I had better get colonoscopy since I hadn't had one in almost 7 years, and at my age I'm told I should have had one at least every 5 years depending on results.

I went for the procedure last month; several days later the doctor's nurse called to ask me to come in to talk with the doctor (not good news by any means).   As it turns out he had removed five polyps and the largest had cancer cells according the pathology report.   That was the bad news.   The good news was the cells were DEAD which means the cancer was in remission. No cancer cells were in the stem and none were found in the wall of the colon.   In order to be 100% sure, the doctor drew blood to take the test that would show if cancer existed anywhere in my body. That test came back negative.

I had been drinking Mangosteen juice since February and that was the only cancer prevention action that I had taken.   I thank the juice for putting my colon cancer into remission and not allowing it to spread through my colon.
Praise the Lord.

P.S. I have had another colonoscopy since then (Oct. '07) and again showed my colon cancer is still in remission.

~Thomas Sarver
Hermitage, TN

Source: Mangosteen Stories

Stomach, Colon, and Prostate Cancer

Marshall Fallin Story

On July 18, 2004, we left Brooke Army Medical Center in despair. Marshall (73) had just been released after undergoing colon cancer surgery. He had cancer in his intestines, his stomach cavity lining, and his colon. He had also undergone treatments for prostate cancer. The Doctors at BAMC told him he only had 4 months to live, and maybe 5 months, if he took chemotherapy. He said to his doctor that he didn't want to take the chemo, and he didn't.

We told our good friend Jim Cobb about this and he said he knew of something which might possibly help. At that point, Marshall could barely walk, was very weak, had no energy, was ashen gray, and literally looked like "a walking corpse." It was like he had one foot in the grave and the other on a banana peel. Marshall was also very depressed, and so was I.

Jim took us to see his friend, Ed Johnson, and they told us all about the scientific research reports they had read about the "Garcinone E Xanthone" in the pericarp of the Mangosteen fruit, and had learned at a recent seminar. They spoke with a doctor who said there were no guarantees, or any claims that could be made, but he said that if he had these conditions, he would follow the doctor's advice, and also take a 25oz bottle of mangosteen extract a day for 21 days, along with a gallon of distilled water every day, and then go on 6oz a day of mangosteen and be re-tested.

Marshall did just that. After the first 21 days, Marshall went to drinking 6oz a day (3oz in the am and 3oz in the pm), of the mangosteen juice, with lots of water. On Nov. 29, 2004, over four months after his diagnosis, Marshall had blood work done, & on Dec. 9, 04 a CT scan was done at Brook Army Medical Center. A few days later, the doctor met with Marshall and me, and said "it really looks good; there are just a few small spots left, with nothing life threatening."

Marshall is now feeling and looking really good. He has his strength and his life back. We walk a mile a day and dance every Friday night.

We are so thankful to God and for Jim and Ed for introducing us to the Mangosteen Juice! This Christmas will be a Very Special Christmas for us, because last July, it definitely appeared that Marshall would not be alive this Christmas. *~Marshall Fallin & Mary Lou Johnson*

Source: Mangosteen Stories

Colon Cancer

Dr.Gary Winebrenner, D.C., Story

I went into the ER in Dec, with severe abdominal pain and felt I had a kidney stone. Indeed I did, but that was the good news. The CT scan they did also showed end stage colon cancer, which had spread to my liver with the left lobe of liver was consumed and the right lobe almost consumed with cancer. There were 12 tumors that had spread to the mesentery of my abdomen, & a large 2x2" pericaval metastasis – (around the vena cava - big vein in the abdomen).

A few days later (Dec 6, 2005) I had colonoscopy revealing the colon cancer in my lower sigmoid colon. I had surgery shortly after to do a colonic resection to remove as much cancer as possible. The surgeon told my wife that I might live maybe 6 more months.
The CA has spread throughout my colon/abdomen and consumed most of my liver.
I asked my oncologist several times what was the likelihood of anyone with this advanced metastatic colon cancer surviving with chemotherapy and he would not answer, just a look.

There is a colon cancer blood tumor marker called the CEA antigen
(normal is 2; above 24 – Metastatic colon ca).   My **1st CEA** was **67 - fatal**.
Another tumor marker was **CA-19** and my blood test was **6324**.

On Jan 5, 2006, I had my 1st chemo treatment. I talked to a Dr. F. Templeman MD who had suggestions. I then I talked to Dr.Les Berenson MD, FACP who discussed the use of Mangosteen juice verses cancer, as well as alkalinizing the body with super greens (green drink) and changing the way I think and learning to empower the mind to be more proactive. He recommended the movie "What the Bleep Do We Know" and "The Secret".
I wanted to live, so it was a full court press.

On **Jan 13, 2006, I started Mangosteen juice and a 21 day challenge**
(1 bottle Mangosteen juice / day for 21 days, plus a gallon distilled water per day).

1 week later Jan 19, my **2nd CEA** test number was **46 down from 67 (30% decrease in 1 week)**! My white cell count was extremely low from the previous chemo, so I couldn't have another round of chemotherapy. **2nd CA-19** test was **5634.**

Two weeks after starting on Mangosteen juice Jan 26, my **3rd CEA** test had decreased to **24.** **3rd CA-19** test was **4510.** This was before my 2nd round of chemotherapy, which I did later that day.

My 3rd week my **4th CEA** decreased to **9** (My **4th CA-19** test was **2375**. (Feb 8, 2006)
(Again this was before chemotherapy which I did the next day.
Four weeks later my PET / CT scans showed all tumors/masses are reduced, most gone and basically inactive at this time. My final CEA was 2.4 all being normal.

At this point I haven't told my doctor I was taking the Mangosteen juice, because oncologists often tell patients to not take any antioxidants and I knew there was little likelihood of an oncologist taking the time to explore this "all natural, functional health beverage and fruit juice" called the mangosteen. Today I believe I'm alive because of this botanical, and today I continually use it in my practice for any patients with pain & inflammation.

~Dr.Gary Winebrenner, D.C.
Chiropractic Physician
Granite Falls, WA.

Source: Mangosteen Stories

Colon Cancer

Richard Old Story

I want people to hear my story. It started in January of 2004. I went to the Doctor with a painful stomach. He misdiagnosed the problem and simply gave me some pills. That was a Friday.

On Monday at work, I had new symptoms, air and other stuff coming out of my penis. A call to the Doctor came back with *"Oh, that's not good"* and an appointment with a second Doctor who saw me the next day. He also said *"Oh, that's not good"*, (must have gone to the same school). But he did examine me and found colon cancer.
He said it was bad. I took a lot of tests that day and the testers said it would take a week or so to hear back from the doctor.

He called the next day and scheduled me for surgery that Sunday with the surgeon voted the best colon-rectal surgeon in Kansas City. After surgery, the surgeon said he could not take it out now and would schedule me for radiation and chemotherapy to try to shrink the melon size tumor so he could attempt to take it out at a later date, although he did say I would probably lose my bladder and prostate. That's two more Doctors. He also hooked me up with a specialist for urinary tract surgery.

> Note: The cancer, above, had spread from the colon to the bladder, prostate, and spinal column. The doctors concluded that they dared not try to remove the tumor, and cause catastrophic damage (fatal damage), they would try to shrink it first.

The chemo and radiation came and went and the surgeon got sadder and sadder every time I saw him. He said he might not be able to take it out, as it was not shrinking. I checked this out on the Internet and found that I would have about a year to live. I was 54 and just met my life partner 4 years ago, (married 3 years ago) & I wasn't willing to let that go...yet.!

A, (GOD send), good friend told me of a juice that might help and I went to the surgeon and asked if I could hurt the radiation or chemo and he said I couldn't hurt them and I should try anything and everything that I could think of as they weren't shrinking the tumor. I drank a lot of [mangosteen juice] and 3 weeks later the Surgeon smiled and said, "it's shrinking". At that point I had known him for 4 months and this was the first time my wife (Virginia) and I saw him smile. Two weeks later he said it had appeared to separate from the bone, which meant he could at least remove it, even though that meant sacrificing the bladder and prostate (yes he was smiling again). That meant that I would be able to spend a lot more time with the love of my life.

Now the surgery, (Virginia, said I would be just fine and I believed her), I slept through the whole thing but when I awoke and saw my wife grinning from ear to ear (and she has the prettiest smile) I knew it was good news-but I didn't understand how good until I talked to the surgeon. He was like a kid with a new present at Christmas, and said, *"this was the worst case of colon-rectal cancer I have ever worked on and it turned out with the best results I have ever had"*. He also said that radiation and chemo cannot shrink a tumor from melon size to that of a walnut and he also said he does not know how it pealed it self off of the bladder and prostate. The hole in the bladder was healed up and was in great shape and that did not make sense to him. He said this was one of those, once-in-a-practice you can only hope for situations. Needless to say he is now studying [mangosteen juice] for use in his practice.

~Richard Old

Source: Mangosteen Stories

CHAPTER 16

Actions You Can Take Right Now To Heal From Colon Cancer

If I or a loved one were ever diagnosed with Colon Cancer, I would recommend the following:

❏ As a critical first step, consider doing a 30-day **detox**. Consider doing a **mucoid plaque** cleanse as well (colon cleanse), and a **parasite cleanse**.

❏ Change to a more **organic, cleansing** and **alkalizing** lifestyle. Eat a diet that is 70-80% "greens". Some excellent alkaline-forming foods are: lemon juice, most raw vegetables, wheatgrass, barley grass, wheatgrass, figs, lima beans, olive oil, honey, miso, green tea, most herbs, sprouted grains, and sprouts (see full list of alkaline foods here: www.rense.com/1.mpicons/acidalka.htm). Consider growing and juicing every day **your own wheatgrass**. You can buy a simple wheatgrass-growing kit. This will do wonders for your health. You can also use Dr. Young's 'Supergreens' products, available at www.phmiracleliving.com.

❏ **Cut out sugar from your diet.** Sugar metabolizes to *acid* and sugar feeds cancer. Sugar leads to cancer of the breast, ovaries, prostrate, and rectum, among many other diseases.

❏ **Cut out dairy products from your diet.** Higher dairy intake has been linked to **cancer risk**, acne, food allergies, type 1 diabetes, and higher rates of multiple sclerosis.

❏ Eliminate from your life the toxicities listed in this book, including **ALCOHOL, CIGARETTES, COFFEE, TOXIC PERSONAL CARE PRODUCTS and SOAPS,** and **FLUORIDE**.

❏ Consider starting one of the natural cancer remedy protocols listed in Chapter 14.

❏ Study the health advice contained in **Chapters 28 to 36** in this book.

❏ Get rid of your **DENTAL AMALGAMS** (mercury, heavy metals) and **ROOT CANALS**, using the precautions mentioned in this book.

According to Amalgam.org:

"Mercury is a common cause of chronic conditions related to intestinal dysfunction, such as ulcerative colitis, IBS, Crohn's, and psoriasis. When intestinal permeability is increased, food and nutrient absorption is impaired. Dysfunction in intestinal permeability can result in leaky gut syndrome, where larger molecules and toxins in the intestines can pass through the membranes and into the blood, triggering immune response. **Progressive damage can occur to the intestinal lining,** *eventually allowing disease-causing bacteria, undigested food particles, and toxins to pass directly into the blood stream.*

[...] **Mercury causes significant destruction of stomach and intestine epithelial cells,** *resulting in damage to stomach lining which alters permeability and adversely alters bacterial populations in the intestines causing leaky gut syndrome with toxic, incompletely digested complexes in the blood and accumulation of heliobacter pylori, a suspected major factor in ulcers and stomach cancer and Candida albicans, as well as poor nutrient absorption.*

[...] Replacement of amalgam fillings and metal detoxification have been found to significantly improve the health of most with conditions related to bowel dysfunction and leaky gut syndrome.

Other common causes or factors in leaky gut and the related conditions include food allergies and intolerances; drugs (NSAIDs, aspirin, stomach h2 blockers, steroids, etc.); dysbiosis **(overgrowth of organisms** *due to antibiotic use and/or low probiotic levels);* **alcohol consumption;** *synergistic toxic exposures and chemical sensitivity; chronic infections; and* **inadequate digestive enzymes.** *[...]* **food additives** *or* **processed foods** *that contain* **glutamate (MSG), aspartame, high-fructose corn syrup,** *dyes, etc. are common causes of leaky gut syndrome.*

[...] In addition to improvements in many patients after amalgam replacement and detoxification, **diet and nutritional measures** *are usually effective at improving Crohn's Disease. The 4-R program has seen good success in many patients. The program removes all foods where there is suspicion of allergy that might produce inflammation.* **Common allergens include wheat/gluten, dairy, eggs, peanuts, tomatoes, corn, and red meat.**

Additionally, **elimination of gastrointestinal parasites, undesirable bacteria, fungus, and yeasts** *are carried out. Sometimes a treatment such as nystantin is used to eliminate yeast. Then vital nutrients are replaced by dietary measures and supplementation of a good multivitamin and mineral,* **minerals found deficient such as iron, magnesium, calcium, selenium, zinc, iodine and vitamins, such as B-complex, B6, B12, and folic acid.** *Next the intestines are re-inoculated with friendly bacteria (Lactobacillus acidophilus* *and Lactobacilus bulgaricus.) Finally, measures are taken to repair the intestine to correct for the increased permeability. This is done by adding nutrients such as glutamine, pathothenic acid (B5), zinc, FOS, and vitamin C. DHEA and Butyrate have also been found effective in many patients at reducing inflammation.*

Supplements and other treatments that reduce intestinal permeability have also been found to be protective against and improve these conditions. **Glutamine, berberine, probiotics, and vitamin D** *have been found to decrease intestinal permeability and protect against effects caused by leaky gut syndrome. Butyrate has been found to inhibit inflammation and carcinogenesis in the intestines and low butyrate levels are found in colon cancer, ulcerative colitis, and Crohn's disease.*

Supplementation with **chlorella** *has been found to result in beneficial effects when used in patients' chronic conditions such as ulcerative colitis, hypertension, or Fibromyalgia. Doctors have suggested that the mechanism by which chlorella improves treatment of such conditions is* **metal detoxification**, *which is the main mechanism of action of chlorella and has been found to greatly improve intestinal function."*

Source: http://amalgam.org/education/scientific-evidenceresearch/mercury-food-intolerances-connections-ulcerative-colitis-ibs-crohns-skin-conditions

❑ **Get tested for mercury and heavy metal levels** in your body.

❑ <u>Do a bioresonance test</u> to find out your food sensitivities. For example, I found that my food sensitivities (foods that cause INFLAMMATION in my body) included: All Dairy; Potato, Tomato, Aubergine, Peppers, Mushrooms; All Gluten: Wheat, Bread, Pasta, Oats, Barley, Rye; Yeast; Sugar; Vinegar; Lemon and Grapefruit (due to over-consumption for many years); Chocolate, Cocoa, Tea, Coffee; Alcohol. Find a local practitioner. This will change your life!

❑ Get your hormone levels tested, for estrogen imbalances. Remove xenoestrogens from your environment, food, water, and personal care products! Balance your progesterone and estrogen levels. This is extremely important!

❑ **Cesium Chloride/DMSO/MSM** is one of the most popular alternative cancer treatment for patients who have been *"sent home to die"*. It is often combined with other treatments, such as DMSO, hydrogen peroxide (H2O2), ozone (O3), etc.

Unfortunately, conventional treatments such as toxic chemotherapy, radiation, and surgery have often wiped out the patient's immune system and critically damaged one of more of their vital organs by that stage... And yet, Cesium

Chloride manages to achieve an astonishing 50% survival rate on patients who were given "just weeks to live."

The protocol described here is considered to be "High pH therapy for cancer", just as Baking soda with lemon juice aims to achieve. Cesium Chloride is **an extremely alkaline mineral**. This treatment can help *all* cancer patients, but has proven particularly effective for Sarcoma, Carcinoma with bone metastasis, and Colon Cancer (a 97% improvement).

❏ Get a 'whole-house' **water filter,** to protect yourself and your family from fluoride, chlorine, drugs and other toxic compounds in the water supply.

❏ Invest in some high quality **nutritional supplements** (see Chapter 28).

❏ Get a good **Iodine** supplement. Iodine deficiency leads to cancers of the breast, prostate, ovaries, uterus, thyroid, and many more.

❏ Eat Brazil Nuts every day – they are extremely high in **selenium**.

❏ Consider growing and juicing every day your own **wheatgrass**. You can buy a simple wheatgrass-growing kit and a small wheatgrass juicer.

❏ **Ellagic acid** is a naturally occurring substance found in almost 50 different fruits and nuts (like red raspberries, strawberries, blueberries, grapes, pomegranates, and walnuts). The Hollings Cancer Institute at the University of South Carolina conducted a nine-year study on 500 cervical cancer patients. The study, published in 1999, showed that **ellagic acid stops mitosis (cell division) within 48 hours and induces apoptosis (normal cell death) within 72 hours**, for breast, pancreas, skin, colon, oesophageal, and prostate cancer cells. Additionally, ellagic acid has been shown to induce cervical carcinoma cell death (apoptosis) within 72 hours.

❏ **Keep hydrated,** with water, so that your bloodstream can bring oxygen and nutrients to your cells more efficiently and for your liver and kidneys to detoxify your body more easily. **Drink 3 litres of spring water or distilled water a day** for 30 days (this is the equivalent of two 1.5-litre bottles a day). Have a glass of water every 15 minutes.

❏ **Black seed extract** suppresses colon cancer growth. Animal research has found that black seed oil has significant inhibitory effects against colon cancer in rats, without observable side effects.

❏ Apply Dr. John Bergman's advice for eliminating 97% of so-called 'autoimmune' diseases: Get deep, **restful sleep** every night; Go to sleep early; Change your diet to one of whole, **organic foods**; Get lots of **Vitamin D3** (at least 3000 IUs per 100lbs of weight per day); Consume good **Omega 3 fats**; Consume high **antioxidant** foods, e.g. organic blueberries, cranberries, blackberries, raspberries, strawberries, cherries, beans, and artichokes; Consume **resveratrol** – red wine, whole grape skins, grape seeds, raspberries, mulberries; Use **Coconut oil**; Get Lugol's Iodine; Get Vitamin C with Bioflavinoids; Get lots of fresh organic veggie juice; **Exercise regularly**.

Do NOT consume GMOs; Do NOT consume Non-Organic Grains; Do NOT consume Commercial Dairy; Eliminate chemicals and toxins from your life, e.g. toxic household cleaners, soaps, personal hygiene products, air fresheners, bug sprays, lawn pesticides, insecticides, etc.; Avoid pharmaceutical drugs.

❑ Stop using refined **vegetable oils**. Vegetable oils contain very high levels of polyunsaturated fats (PUFAs) that are highly unstable, oxidize easily, and cause inflammation and mutation in cells. That oxidation is linked to all sorts of issues from **cancer**, heart disease, endometriosis, to Polycystic Ovarian Syndrome (PCOS), and more.

❑ **Exercise** every day. Sweat. Go for a walk every day. Use a rebounder. Use a sauna. Sweating is powerful way to cleanse your body from accumulated toxins. Some modern industrial toxins and pesticides can leave your body only through the sweat glands.

❑ Use **Chlorella and MSM** every day, to help remove heavy metals them from the body. I add a teaspoon to my morning glass of water with lemon juice, together with aloe vera juice and iodine.

❑ Supplement every day with a good **multivitamin and mineral supplement**. Vitamin D, Glutamine, and berberine are also recommended for patients with Colon Cancer.

❑ **Nettle leaf** is effective at reducing symptoms of the digestive tract ranging from acid reflux, nausea, Irritable Bowel Syndrome, colitis, Coeliac disease and even Colon Cancer.

❑ **Carnivora™** has been successful in treating Arthritis, Lyme disease, hepatitis C, Crohn's disease, lupus, chronic fatigue syndrome, ulcerative colitis, and multiple sclerosis.

❑ Get plenty of beneficial bacteria either through **fermented foods** or probiotics in your diet, as this will help to heal your intestinal tract. Fermented foods, if properly fermented, can contain 100 times more probiotics than a supplement. according to Dr. Joseph Mercola. Personally, apart from eating Sauerkraut (fermented cabbage) from time to time, I use "Udos Beyond Greens" in my daily Green Juice smoothie, to add digestive enzymes to my diet.

❑ Dr Joel Wallach advises :

"Eliminate fried food, margarine, and offending foods based on the pulse test (i.e. wheat, milk, soy). Get on a gluten-free diet (no wheat), and drink eight to ten glasses of water each day. Supplement your diet with the baseline nutrition supplement program (the 90 essential nutrients and Vitamins the human body needs), plus pancreatic enzymes, folic acid, and betaine HCl."

❑ Remove toxic household and personal care from your environment. For example: **Perfluoroalkyl substances (PFASs) have been linked to** ulcerative colitis, liver toxicity, disruption of the immune and endocrine systems, neonatal toxicity and death, tumours in multiple organs, testicular, colonic and kidney cancers, hypothyroidism, reduced hormone levels. They are in a variety of products, including car and plane electrical wiring, pizza boxes, microwave popcorn bags, sleeping bags, water-repellant and stain-repellant clothing, non-stick cookware, electronics (like cell phones and hard disk drives), backpacks, footwear and even hospital equipment (it can be found in stents, needles, pacemakers, hospital gowns, and divider curtains); items treated with flame-retardant chemicals, which includes a wide variety of baby items, padded furniture, mattresses, and pillows. (source: www.naturalsociety.com)

❑ Consider using **Aloe Vera**. Aloe Vera is known to help heal wounds, burns, abrasions, and skin conditions (the healing properties of the Aloe Vera plant are mentioned eight times in the Bible). Patients with colitis and many bowel issues such as IBS have reported great results from supplementing their diet with glyconutrients that are derived from the Aloe Vera plant.

❑ Eat small amounts of meat, and **only from clean, organic sources**.

❑ Do *not* eat processed meat or 'mass-produced' meat. According to Dr. Robert O. Young, in his book *Sick and Tired*:

*"Especially in the United States, animals are super-fattened with hormones. **Hormone residues (and mycotoxins) tend to accumulate in the fat layer.** Research has noted the nationwide **correlation between consumption of animal fat and the mortality rate from prostate cancer.** This has raised the hypothesis that dietary animal fat increases risk of this malignancy, and they found the association due primarily to animal fat, as opposed to vegetable fat.*

*Noting that breast cancer was rare in Japanese women prior to World War II, researchers investigated the relationship of various elements of the Western dietary invasion of Japan to the incidence of breast cancer. Results indicated that Japanese women with Westernized dietary habits have **a higher risk of breast cancer when they eat large amounts of meat.** A correlation between certain foods and the risk of thyroid cancer has also been shown. In this study, cancer cases tended to consume significantly **larger***

amounts of poultry, cooked ham, salami, bacon, and sausages. *Significant direct associations were also observed with* **cheese, butter, and oils** *other than olive oil. Olive oil is generally free of mycotoxins."*

[...] *"Yet another study in 1993 verified the hypothesis that the type of dietary fat consumed may influence the occurrence of endometrial cancer,* **ovarian cancer,** *and stomach cancers. Cancer cases consumed more animal-derived fats, and in particular used more butter in cooking, ate more bacon and ham, and drank more whole milk. A population-based case-control study carried out in Sweden in 1982-84 found a number of dietary factors in association with pancreatic cancer. In this case, risk increased with higher consumption of* **fried and grilled meat,** *as well as* **margarine** *on* **white bread."**

BUT while I recommend cutting out processed meat from one's diet, I still advise people to eat *some* meat, from clean sources. Stewart Swerdlow states:

"We have made it very clear over the years that humans are omnivores, not herbivores. Plants on farms also suffer and have feelings. Plants and animals are here for a purpose of nourishing all above them on the food chain. Human DNA is made up of animal protein bases. We need that to repair and grow our cells. Otherwise, it is like a copy machine running out of ink.

Vegetarians weaken and die eventually sooner than others. [...] This has also been shown in studies in Russia, South America and Asia.

The proteins from plants is good for us, but not enough. **The woman who brought macrobiotic vegetarianism to the US is dead from ovarian cancer at a young age because her body was not strong enough to fight it off.** *Humans need animal proteins. You need like material to build the body."*

❑ Avoid pesticides. Eat organic. Detoxify regularly, if you have been exposed to pesticides. Diazinon in insecticides was associated with cancer (it doubled the risk), and authors of one study observed increased risk with Organophosphates use for breast, thyroid and ovarian cancers.

❑ Get to **the root cause** of what is causing your Colon Cancer. Do some self-analysis. Learn to let go and *forgive*. Get some healing. Get some counselling, therapy, of use the Emotional Freedom Technique. Look into changing your mindset, as per Richard Moat's work.

❑ Focus on and visualize yourself being healthy and vibrant. **Visualize and focus on a mental picture of yourself being healthy, vibrant, and happy**. **Visualize** yourself as HEALTHY, VIBRANT, STRONG, HAPPY, SMILING, ENJOYING LIFE. Use **affirmations** daily, such as *"Every day in every way I am healthier and stronger"*, *"Every day in every way my bones are healing and getting stronger"*. Use **subliminal message technology** (software that flashes messages on your computer screen) to program your subconscious mind for success, thousands of times a day, effortlessly.

❑ **Write down 100 Reasons WHY You MUST Regain Your Health!** This will give you the motivation necessary to see this through, will transform your Hierarchy of Values (in life, we get what is HIGHEST on our hierarchy of values), and will reprogram your subconscious beliefs regarding health. You will automatically make better choices, without having to consciously think about it.

If you have any questions, or would like some help in implementing the advice contained in this book – after you have consulted with your primary healthcare professional – get in touch with us at info@TheNewBiology.co.uk.

Part III

THE NEW BIOLOGY

CHAPTER 17

Good Health Begins Before Birth

As you embark on your healing journey, it is sometimes useful to find out from you parents about your birthing conditions. Were you born via caesarean? Was it a long birth? What was the state of mind of your mother? Were you breastfed? Were you vaccinated? Were you often ill as a child?

If you are considering becoming a parent for the first time, it is also important to be aware of how good health begins in the womb, to get your child off to the best start in life. One of the most important things is *the state of mind* of the mother. Is she happy? Is she looking forward to her child? And secondly: the *nutrition* the mother is receiving during conception and during her pregnancy is *critical*.

Mineral Deficiencies Can Lead to Miscarriages And Birth Defects

Dr. Joel Wallach states that there are 90 essential nutrients required by our bodies for optimal health and longevity, but most of these are mostly absent in our modern diet. He was nominated for the Nobel Prize in Medicine in 1991 for his stunning discoveries in the use of trace minerals *to prevent diseases in new-born babies*. It is very important that expectant mothers supplement their diet.

In 1977 Dr. Wallach discovered that Cystic Fibrosis in monkeys was due to a nutritional deficiency – specifically, a lack of *selenium* in their diet. He also found that Vitamin A deficiencies in children caused keratitis, corneal ulcers, and blindness. Calcium deficiency caused arthritis and Multiple Sclerosis in adults. Iodine and copper deficiencies caused miscarriages and Goiter. Infants were born with spina bifida and serious cleft palates as a result of folic acid or zinc deficiencies. Beriberi with resultant congestive heart failure was the result of a thiamine or vitamin B1 deficiency. He states that in most instances "genetic defects" are simply mineral deficiencies that leave a repeatable 'fingerprint' on a specific gene. **Mineral deficiencies are the root cause of most diseases mistakenly thought to be "genetically transmitted".**

211

Dr. Wallach writes: *"The Amish families that did not supplement with vitamins and minerals had younger children with congenital birth defects such as cleft palates, spina bifida, Down's syndrome, PKU, autism, ADD, clubbed feet, hernias, muscular dystrophy, and heart defects. The Amish also breastfed their babies. If they didn't supplement the mother, she would become more and more depleted of minerals with each succeeding child. As a result of this pattern, the younger children tended to have the birth defects and middle aged mothers tended to have a variety of degenerative diseases including lupus, arthritis, Multiple Sclerosis, high blood pressure, diabetes, and heart disease."*

The Benefits of Vitamin D for Pregnant Mothers

New studies show that sufficient vitamin D levels can reduce your risk of having a premature delivery. It can also help protect your newborn baby from other health problems. U.S. researchers Drs. Hollis and Wagner revealed that:

❑ Mothers who took 4,000 IU's of vitamin D a day during pregnancy had their risk of premature birth reduced by 50%.

❑ Women taking high doses of vitamin D had a 25% reduction in infections, particularly respiratory infections such as colds as well as fewer infections of the vagina and the gums.

❑ The "co-morbidities of pregnancy" were reduced by 30% in the women who took high doses of vitamin D (Including diabetes, high blood pressure, and pre-eclampsia).

❑ Babies getting the highest amounts of vitamin D after birth had fewer colds and less eczema

❑ They found that over 87% of all newborns and over 67% of all mothers had severe vitamin D deficiencies (levels lower than 20 ng/ml), and concluded that it is absolutely imperative that pregnant women maintain a blood level of between 50 and 70 ng/ml of Vitamin D.

❑ A different study on vitamin D deficiency in newborns with acute lower respiratory infection confirmed a strong correlation between newborns' and mothers' vitamin D levels.

❑ In addition, numerous other studies have found that <u>Vitamin D may protect against a number of birth defects and autism</u>.

Detoxify and Cleanse Your Inner Terrain *Before* Getting Pregnant

Make sure you are eating organic, use natural cleaning and beauty products, and as little makeup as possible. Avoid fluoride *at all costs*. Fluoride is linked to infertility, birth defects, low IQ, and cancer. <u>Detoxify thoroughly *before* you even begin trying to conceive a baby</u>. Due to toxic chemicals in pesticides, personal care products, and food additives, many babies are born today with more than 200 chemicals in their blood, many of which are highly carcinogenic. A study by EWG found that blood samples from newborns contained an average of 287 toxins, including mercury, fire retardants, pesticides, and Teflon chemicals. 180 of these chemicals cause cancer in humans, 217 are toxic to your brain and nervous systems, and 208 cause birth defects or abnormal development in animal tests! Experts believe rising rates of birth defects, asthma, neuro-developmental disorders and other serious diseases in American children are a result of these early chemical exposures.

Pharmaceutical Drugs Are NOT Safe During Pregnancy

Furthermore, for the love of God, do NOT use pharmaceutical drugs during pregnancy. <u>Most medications are not tested for safety during pregnancy</u>, and can cause serious birth defects.

It is estimated that 14 percent of US pregnant women use antidepressants. Unfortunately, the use of the antidepressant Paxil (paroxetine) was associated with <u>an increased risk of five birth defects</u>, including heart defects and anencephaly, which is abnormal brain and skull formation. The use of Prozac (fluoxetine, made from fluoride) was associated with two birth defects, including heart wall defects and abnormal skull shape. <u>Birth defects occurred two to three times more often</u> in babies born to women taking the drugs. More worrying still… these drugs have found their way into the US water supply! *Are they trying to medicate the entire US population with antidepressants against their will?* Or are the drugs in people's urine not being removed by water treatment methods? I would certainly not be surprised if it's both!

The Dangers Of Wi-Fi and Cell Phone Radiation

Direct exposure to the radiation emanated by cell phones while in the womb and thereafter can profoundly affect the health of children. Spiritual channeller Barbara Marciniak says: *"A pregnant mother who is carrying cell phones, who is sitting in front of television or who is going to movies, watching violent movies and having wireless signals all around… and every doodad in the house is electric… all of this is bombarding the foetus. It cannot survive it. It is not a nourishing environment. So you are going to see a huge increase in diseases. There is going to be an awakening… 'we can't keep doing this to ourselves'… 'We can't do this to our children and grandchildren anymore…'"*

The president of Environmental Health Trust, Devra Davis, says *"Radiation from Wi-Fi can cause diminished reaction time in children, decreased motor function, increased distraction, hyperactivity and inability to focus."* Furthermore, foetuses react very negatively to **ultrasounds** and this can lead to developmental problems later on. This is why we only agreed to two *very brief* ultrasounds when my wife was pregnant.

The Benefits of Hypnobirthing and Natural Births

If you are a woman, I highly recommend going on a **Hypnobirthing** course, to prepare you for a natural and pain-free childbirth experience *without* the use of drugs nor the need for a caesarean. A friend of mine teaches Hypnobirthing in Europe, and 87% of her 900+ students so far gave birth naturally, <u>without any drugs whatsoever</u>, in just 4 to 8 hours, and were out of the hospital within a day or two. Your body is *designed* to do this!

In the animal kingdom, when a female is about to give birth, she finds a dark, quiet place, where she feels *safe*, and she gets into a trance-like (or 'meditative') state. The contractions get progressively more intense, but they allow for resting time in between. These contractions naturally 'eject' the baby from the female's body. She doesn't need to 'push like crazy', in contrast to what we see on TV.

When my wife gave birth a year ago, I insisted that the clinic's room was dark, I put some soothing music on and some candles, I placed big fluffy pillows on the ground, and I instructed the nurses: *"You can check on her now at the start, but then leave us alone for a few hours. I will come get you when it's time. If any one of you comes in before and gets her out of 'state', I'll rip your heads off."* OK, so I didn't *say* that last bit, but it was something to that effect. They were surprised, but they smiled and left us to our own devices. Usually nurses and doctors pop in and out of your room every few minutes, it's loud, it's bright, they're attaching machines and IV drips to your body, scanning, testing, performing ultrasounds… it makes it incredibly *stressful* for the mom-to-be. How can she *possibly* relax and let her body do what it's meant to do?!

We had written down our birth plan, which we gave to them, and we had also written down how that day was going to unfold. We wanted to program it into our subconscious: *"When the waters break, we calmly drive to the clinic, and we have a lovely and calm journey on the way. We are so happy and we are looking forward to meeting our baby. I don't ask any questions (as this would stimulate her neo-cortex and get her out of 'state') as she goes through her Hypnobirthing relaxation and visualization techniques. The nurses and doctor will be very helpful, lovely, and friendly, and they will acquiesce to our birthing wishes. Our baby will be born within a few hours…".* You get the idea. We *programmed* this, and guess what: that's exactly how it happened! My wife gave birth naturally, without the need for pain-relief drugs nor an epidural, with no Pitocin, and no caesarean. She felt strong 'pressure' towards the end, but nothing more. *"Like a strong period pain"*, is how she puts it.

Babies Born by Caesarean Suffer More Chronic Disorders

Babies born by caesareans are born in *trauma*. They are traumatized from the start of their lives. Studies show that their health suffers from it *throughout* their lives. In a huge study conducted by Danish scientists in 2014, results proved that <u>people born by caesarean suffer from chronic disorders such as asthma, rheumatism, allergies, bowel</u>

<u>disorders, and leukaemia more often</u> than people born naturally. *"It is clear that caesarean-born children have worse health"*, concluded Dr. Jan Blustein. It was perhaps not surprising to find out that doctors earn more by performing such a surgery than in the case of a natural birth. They can also plan their schedule better, by scheduling a caesarean at a given time on a specific day, rather than be on call 24/7 throughout the night and on weekends.

Hospital births are extremely traumatic. My wife assisted a few births in a hospital, and she said it was akin to witnessing a rape... Both she and the mother were left traumatized, to say nothing of the child. One doctor took the birth plan that was handed to him, bunched it up and threw it on the floor angrily, yelling to the terrified mother, *"Who do you think you are, telling me how to deliver a baby!"*

We were lucky in that we could afford a private clinic, but not everyone gets that chance. I believe that hospital births are *that* traumatic and stressful *by design*. Why? Because <u>traumatizing a child at birth fragments its mind, and makes it much more receptive to mind control techniques</u> and programming (brainwashing) by the state. It creates a human being that constantly seeks reassurance and acceptance, by <u>conforming to the prevailing status quo</u>, *doing what it is told*.

Under the traumatizing and stressful conditions of a hospital birth (bright lights, loud noises, IV drips, ultrasounds, constant interruptions, chemicals, caesareans...), the mother is in *no* state to give birth naturally. Stress kicks in, which means she is in 'fight-or-flight' mode – the exact *opposite* in fact of what her body requires to give birth naturally. So the doctor says *"The baby is not coming. We need to give you Oxytocin to accelerate the contractions."* Well, *of course* the baby is not coming. You've interrupted the birthing process entirely! And that "oxytocin" is not REAL oxytocin. It is a chemical called 'Pitocin', *which harms the baby*, and which makes the contractions become violently strong, coming all at once (no resting time in between), and very painful. And this usually *still* doesn't induce labour. And that's when they hit you with, *"We need to perform a caesarean. The baby is in distress."* The hospital and doctor make more money the more drugs and surgeries they sell to you. The baby is in distress because of the mother's stress levels, the chemicals injected into her, the ultrasounds...

According to the Russian psycho-genetic therapist Galina Šeremetěvová, "If a child is born by caesarean, they simply can't handle problems later in life. If a birth is generally long, but goes well in the end (a natural child birth), the child has a feeling of safety and security when in contact with problems later in life. A complicated and difficult birth imprints in the human psyche the feeling of pessimism and failure. The child grows up to feel like "oooh, life is so hard... everything is a problem... life is too complicated for me to be successful." He will feel powerless and unworthy, and will always run away from more complicated situations or problems. Also, a lot of children born with caesareans have a lot of tension in their intestines. If you choose anaesthetics, it has a really deep effect on the psychology of the child: "The only way how to deal with problems is the escape through drugging myself". Could today's epidemic of drug use be partially because of epidurals used at birth?"

You will find vastly different approaches to childbirth, depending on where you live. For example, in Europe alone, Cyprus has an astonishingly high 68% caesarean birth rate, compared to 7% in Finland, Norway, and the Netherlands, and 9% in England. Take the time to find a clinic and obstetrician that will provide with you with the best childbirth experience possible. 'Conscious parenting' and 'Contact Parenting' are important topics to cover when it comes to raising a healthy child, but these are outside the scope of this book. I do strongly urge you to look into these. *If you have questions about Hypnobirthing or Conscious Parenting, send us an email at info@thenewbiology.co.uk*

Recently 'Oxytocin' injected into women during childbirth ('Pitocin') <u>was linked to thousands of cases of cerebral palsy</u>. In the UK, 70% of claims against the NHS relating to births were about Pitocin.

The Benefits Of Breastfeeding Your Child

Breast Milk contains over over 200 compounds that fight infection, help the immune system mature, aid in digestion, and support brain growth. Formula milk, on the other hand, lacks many of the nutrients and antibodies that breast milk provides. Breast milk contains the right amount of nutrients essential for brain and nerve development, and breast milk can protect the baby from many diseases and potential infections. I have also been told that a mother's body *knows to produce the specific nutrition that the baby needs* in her breast milk every moment, from holding the baby close to her. How is this even possible? Aside from esoteric explanations, it is said that babies leave stem cells inside the mother, which *communicate* with the cells in the baby. This is how some scientists explain the strong bond and almost telepathic connection mothers have with their children. Furthermore:

❑ Children exclusively breastfed for the first 6 months are **14 times more likely to survive** than those who are not (check out ***"101 Reasons to Breastfeed"*** on www.notmilk.com/101.html).

❑ Breastfeeding leads to reduced risk of asthma, allergies, obesity, and childhood cancer.

❑ **Bottle-feeders suffer more breast cancers and ovarian cancers**, and their babies suffer more childhood cancers (like leukaemia) and bowel cancers later in life.

❑ Breastfeeding reduces the risk of baby girls eventually developing breast cancer by 25% (*"Exposure to breast milk in infancy and the risk of breast cancer"* Freudenheim, J. 1994)

❏ A baby breastfed for one month has a **reduced risk of childhood leukaemia by 21%.** This risk reduction becomes 30% after 6 months. (Robison, L. at University of Minnesota, 1999)

❏ Breastfeeding reduces maternal risk of premenopausal breast cancer by 59% (Stuebe at University of North Carolina, published in the Archives of Internal Medicine, Aug. 2009)

❏ Babies fed formula milk are 6 to 20 times as likely to develop serious bowel disease.

❏ Breast fed babies tend to be smarter than babies who were fed with formula.

❏ ***"Formula Feeding Doubles Infant Deaths in America"*** – A study published in the journal Pediatrics, (May 2004), titled *"Breastfeeding and the Risk*

❏ *of Postneonatal Death in the United States,"* reports 56% more infant deaths for those receiving mostly formula.

❏ A large-scale study taking place in poor areas of Ghana, India, and Peru found a shocking **10.5 times the number of deaths for those not breastfed** versus the babies who were exclusively breastfed.

❏ Most baby milk formulas are actually filled with some pretty dangerous chemicals, which is why we recommend the brand or organic baby milk brand **Holle.** Mike Adams of NaturalNews.com states: *"Chemical and bacterial contaminants can come into play when bottle feeding infants. Mixing powdered infant formula with water from the tap, or even bottled drinking water, can open the door to numerous water contaminants, including chlorine byproducts, pesticides, lead, solvents, arsenic or nitrates from fertilizer runoff. Some formulas may contain excessive levels of metals like aluminium, cadmium, lead or worse."*

Vaccinated Children Are FIVE TIMES More Prone to Disease

In some Western countries, more than *50 doses* of 14 different vaccines are administered to children before they reach kindergarten age, including 26 doses in their first year. One study revealed:

❏ Vaccinated children are about two-and-a-half times as likely (250% more!) to develop **migraine headaches** compared to unvaccinated children.

❏ Vaccinated children are eight times more likely (800% more!) to develop **asthma** and **chronic bronchitis** (respiratory problems).

❏ Vaccinated children are also three times more likely (300% more!) to develop **hyperactivity**, four times more likely (400% more!) to suffer from **hay fever,** and a shocking 17 times more likely (1,700% more!) to experience **thyroid disease**, compared to unvaccinated children.

❑ Vaccinated children are 22 times more likely (2,200% more!) to develop **ear infections**.

❑ Less than 10% of unvaccinated children suffer from **allergies** of any kind. This compares with 40% of children in the USA ages 3-17 reporting an allergy to at least one allergen.

❑ Vaccinated children are 19 times more likely to develop severe **Autism**.

CounterThink

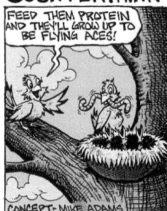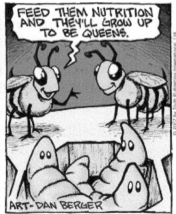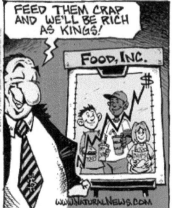

Thanks to Mike Adams and *www.NaturalNews.com* for the cartoon above.

Andreas Moritz, author of ***Cancer is not a Disease – It's a Survival Mechanism***, points out in his book:

❑ Some of the most powerful influences that a child can experience occur while it is still in the mother's womb. It is a scientific fact that what a mother goes through emotionally and physically has a strong impact on the emotional and physical health of her child.

❑ Childhood stress can lead to cancer and human beings experience stress early, even before they are born. Being born by Caesarean section can have traumatic effects on babies.

❑ In addition, not breastfeeding a baby and keeping a baby in a separate room from the mother can cause a biological separation conflict which can even cause crib death. Not sensing and feeling the heartbeat of the mother turns out to be anxiety-provoking for an infant. Prematurely born babies are particularly traumatized by separation anxiety.

❑ Vaccinations cause biological shocks, similar to mini strokes, besides exposing the baby to numerous carcinogenic toxins contained in vaccines.

❑ An inadequate diet that includes sugar, cow's milk, animal proteins, and fried foods, and other junk foods, greatly affects children, too. If mothers drink alcohol, eat junk food or take medication during pregnancy, or were vaccinated themselves, this also has a detrimental effect on the baby's health.

❑ Treating babies for infections with antibiotics is severely damaging to their immune systems.

❑ The poison *fluoride*, added to the municipal drink water in the United States and other countries, has been clearly linked to causing cancer of the bone, and other types of cancer.

❑ Clamping the umbilical cord too early, instead of the required 40-60 minutes after birth, can reduce the oxygenation of the blood in the baby by over 40%, and prevent filtering toxins out of the blood through the placenta. This practice has a severely negative effect on the growth of children.

CHAPTER 18

Dead Doctors Don't Lie, or 'Why Your Body Needs Minerals'

Dr. Joel Wallach was a veterinarian for 30 years and worked as a research veterinary pathologist with The National Institute of Health, performing over 17,500 autopsies on 454 species of animals, and 3,000 on humans. Due to his background and the nature of his work, he was in a unique position to observe how nutritional deficiencies caused specific health problems in animals, as well as humans.

In 1977, he discovered that Cystic Fibrosis in monkeys was due to a nutritional deficiency – specifically, a lack of *selenium* in their diet – which held great hope for children who suffer from this condition. However, when he made his discovery public, flying in the face of the commonly held belief that *"cystic fibrosis is genetic"*, the Institute fired him on the spot. Chagrined and perplexed, he made the decision to go to medical school so he could treat children for cystic fibrosis himself.

He was nominated for the Nobel Prize in Medicine in 1991 for his stunning discoveries in the use of trace minerals to prevent diseases in new-born babies. Thousands of people have attended his lectures on nutrition, and millions have read his book *Dead Doctors Don't Lie*, in which he states:

❑ **There are 90 essential nutrients required by our bodies for optimal health and longevity** (60 essential minerals, 16 essential vitamins, 12 essential amino acids, and 3 essential fatty acids) but most of these are either totally absent or of variable availability in our modern diet. It is important to note that plants can't *make* minerals, they can only take them from the soil. And if the soil is depleted from intensive agriculture practices, then most of these minerals are simply *absent* from our diets, hence the need for nutritional supplements.

❑ **The human genetic potential for longevity is 120 to 140 years**, yet the average lifespan in the US is only 75.5 years. You need to supplement your diet with these essential nutrients, in order to live a long and healthy life.

❑ **Doctors are neither healthier nor do they live longer than the average population**. On the contrary… American doctors actually live only to 62 years old on average, compared to 75.5 years for the average American. Why are you asking them for health advice? "If doctors knew what they were talking about when it came to health and longevity, they should be healthier and live longer than the average American", Dr. Wallach concludes.

❑ To make farming, agriculture, and animal husbandry predictable and profitable industries, **farmers and ranchers learned to add vitamins, minerals, and trace minerals to animal feeds, to prevent disease, eliminate infertility, prevent birth defects, reduce losses from death**, and reduce veterinary bills, all of which were counterproductive. They found you could <u>prevent up to 98% of the birth defects in animals by supplementing the female with the proper nutrients prior to conception</u>. In most instances, "genetic defects" are simple mineral deficiencies that leave a repeatable 'fingerprint' on a specific gene on a specific chromosome. Mineral deficiencies are the root cause of most diseases mistakenly thought to be "genetically transmitted". Dr Wallach states: "We went to a great deal of trouble to make sure that livestock had optimal amounts of vitamins, minerals, and trace minerals in their feed. No one seemed too worried about the need to give humans these same vital supplements!"

❑ It is very important that mothers and expectant mothers supplement their diet: "The Amish families that did not supplement with vitamins and minerals had younger children with congenital birth defects such as cleft palates, spina bifida, Down syndrome, PKU, autism, ADD, clubbed feet, hernias, muscular dystrophy, and heart defects. The Amish also breastfed their babies. If they didn't supplement the mother, she would become more depleted of minerals with each succeeding child. As a result of this pattern, the younger children tended to have the birth defects and middle aged mothers tended to have a variety of degenerative diseases including lupus, arthritis, Multiple Sclerosis, high blood pressure, diabetes, and heart disease."

❑ Studies of the vegetation and water analyses in South Africa proved that **the healthier and larger animals came from areas that were mineral-rich**. Wild animal populations avoided mineral-poor water, forage, and soils. Giraffes sometimes eat antelope bones. Elephants, rhino and other animals spent a great deal of time eating clay termite nests (minerals are brought up from hundreds of feet underground by these insects) and they also eat crushed limestone road beds for calcium and trace minerals.

❑ Many "deficiency diseases" occur when single and multiple nutrients are missing from an animal's ration. **Calcium deficiency** alone can result in as many as 147 different diseases ranging from Multiple Sclerosis to osteoarthritis.

❏ **Selenium deficiency** causes infertility, miscarriages, cystic fibrosis of the pancreas, Sudden Infant Death Syndrome in animals, liver cirrhosis, stiff lamb disease, white muscle disease, muscular dystrophy, anaemia, Alzheimer's, and cardiomyopathy. In each case, selenium supplementation prevented the disease and in many cases *reversed* existing diseases.

❏ In humans we deal with fibromyalgia, muscular dystrophy, liver cirrhosis, and cardiomyopathy by treating the *symptoms* with muscle relaxants, prednisone, liver transplants, pacemakers, and heart transplants – none of which cure fibromyalgia – instead of actually addressing the nutritional deficiencies that *cause* fibromyalgia in the first place.

❏ **Copper** is required as a cofactor to manufacture hair pigment, and a copper deficiency in human beings presents itself first as greying hair. Additional symptoms include crow's feet, skin wrinkles, varicose veins, haemorrhoids, liver cirrhosis, and aneurysms. When humans supplement with plant derived colloidal copper, their original hair colour can come back.

❏ While working in a nature reserve in Botswana, Africa, Dr. Wallach also treated the local children, and found that nutritional deficiencies were very common. **Vitamin A deficiencies** in children caused keratitis, corneal ulcers, and blindness. **Calcium deficiency** caused osteomalacia in children and arthritis and Multiple Sclerosis in adults. **Iodine and copper deficiencies** caused Goiter in adults and miscarriages. Infants were born with spina bifida and serious cleft palates as a result of folic acid or **zinc deficiencies**. Beriberi with resultant congestive heart failure was common, the result of a thiamine or **vitamin B1 deficiency**.

❏ Dr Wallach has had great results in treating Arthritis, by supplementing his patients' diets. He points out that traditional medical treatments rarely solve the problem, and can come with dreadful side effects: "Painkillers and anti-inflammatory drugs are the arthritis treatment of choice, though their dangerous – even deadly – side-effects are rarely mentioned. None prevent or cure arthritis. Aspirin doesn't fix arthritis and can cause gastric bleeding and death. Tylenol™ doesn't fix arthritis and causes 50,000 cases of kidney failure each year, 10% of which cases (5,000) are serious enough to require a kidney transplant. Ibuprofen, Advil™, and Aleve™ don't fix arthritis either, but they can cause liver damage in up to ten percent of users, some even requiring a liver transplant. Prednisone and cortisone don't fix arthritis and they suppress your immune system, leaving you open to diseases far worse than arthritis. And when prescription drugs don't work anymore to relieve pain and inflammation, the only thing left for you medically is joint replacement surgery. These surgeries rarely work out well."

❑ He goes on to say that Arthritis is like a "warning signal" from your body, that you are deficient in essential minerals. The drugs and painkillers only serve to *hide* these warning signals, while the underlying problem gets worse. He recommends supplementing one's diet with 2000 mg/day of calcium, 800-1000 mg/day of magnesium, Vitamin C 1000 mg/day, Vitamin B6 (100 mg twice a day), Vitamin B3 (450 mg twice a day as time-release capsules), Vitamin E at 1000 IU/day, 2 mg/day of Copper, 300 mg/day of Selenium, 50 mg of Zinc three times per day, and 1000 mg cartilage (collagen, glucosamine sulfate and chondroitin sulfate) three times per day. Oral food grade H2O2 is very helpful too. He says: "I have seen tens of thousands of people who have had a regrowth of cartilage, ligaments, tendons, connective tissue, bone foundation, bone matrix. It doesn't matter if they are 20 or 90 years old, I've seen people 97 years old regrow cartilage and bone, even if they had bone to bone arthritis. If there's blood supply to that joint and that bone, they will regrow bone and cartilage."

❑ He shares the following story about how the mainstream medical establishment reacted to his "heretic" views on Arthritis: "The Harvard Medical School wanted to prove me wrong, so they took 29 arthritis patients who had not responded in any way to medical treatment for arthritis over 15 years. They took them off their medication, it wasn't working anyway, lined them up for joint-replacement surgery, and for 90 days before their surgery they gave them heaping tablespoon of ground up chicken cartilage in their orange juice every morning for 90 days. They were sort of chuckling in their beer saying "nothing is going to happen". Well, in 10 days these people had complete relief of pain inflammation that they hadn't had in 15 to 20 years. In 30 days they could open up a new pickle jar that had never been opened without pain to the fingers, wrists, elbows and shoulders. In 90 days, 28 of the 29 were clinically cured. Now this is from the Harvard Medical School. That meant that they had complete return of the range of motion, all of the pain and inflammation was gone, and you would think they would call me up, these professors from Harvard Medical School, and say "Look, Wallach, we have to apologize to you." Here's what they actually said: "After 3 months it was clear that the drug was beneficial." Chicken cartilage had become a drug in 90 days! And you, too, for $3500 a month, can get Harvard Medical School's chicken cartilage in a capsule for arthritis (this actually costs just 30 cents a day...). And of course, cartilage or gelatine, has chondroitin sulfate in it, glucosamine sulfate, collagen, these are all the basic raw materials to rebuild cartilage and bone, the things I have been telling my patients about for 20 years."

❑ Regarding weight loss, Dr. Wallach explains that huge numbers of Americans are obese because of *a lack of minerals in their diet,* which leads to overeating and constant snacking.

❑ "A good farmer knows that when a horse cribs, the animal really has a craving for minerals. The farmer supplements the animal's diet with minerals to save the animal's life, save on veterinary bills, and save from having to rebuild the fence, because a mineral deficient animal will literally eat the fence looking for minerals. [...] **The "munchies" is a plague that shows America as a whole is so minerally deficient...** exhibiting symptoms of mineral craving once known primarily among expectant mothers. Unfortunately, our bodies temporarily interpret sugar and salt intake as a fulfilment of the cravings for essential minerals."

❑ He observed that overweight people have similar cravings and binge eating habits as pregnant women. They craved salt, fried foods, sugar, spicy foods, and even non-food items such as clay, hair, finger nails or they chewed on paper. The common thread between the "cribbing" behaviour displayed by pregnant women and the obese patient is *a deficiency of minerals.* As a result, Dr. Wallach's weight loss programs contained complete mineral supplementation programs, personalized to each individual following a hair analysis.

❑ Children will often eat lead paint and one study reported that 25% of children eat earth, because their bodies are screaming for minerals for their mineral starved bodies.

❑ He describes how thousands of Americans flee the US medical system to visit alternative medicine clinics abroad: "The orthodox medical profession viciously attacked the philosophy of alternative medicine as quackery, yet people came to Mexico by the tens of thousands for this "unorthodox" treatment. Terminally and chronically ill patients, including cancer patients, diabetics, arthritics, stroke patients, and Alzheimer's patients poured into Mexico. They fled the U.S. by the tens of thousands. They were fleeing from the orthodox medical doctors with their "Cut, Burn, and Poison" treatments that rarely cured anything! First of all, the orthodox medical approach was **expensive**; second, **it didn't cure anything**; and third, medical treatment itself could be **dangerous and life threatening**!"

❑ In a January 1993 news release, Ralph Nader declared that *"doctors kill 150,000 to 300,000 Americans each year in hospitals alone, as a result of medical negligence."* On November 5, 1996, the Rand Corporation and Harvard Medical School jointly published a survey showing that **doctors kill 180,000 Americans each year in hospitals alone as a result of *medical negligence*.** It further demonstrated that 1.3 million people are *injured* each year from medical

225

negligence. In March of 1998, the CDC stated that two million *infections* occur each year in hospitals alone as a result of medical negligence. But doctors rarely admit to any wrongdoing: *"Doctors as a group are too arrogant to admit they could have been so wrong.*

❑ Dr. Wallach shares the story of Inge Reagen, a woman in her fifties who suffered for 12 years with **Multiple Sclerosis, osteoarthritis**, bone spurs, **ankylosing spondylitis, fibromyalgia**, and high blood pressure. Inge had 9 doctors, including orthopaedic surgeons, rheumatologists, an internist, an endocrinologist, and a podiatrist. To pay all these doctors she spent the life insurance proceeds after her husband died, refinanced her house, *and* spent $250,000 to install wheel chair ramps, elevators, and special plumbing to accommodate her wheel chair.

Her son Rudy would pick her up out of bed every morning, strap her in the wheel chair, feed her, and then head out to work. Every evening he would return from work and reverse the process. This went on day after day, *every* day, for twelve years.

Inge had cervical vertebrae fused. She'd had several finger joints replaced. The surgeons wouldn't replace her hips, knees, and shoulders because her bones were too "crumbly". She kept complaining about hip and knee pain so the surgeons suggested amputating her legs.

Inge started on Dr. Wallach's 'Pig Arthritis Formula' supplementation protocol. In six weeks she was able to slip out of the wheelchair and into a walker by herself. After several more weeks he was able to walk with the use of a cane. A few weeks later Inge was able to function at 100 percent without pain nor restricted motion.

CHAPTER 19

Longevity Secrets: How to Live to 100 and Beyond

In Dan Buettner's 2008 book *"The Blue Zones: Lessons For Living Longer From The People Who've Lived The Longest"*, he lists the characteristics of five communities throughout the world that have the highest concentrations of centenarians – people who live to 100 years of age or beyond.

These include:

- ❑ The Barbagia region of Sardinia in Italy
- ❑ Okinawa in Japan
- ❑ The community of 7th Day Adventists in Loma Linda in California
- ❑ The Nicoya Peninsula in Costa Rica
- ❑ The Greek island of Ikaria

These communities live long and healthy lives, and they rarely experience the diseases that are decimating the populations of Western countries. Let's have a look at what they have in common.

The Barbagia Region of Sardinia in Italy

The inhabitants of the mountainous Barbagia area of inner Sardinia consume a diet that is largely plant based with an emphasis on beans, whole wheat, garden vegetables and Connanau wine. They don't do stressful or strenuous work but get enough low-intensity physical activity on a *daily* basis. They include mastic oil in their diets. They consume a lot of natural, unprocessed goat's milk and cheese, rich in calcium, vitamin B6, vitamin A, potassium, and niacin (Vitamin B3). They have a great sense of humour. Closeness of family is one of their top priorities in life.

Okinawa in Japan

Okinawa comprises of 150 islands in the East China Sea between Taiwan and Japan's mainland. It's known for its tropical climate, broad beaches and coral reefs. Its inhabitants embrace *ikigai*, a Japanese concept meaning *"a reason for being" (everyone, according to the Japanese, has an ikigai. Finding it requires a deep and often lengthy search of self)*. They lead purpose-driven lives that make them feel wanted and needed, which explains their zest to *get up and go* every morning.

Their tradition of 'moai' (Japanese for "meeting for a common purpose"; social support groups) provides them with a secure and stable social network, giving them financial and emotional support throughout their lives.

The people rely mainly on a plant based diet, high in nutrients and low in calories. They consume Goya, a bitter melon that is high in antioxidants and other compounds that lower blood sugar. Their diets are rich in soy products, such as tofu and miso soup (note: non-GMO soy).

They grow medicinal herbs such as mugwort, ginger, and turmeric, which help protect them against illnesses. They garden, *a lot*. This is their number one source of their daily physical activity, which explains why they're fit and healthy, even in old age. It provides them with a way of managing stress and puts fresh vegetables on the table. They get out into the sun enough, getting plenty of vitamin D. Okinawans are walkers of note and spend a lot of time doing this particular activity.

The Loma Linda 7th Day Adventists Community in Southern California

The Seventh Day Adventists community of Loma Linda in southern California regularly find some sanctuary in time, to re-focus on family, God, camaraderie and nature. This helps them manage their stress levels, strengthens their social networks and provides them with consistent exercise.

They keep active and only eat what they need to in order to nourish their bodies. Their diet includes a lot of nuts and seeds. They follow the rule of *"Eat breakfast like a king, lunch like a prince, and dinner like a pauper,"* and follow a mainly vegetarian diet.

They spend a lot of time with like-minded people. The Seventh-Day Adventists church encourages its members to volunteer, which help them to stay active and find *purpose* in life by helping others.

The Nicoya Peninsula in Costa Rica

The inhabitants of the Nicoya Peninsula in Costa Rica have a *"plan de Vida"* which means they have a strong sense of purpose in life, so they feel needed and they want to contribute to the greater good.

They eat light dinners early in the evenings. They keep their focus on family, living in family groups that provide them with support and a sense of purpose and belonging.

They keep hard at work, enjoying physical forms of work because they find joy in everyday physical chores. They really love to get out into the sun, which boosts their vitamin D levels naturally.

The Ikaria Island Blue Zone in the Aegean Sea

The inhabitants of Ikaria consume a lot of goat's milk, which provides them with a great source of calcium, potassium and tryptophan. They follow a Mediterranean diet, consuming a lot of fruits and vegetables, whole grains, beans, potatoes and olive oil.

They exercise daily by gardening, walking over to the neighbours' houses, and doing yard work.

They make family and friends a priority, fostering social connections, which in turn benefits their overall health and longevity. They love drinking herbal teas rich in antioxidants. They include rosemary, sage and oregano in their diet. They regularly take mid-afternoon naps. The Ikarians also fast occasionally, helping the body cleanse itself.

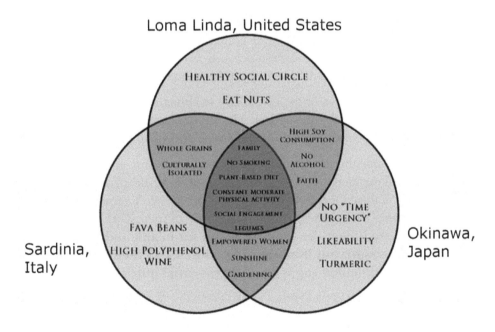

Venn Diagram of longevity clues from Okinawa, Sardinia, and Loma Linda (source: Wikipedia)

According to Dan Buettner, the nine lessons for longevity to derive from the Blue Zone communities' lifestyles are:

- ❏ Do moderate, regular physical activity. Keep active.
- ❏ Have a strong sense of *life purpose*.
- ❏ Reduce or eliminate your stress.
- ❏ Have a moderate calorie intake (this is helped, of course, by consuming nutrient-dense food). The centenarians from the Blue Zones follow diets of no more than 2000 calories per day.
- ❏ Consume a mainly plant-based diet.
- ❏ Moderate alcohol intake, especially wine.
- ❏ Engagement in spirituality or religion. Give thanks for your food.
- ❏ Have a strong engagement in family life.
- ❏ Have a strong engagement in social life.

The Importance of Mineral-Rich Diets

In his book *Dead Doctors Don't Lie,* Dr. Joel Wallach points out that the longest living populations in the world consume *mineral-rich* and *nutrient-dense* foods. He states that the genetic potential or upper limit for longevity for human beings is 168 years.

The US has the most expensive and "advanced" healthcare system in the world, and yet Americans only live to 75, on average. He advises people to *avoid* going to the doctor, if at all possible, because "Given half a chance they will kill you."

He advocates consuming the 90 essential nutrients in optimal amounts each day to warrant that you will properly develop, maintain, and repair your body: "Nothing works in the body without mineral cofactors – nothing! Vitamins, DNA, RNA, chromosomes, enzymes, hormones, energy, not even oxygen works without mineral cofactors. **Minerals are in fact the limiting factor for health and longevity – they are in fact the long sought out 'fountain of youth'. [...] Potentially 900 diseases are preventable by supplementing with all 90 essential nutrients.**"

Dr. Wallach warns against *intense* exercise, as athletes who do not take supplements are at risk of sweating out their essential minerals, such as copper, selenium, chromium, vanadium, calcium, magnesium, and sulphur. "The great distance runners, Jim Fixx and Dr. George Sheehan, believed that exercise was the elixir of health and the foundation for longevity. To that end they ran and jogged almost every day of their adult lives. Neither took vitamin or mineral supplements. Jim Fixx died at age 52. Dr. Sheehan died of prostate cancer at the age of 76."

Many of the long-lived populations are peoples who fled persecution and looked for refuge in desolate high mountain valleys ranging from 8,500 to 14,000 feet in elevation. These regions typically have 60 to 72 minerals in the parent rocks and soil, and have an arid climate, with less than two inches of precipitation per year (this avoids "washing away" those vital minerals from the soil). These regions also typically depend on glaciers as their permanent source of water. As a result, many live to be 120 to 140 years of age, with some extraordinary individuals living to be 150 to 160.

"Glaciers literally weigh millions of tons. As they move up and down the mountains' slopes in synchrony with the seasons, they grind up tens of thousands of tons of rock into rock "flour" each year.

This rock flour containing 60 to 72 minerals comes out from under the glacier suspended in the water by turbulence and small particle size. This rock flour suspension is known as "glacial milk".

Not only do these age beaters drink the "glacial milk," they irrigate with the mineral-laden glacial milk or have fields on the flood plains that get replenished with mineral-laden silt every spring when it floods. Their grains, vegetables, fruits, and nuts convert the inorganic elemental minerals in the fields to plant derived colloidal minerals. It is the plant derived colloidal minerals in their grains, vegetables, fruits, and nuts that are the common threads giving the age-beaters their health and longevity", writes Dr. Wallach.

Dr. Wallach lists the following cultures whose peoples routinely live to their maximum genetic potential of 120 to 140 years of age:

❑ The Himalayan Tibetans from the northwest of China

❑ The Hunzakut from the Karakarum Mountains of eastern Pakistan

❑ The Russian Georgians from the Caucasus Mountains (and their sister cultures of Armenia, Azerbaijan, Abkhazia, and Turkey)

❑ The Vilcabamba from the Andes of Ecuador and Titicaca's of the Andes of Peru.

The common denominators of these long-lived cultures include:

❑ The communities are found at elevations ranging from 8,500 feet to 14,000 feet in sheltered mountain valleys.

❑ The annual precipitation is less than two inches (minerals are not washed away).

❑ Their water source for drinking and irrigation comes from glacial melt and is known as "glacial milk" because the highly mineralized water is an opaque white in colour.

❑ There is no heavy industry or modern agriculture to pollute their air, water, or food.

❑ Only natural fertilizer including animal manure, plant debris, and glacial milk is applied to their fields. No pesticides nor chemicals pollute their soils and their crops.

❑ Their caloric intake is 1200 to 1900 calories per day, compared to the average American daily calorie intake of 3800.

❑ Western allopathic medicine has not been historically available to these cultures.

It is interesting to point out that these cultures are from "Third World" countries, rather than "*modern*", "*advanced*", "*civilized*" Western nations, and yet they live longer than we do!

Himalayan Health

Dr. Wallach writes: "Tibetans are devout Buddhists. Their staple diet consists of "Tsampa", a smelly hand-mixed paste of lightly toasted barley flour, yak butter, salt and black tea. It is served with turnips, cabbage, potatoes, trout, egg omelettes, and beans. Tibetans routinely drink 30 to 40 cups of black or green tea daily to prevent dehydration, because of the dry air encountered in the high elevations. Each cup of tea is flavoured with a chunk of rock salt the size of a Concord grape and two pats of yak or goat butter. There are tens of thousands of acres of terraces fed and watered by mineral rich 'glacial milk that originates in the Himalayan glaciers and supplies an endless source of minerals to replenish the fields. [...] Li-Ching-Yun reportedly lived to the age of 256, outliving 23 wives. At the age of 250, Li lectured to a thousand medical students in Beijing on the art of living a long and healthy life. His advice: "Keep a quiet heart, sit like a tortoise, sleep like a dog."

Georgian Longevity

"The Russian Georgians of the Caucasus Mountains live in simple stone houses without electricity. They typically drink an eight-ounce glass of vodka with breakfast and have a large glass of wine with lunch. Almost all of the old people are from rural backgrounds or occupations such as farmers, shepherds and hunters. 5,000 of the 500,000 inhabitants are over 100 years of age. They feel that youth is up to 80 years of age, 80 to 100 is middle age and 100 to 160 years of age are the seniors. Studies have shown that only the married individuals attained advanced age, and they still had an active sex life after the age of 100. Women continue to have children after the age of 52. The staple diet of the Caucasus region includes chicken, mutton, beef, goat milk, cheese, yogurt, butter, bread, boiled corn meal mush, red pepper, tea, wine, and salt. Their caloric intake per is 1,900. Their fields have been irrigated with glacial milk for over 2,500 years.

The oldest known person from the Caucasus region in 1973 was Shirali Mislimov. At 167, he still worked in the village tea plantation in the small Azerbaijani village of Barzavu on the Iranian border. His wife was 107 when he turned 168 in May of 1973."

Ecuadorian Centenarians

"Ecuador's star-shaped "Sacred Valley of Longevity" is actually five valleys that converge and sit between two Andean Mountains at 12,434 feet above sea level. They have nine centenarians per 819 of population, or an astounding one centenarian per 100 people! The staple diet of the Vilcabamba Indians includes corn, beans, goat meat, chicken, eggs, milk, cheese, and soup known as "repe" which is made from bananas, beans, white cheese, salt, and lard. Miguel Carpio at age 123 was the oldest living Vilcabamban found on the census – he still smoked, drank wine, and "chased women." The average total calorie intake of the Vilcabamba Centenarians ranges from 1,200 to 1,800 calories per day. Glacial milk-fed Lake Titicaca is 3,200 square miles in surface area."

The Hunza in Eastern Pakistan

"The Hunza consume milk, buttermilk, yogurt, and butter (which they put in their tea). Hunza children are breast-fed until two to four years of age. Cultivated plants included barley, millet, wheat, buckwheat, potatoes, turnips, carrots, beans, peas, pumpkins, tomatoes, melons, onions, garlic, cabbage, spinach, cauliflower, apricots, mulberries, walnuts, apples, plums, peaches, cherries, pears and pomegranates. The Hunza do not cook the majority of their food because of a lack of fuel. Their basic diet is whole grains, vegetables, and fruits. Their farm soils are maintained by organic agricultural practices. Glacial milk is the exclusive water source used for drinking and irrigation purposes. Mutton, goat, yak, beef, poultry, brain, kidney, and liver are eaten as available. A grape wine known as Pani is consumed daily. The Hunza consume 1,800 to 2,000 calories each day. There is a total absence of additives, preservatives, or chemicals in their air, food, and water. No agricultural sprays or chemicals of any kind. No vaccines or antibiotics. Native herbs are used for medicine, seasoning, and food. There are no western style hospitals or doctors in Hunza. All Hunzas work 12 hours each day, seven days each week. [...] For more than 2,300 years the Hunza people have drunk and irrigated their terraced fields with glacial milk, assuring an intake of the more than 60 minerals in the glacial milk of the Ultar Glacier!"

He concludes by stating: "It is the eating of the plants rich in organic colloidal minerals that is the secret of health and longevity of the eight long-lived cultures."

According to Dr. Joseph Mercola, human used to consume **2 to 10 times more nutrition** than we currently do! I, for one, have drastically increased my nutritional intake, to maximize my longevity potential. I invite you to do the same.

Recap – The New Biology

❑ To experience extraordinary levels of health, the key question you should be asking yourself is: *"What do I need to do to ensure optimum health at a **cellular** level?"*

❑ Your cells need **oxygen**, **nutrients** (minerals), and the ability to eliminate their own **waste**.

❑ According to Dr. Joel Wallach, your cells need 90 essential nutrients. Many diseases are actually **'nutrient deficiency diseases'**.

❑ Cancer occurs when cells are denied 60% of their oxygen requirements (they mutate, *to survive*). Cancer is not a disease, it is *a survival mechanism*.

❑ Disease is due to a *deficiency of force*. When the natural strength of the body is depleted, it no longer has the *energy* to remove toxicity, heal itself, and defend itself from disease. Therefore, to be truly healthy **you need plenty of *energy*.

❑ Your body *must* maintain an alkaline inner terrain – **a pH level of 7.36**. Your body will do whatever it takes to maintain that balance. Eat a diet that is 80% alkaline.

❑ An acidic inner terrain destroys your energy levels. When you are overly acidic, your red blood cells (that carry oxygen and nutrients to every part of your body) start clumping together, moving slower, breaking down, and your energy goes 'through the floor'.

❑ An acidic inner terrain leads to **inflammation** and destruction of your cells, arthritis, Multiple Sclerosis, diabetes, cholesterol, weight gain, and a host of other 'diseases'.

❑ The people who live the longest have the following in common: they eat a mainly plant based **nutrient-rich diet** (though they also eat meat), a strong sense of **purpose**, a strong **family and community life**, a focus on **spiritual** matters, moderate daily **exercise**, little to no stress.

❑ Many so-called diseases are nothing more than your body dealing with *how toxic* you are. If you take *a poison* and put it into your bloodstream, your body does whatever it takes to get it *out* of the body in the fastest way possible, using any elimination channel available: **fever** to sweat out the poison, **mucus**, waste coming out **through your skin, diarrhoea**, throwing up, etc. Your body will use up every ounce of energy to *fight* the poison. Your body shuts down your digestive system, restricts blood flow to your brain… so you experience headaches, low energy, fatigue, joint pains, inability to sleep, kidney problems, burping, gas, irritations, etc. hence the importance of *regularly* **detoxifying** *your system* (see Chapter 12, *Cleanse & Purify Your Body*).

❑ To **give your children the best start in life**, do a detox *before* conceiving; take nutritional supplements before, during, and after childbirth; *avoid* taking pharmaceutical drugs during pregnancy; have a natural 'Hypnobirthing' childbirth, without drugs; avoid a caesarean; breastfeed your child as long as possible; avoid feeding your child fluoride and commercially-available formula milk; hold your child close to you and have it sleep in the same room as you for the first 18 months; NEVER give your child ANY vaccines whatsoever.

❑ **What makes your immune system weak**: Vaccinations; Antibiotics; Pharmaceutical drugs; Radiation; Blood transfusions; Poisoned Air, Water, and Food; Stress and Worry; Toxic Cosmetics; Toxic Living Environments; Toxic (Negative) Family Members; Fear.

❑ Disease starts in the mind. Whenever you have an illness, you can determine **the mind-pattern that caused it** from the part of the body that is affected. Illness is your body's way of telling you where you are lying about life. We get ill to teach us to **love**. Learn to let go of the past, forgive, and move on.

❑ **All illness is self-created**. Most people worry themselves *to death*.

Doctors Don't Know How To Live Long and Healthy Lives!

Ironically, most doctors are generally very unhealthy people. Their life expectancy is 6 to 12 years *less* than average people.

They know very little about nutrition and about "being healthy", having received just 3 hours of training on nutrition in medical school, out of 3,500 hours of medical training, and they tend to ingest more drugs.

Why are you asking *them* for health advice?

Dr. Leonard Coldwell states: *"Doctors statistically have the shortest lifespan, highest drug and alcohol abuse rate, highest suicide rate second to psychiatrists… and yet we go to doctors to ask them how to live a long and healthy and happy life? We should rethink this."*

CHAPTER 20

These Five 'Acid Addictions' are Destroying Your Health

In order to regain your health, you must cut out the self-destructive habits that are so prevalent in the Western world, and it starts with throwing away that pack of cigarettes.

Acid Addiction #1 – SMOKING

Cigarette smoke <u>contains over 4,000 chemicals, including 43 known cancer-causing compounds</u> and 400 other toxins. These include nicotine, tar, and carbon monoxide, as well as DDT, formaldehyde, ammonia, hydrogen cyanide, and arsenic. It's no surprise that **Tobacco has killed over 100 million people in the 20th century.**

You simply *cannot* **smoke AND be healthy**. Do whatever it takes to quit. Just look at what it does to your lungs and brain. If the pictures below don't convince you, nothing will!

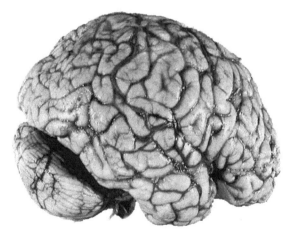

Brain of a smoker

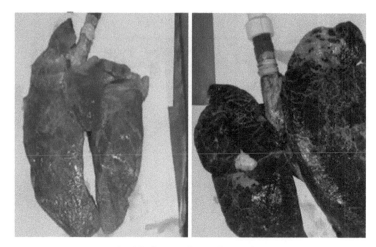

healthy lungs vs lungs of a smoker

Acid Addiction #2 – COFFEE

Coffee is *pure acid*, and it is a powerful nerve toxin. This acid addiction turns your bloodstream to *sludge*. Coffee is one of the most acidic things you could consume, and does *not* give you energy. It is a nerve toxin that *spikes your adrenaline* because your body is *fighting to get rid of this poison*, so you feel like you're "buzzing", briefly, and then you 'crash' because coffee actually *robs you* of energy. Do you really think coffee brings your body any nutrition whatsoever? It does not!

Caffeine *increases* catecholamines, your stress hormones. The stress response elicits cortisol and increases insulin. Insulin increases inflammation and this makes you feel lousy, not to mention it increases your risk of mortality related to cardiovascular disease. The acidity of coffee is associated with digestive discomfort, indigestion, heart burn, GERD, and imbalances in your gut flora. Coffee, filled with milk and sugar, is the epitome of food lacking nutrition and it makes you feel lousy, too! Coffee drinkers are at risk of having lower levels of serotonin, which is necessary for normal sleep, bowel function, mood, and energy levels. That's right; caffeine can disrupt sleep and promote anxiety and depression. Coffee also interferes with the detoxification process of the liver. Coffee is so acidic that it depletes your body of vital minerals such as calcium, magnesium and potassium – your body leaches these alkaline elements from your bones when you drink coffee! Coffee is totally destructive for your body! The only reason you drink coffee is because you've been conditioned to do so. You take this toxin in every day because of a social hypnosis. *Wake up and quit this toxic addiction!*

Acid Addiction #3 – ALCOHOL

Alcohol destroys your ability to digest anything else. It irritates and alters your body, and radically destroys the amount of oxygen flowing to your brain. You get "drunk" because of the low levels of oxygen reaching your brain. This happens because your body is actively trying *to restrict the flow of toxic alcohol-soaked blood* to the brain, in order to preserve it from this destructive poison. Before you even swallow down that Jack Daniels, the alcoholic vapours have seeped through your palate and into your brain, causing immediate damage. Drinking alcohol weakens your immune system; it damages your brain, your central nervous system, your liver, your pancreas, your gallbladder; it increases your odds of diabetes and liver cancer; it can lead to strokes, cause ulcers in the oesophagus and stomach, and wreak havoc with your digestive system. Over the long term, drinking can actually shrink the frontal lobes of your brain and cause dementia. Alcohol makes it harder for your digestive tract to absorb nutrients and B vitamins. Alcoholics often suffer from malnutrition. Erectile dysfunction is a common side effect of alcohol abuse in men. It can also inhibit hormone production, affect testicular function, and cause infertility. While an occasional glass of pesticide-free and sulphites-free quality red wine is OK, I don't recommend that you drink *any* alcohol unless you are at a level of peak physical health, by doing everything else we recommend in this book.

By the way, most American beer is laden with high fructose corn syrup, artificial flavours and toxic ingredients such as airplane de-icing liquid, caramel colouring, propylene glycol, MSG (an *excitotoxin* that can cause brain damage, nervous disorders, and cause radical hormone fluctuations), GMO's, fish bladders, stabilizers like carrageenan that are linked to intestinal inflammation, and a host of other carcinogens.

A lot of the American beer companies are not even doing fermentation anymore, which essentially means, you are not even drinking beer. MillerCoors is not even using real hops. They have a patent on something called *tetrahops*, which is a synthetic chemical that mimics hop flavour (and which is significantly *cheaper* to produce). The caramel colouring often used is a carcinogen proven to cause liver tumours, lung tumours, and thyroid tumours in rats and mice. But it doesn't matter, since advertising will make the consumers buy anything. *Shockingly, beer manufacturers are not obliged to list all their ingredients on their packaging!*

Stay away from alcohol – you don't really know *what* they put in those products anyway – *and for that matter, stay away from ALL processed foods!*

Acid Addiction #4 – SUGAR

Nancy Appleton, Ph.D., author of *"Lick The Sugar Habit"*, lists **124 ways how sugar can ruin your health**, based on research published in medical journals and other scientific publications, including:

- Sugar metabolizes into acid in your body. Viruses, bacteria and cancer cells, thrive in an acidic environment (sugar feeds cancer)

- Sugar upsets the mineral relationships in the body

- Sugar causes chromium deficiency, copper deficiency, and interferes with absorption of calcium and magnesium

- Sugar leads to cancer of the breast, ovaries, prostrate, and rectum

- Sugar causes premature ageing

- Sugar suppresses the immune system

- Sugar causes hyperactivity, anxiety, difficulty concentrating, and crankiness

- When children were put on a low sugar diet, there was a 44% drop in antisocial behaviour

- Sugar contributes to: Arthritis, Asthma, Gallstones, Heart Disease, Candida, Multiple Sclerosis, Haemorrhoids, Varicose Veins, Multiple Sclerosis, Gout, Cholesterol, Food Allergies, Diabetes, Eczema, Parkinson's, Alzheimer's, Increased Kidney Size, Kidney Stones, Damage to the pancreas, Pancreatic Cancer in women, reduced eyesight, reduced ability to learn in children, and more.

It is particularly worrying how the food industry now puts sugar in almost *all* processed foods. It is **a $50 billion dollar a year industry**, that is using the same techniques as *the tobacco industry* to keep the public ignorant of its effects on your health. In Damon Gameau's excellent documentary *That Sugar Film,* he exposes how *sugar* is killing millions of people a year, and how food manufacturing companies conspire to keep this out of the headlines. According to this documentary, the average Australian consumes *40 teaspoons of sugar a day* (that's roughly 160 grams of sugar a day). An Australian family of four consumes SIX KILOGRAMS OF SUGAR a week (mostly hidden in day-to-day processed food like breakfast cereals, soups, fruit juices, iced tea, energy drinks, sauces, yoghurts). In fact, 80% of the items on supermarket shelves contain sugar!

I was shocked to find out that **Breakfast cereals** *are typically 26% to 46% SUGAR, they are often made from Genetically Modified Organisms, they contain no real nutritional value, and the synthetic vitamins and minerals they add back can't be absorbed by your body!* I grew up on this stuff! Damn!

In the 1970s, a British doctor named John Yudkin believed *sugar* was to blame for the explosion in heart disease throughout the Western world. He stated: *"I'd be very happy if everybody ate just four pounds of sugar a year... They eat a hundred pounds!"* That's 45 kilos of sugar a year... and that was in the *seventies!* Nowadays it's much, much worse. In the last 20 years, the amount of sugar each person consumes yearly in the United States has soared from 26 pounds per person to more than 150 pounds per person (a whopping 80 kilos of sugar a year!).

After just 18 days of eating as much sugar as the average Australian (40 teaspoons a day), apart from feeling moody and tired, Damon Gameau's liver cells showed signs of being damaged or dying, and he had the signs of a fatty liver. Damon explains what happens to our body when we consume sugar:

"After sugar enters the body, it splits into two parts... fructose and glucose. Both of which make their way to the liver. Once in the liver, the glucose is dealt with efficiently. It's either used immediately for energy or it's stored for later, like a spare battery. But the **fructose** half of sugar is very different. The **liver doesn't have a system to regulate the fructose** because it was so rare in nature, so it hoovers it out of the bloodstream whether it needs it or not. And if all our spare batteries are full, then **it rapidly turns it into fat**. Some of that fat is going to stay in the liver and you're going to have increased risk for insulin resistance and diabetes. What also happens is that this fat in the liver is then sent out into the bloodstream as triglycerides, which can lead to excess weight plus blocked arteries and heart disease. Now, when we're eating lots of sugar and other carbohydrates like bread and pasta, we're producing lots of glucose. A hormone called insulin is released, which is like a key that helps to open our cells' doors so they can absorb all the glucose, remove it from the bloodstream and burn it for energy. **The more glucose in the blood, the more insulin is released**. But the key point for us is that while this insulin is in the blood dealing with all the glucose, it tells our fat cells to hold on to the fat. It actually turns off our fat-burning processes. So when we're eating lots of sugar, we're putting fat into our bodies via the fatty liver. Plus, because of all the glucose, we maintain the level of insulin, which tells our fat cells to hold on to the fat. We can't burn off fat when insulin is around dealing with all the sugar! This is what may be happening to a huge number of the population."

Food scientist Howard Moskowitz showed Damon his recent creation of a new soda flavour for 'Dr Pepper'. He started with 61 levels of sweeteners in the formulation, subjected that to more than 3,000 consumer taste tests, then took that data to come up with *the optimum level of sweetness* that was guaranteed to send their new soda flying off the shelf. This optimal amount of sugar is referred to as 'the bliss point'. *"You can't underestimate the amount of scientific effort that these companies will put into maximising the allure of their products"*, one journalist stated.

Creating 'bliss points' in food products is exploiting the biology of children, creating the expectation in them that *"everything they eat should taste sweet"*. This makes it harder for parents to turn their kids onto broccoli or cauliflower... *"The food companies have always known... that adding sweetness (sugar) can make anything palatable."*

COUNTERTHINK

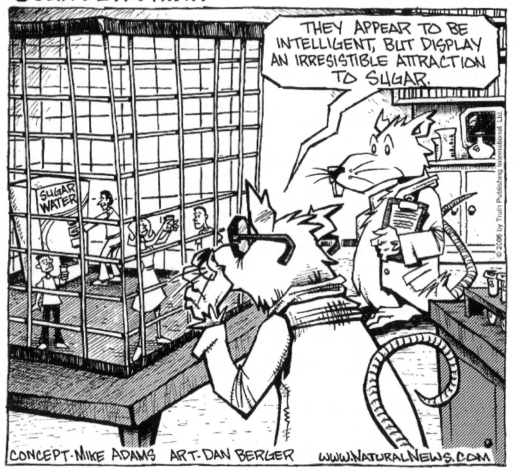

THEY APPEAR TO BE INTELLIGENT, BUT DISPLAY AN IRRESISTIBLE ATTRACTION TO SUGAR.

CONCEPT-MIKE ADAMS ART-DAN BERGER WWW.NATURALNEWS.COM

Thanks to Mike Adams and *www.NaturalNews.com* for the cartoon above

Sugar loads have the same reward areas as nicotine, cocaine and sex, but it doesn't last long (some might argue that neither does sex...). No wonder people get addicted to sugary snacks and treats. We live in an era of instant gratification; nobody wants to wait for anything, and maybe that is why people can't even imagine a life without sugar. Our brains respond to the chemical effect of sugar in the same way as they respond to *love*. ***"If we're feeling upset, what do we do? We have some sugar.*** *If there's not enough sweetness in our life, not enough love, "Oh, I'll just have some chocolate".*" But the effects on our health can be dire.

Chronic diseases related to obesity and diabetes... heart disease, many cancers, gout, hypertension, high blood pressure, possibly Alzheimer's disease... The food industry and the sugar industry have been suppressing the truth about the effects of sugar since the 1970s, similar to what the tobacco industry did to stall or fight off public health actions that would curtail smoking. For example:

- The Sugar Association hired a PR company.

- They paid scientists to do studies. The reviews that say, *"There is no evidence that sugar is associated with metabolic disease of any kind"* are funded by the sugar industry.

- They paid off professional organisations like heart-related and cancer-related organisations.

- They put out deceptive statements in the press, to ensure that sugar wasn't vilified and to make the science look "ambiguous".

- They lobbied the US government. They sent out 25,000 copies of an official-looking "scientific study" titled *"Sugar in the Diet of Man"*, with no mention on it that it was paid for by the sugar industry.

- They characterise science that proves the link of sugar to metabolic diseases as *'junk science'*.

- They state obesity is caused by "too many calories and not enough exercise", which implies that a calorie of sugar is no different than a calorie of broccoli, and that anyone overweight is simply lazy or greedy… rather than admit that sugar is causing the obesity epidemic.

Jack Tatem, president of the Sugar Association's presenting to his board, said, *"Look, this is the lifeblood of our organisation. If anyone ever links sugar to these diseases, we're dead. So our job, what we have to do… is make sure that there's no consensus."*

Damon Gameau, at the end of his 30-day experiment with consuming as much sugar as an average Australian, stated: *"I can function. But, uh… I'm not nearly as efficient as I was, my fuse is a lot shorter. I'm exhausted. And I think that's how a lot of people live their lives. People are up and down all day, but it's just their reality, so they accept it and they've never experienced anything different. If you've always lived this way, you have no idea what life can be like. They eat sugar all the time and they're fuzzy and their mind is cloudy all the time."* Check out www.ThatSugarFilm.com.

ADHD is a sham. Take children off sugar, processed foods, white flour, switch your kids to a more alkaline diet, and you'll be amazed at the difference this will make. Doctors are prescribing drugs such as Ritalin for a disorder that does not exist.

Acid Addiction #5 – SOFT DRINKS

You *must* eliminate soft drinks from your life. They contain *huge amounts of sugar and no nutrients whatsoever*. Sugary soda is bad for your teeth, but the combination of sugar with phosphoric acid and carbonic acid makes soft drinks downright *Weapons Of Mass Destruction* when it comes to your dental health. Also, due to their extremely high sugar load which is ingested quickly, sugary drinks such as colas and fruit juices are *the single most fattening thing* in our modern diet. This massive and rapid sugar intake turns to fat in the liver.

Soft drinks damage the liver. Fructose in drinks appears to dramatically increase the dangerous fat around the belly and organs (visceral fat). Furthermore, the pancreas must make even more insulin to remove the glucose from the bloodstream, so insulin levels in the blood shoot up (this is known as insulin resistance, a step towards Diabetes and heart disease). There are also strong links between the consumption of soft drinks and cardiovascular disease, and even cancer. Soft drinks are linked to a 75% increased risk of gout in women, and almost a doubling of risk in men.

Not only do sugary drinks wreak havoc on metabolic health, they appear to be seriously harmful for your brain as well, as soft drink intake has been linked to Dementia. Furthermore, two preservatives commonly added to sodas (ascorbic acid and sodium benzoate) react to produce **benzene**, which is extremely carcinogenic.

The acidity in Coca Cola literally *leaches* calcium, magnesium and zinc out of your body. One study following 40,000 men for two decades found that those who drank one sugary drink per day had a 20% higher risk of having a heart attack, or dying from a heart attack, compared to men who rarely consumed sugary drinks. Another study found that those who drank two or more sugary sodas per week were 87% more likely to develop pancreatic cancer than those who did not drink soda. One diet soda a day increases leukaemia risk by 42%, multiple myeloma risk by 102%, non-Hodgkin lymphoma risk by 31%, and increases the risk of heart attack and strokes by 44%, according to a 2012 University of Miami study. Soft drinks can also cause premature ageing, as well as chronic kidney disease and cardiovascular calcification.

Pregnant women were warned against drinking diet fizzy drinks after a study done in Denmark on 60,000 women. Women who drank artificially sweetened soft drinks, were found to be more likely to give birth prematurely. It was thought that the chemicals in the artificial sweeteners changed the wombs of the women. Postmenopausal women with high intakes of sugary soda also appear to be at greater risk for cancer in the inner lining of the uterus, called endometrial cancer.

A 2015 study claimed that soft drinks cause 184,000 deaths a year.

CHAPTER 21

Avoid These 6 Deadly Foods At All Costs

Toxic Food #1 – Aspartame

Aspartame is an "excitotoxin" that stimulates your neural cells to death. There are over 900 published studies revealing the damaging effects of Aspartame, including obesity, brain tumours, and Alzheimer's disease. *"The ingredients in aspartame stimulate the neurons of the brain to death causing brain damage of varying degrees"* according to Dr. Russell Blaylock.

Aspartame is most commonly used as an artificial sweetener in low-calorie and sugar-free drinks, snacks like cereals, granola bars and protein bars, chewing gum, crisps, flavoured water, low-fat yogurt, pudding, gelatin and fruit cups, some ketchups, dressings, sauces and marinades. In fact, since 1981 **it has been used in more than 6,000 products** by 250 million people worldwide.

According to Dr Joseph Mercola, Aspartame is the number one source of side effect complaints to the FDA and Aspartame consumption is linked to 91 documented symptoms, including headaches and migraines, muscle spasms, irritability, heart palpitations, tinnitus, dizziness, irregular heartbeat, breathing difficulties, seizures, rashes, insomnia, anxiety attacks, memory loss, nausea, depression, vision problems, joint pain, numbness, and fatigue.

Aspartame can also trigger or worsen health conditions such as brain tumours, Alzheimer's, Diabetes, Multiple Sclerosis, lymphoma, Chronic Fatigue Syndrome, depression, Parkinson's, peripheral nerve cancer, epilepsy, and Fibromyalgia. It is believed that many mental institutions are full of patients who are nothing but aspartame victims. It triggers a range of birth defects from autism to cleft palate, it can cause miscarriages, and it is an endocrine disrupting agent that can cause infertility.

Initial tests of the substance in 1971 by the neuroscientist Dr. John Olney came up with disturbing results: aspartame produced microscopic holes and tumours in the brains of mice and epileptic seizures in monkeys. Searle's own researchers confirmed Dr. Olney's findings in a similar study. However, Searle moved to squash this research, and pressed on with seeking FDA approval, submitting over 100 studies they *claimed* supported the safety of aspartame. A 1976 FDA investigation of Searle's laboratory practices found their testing procedures full of inaccuracies and *"manipulated"* test data, with the investigators commenting that they *"had never seen anything as bad as Searle's testing."* A governmental task force the following year revealed that Searle had falsified data by submitting inaccurate blood tests. Following a third investigation, Searle was forced to admit that <u>uterine tumours found in test animals were due to aspartame</u>.

The FDA formally requested criminal charges be brought up against Searle for misrepresenting findings and *"concealing material facts and making false statements"* in aspartame safety tests, but in 1980 the C.E.O. of Searle, Donald Rumsfeld, was part of Ronald Reagan's transition team as the latter was elected President. According to a former Searle salesperson, Rumsfeld told his sales force that *"no matter what, he would see to it that aspartame would be approved that year."*

He got his wish, and the mass poisoning of the unsuspecting population began. When **Monsanto** bought out Searle in 1985, Donald Rumsfeld received a $12 million bonus.

Toxic Food #2 – Genetically Modified Organisms (GMO)

Scientists are inserting *human genes* into corn, rice, and sugarcane; *jellyfish genes* into corn; *fish genes* into tomatoes and strawberries; and even *spider genes* into goats. We are told that plants have to be genetically modified to *increase crop yield and feed the planet*. Nothing could be further from the truth. GMO crops actually produce a lower yield, and they couldn't care less about the starving Third World populations. **The primary reason for GMO plants is to allow them to *withstand and absorb more poison* –** deadly doses of poisonous herbicides, fungicides, and insecticides. Nearly all GMO crops are described as "pesticide plants" because they either tolerate doses of weed killer (such as Monsanto's Roundup®) or produce an insecticide-like *Bt toxin*. These poisons are then carried into our food supply. An estimated 75% of foods in US grocery stores are made from GMO derivatives (the main GMO foods are soy, corn, cotton, canola, and sugar beets).

In an interview at the European Parliament, Professor Andres Carrasco (Argentine government scientist) reported that <u>childhood cancer increased by 300% and babies with birth defects by 400% during the past decade in parts of Argentina where GMO soy is grown</u> to supply European farmers with cheap GM animal feed. His studies show <u>glyphosate exposure can cause defects in the brain, intestines, and hearts of foetuses</u>. Moreover, the amount of Roundup® used on GMO soy fields was as much as 1,500 times greater than that which created the defects!

The Committee of Research and Information on Genetic Engineering (CRIIGEN) studied three different types of GMO corn, and found *"adverse impacts on kidneys, liver, and detoxifying organs, as well as different levels of damages to the heart, adrenal glands, spleen and haematopoietic system."*

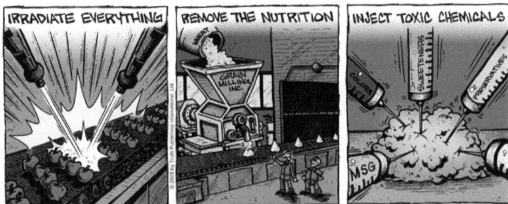

Thanks to Mike Adams and *www.NaturalNews.com* for the cartoon above

Researchers at the Russian Academy of Sciences found that GMO soy caused **sterility** in 3rd generation hamsters. In 2005 Dr. Irina Ermakova from the Russian National Academy of Sciences reported that over 50% of the babies from mother rats that were fed GMO soy died within three weeks. Her boss told her to do no more GMO food study on animals, her documents were burned on her desk, samples were stolen from her laboratory, and one of the colleagues tried to comfort her by saying, *"well maybe the GM soy will solve the overpopulation problem on earth."'*

According to Jeffrey M. Smith, author of *Seeds of Deception*, *"GM foods are particularly dangerous for pregnant moms and children. After GM soy was fed to female rats, most of their babies died – compared to 10% deaths among controls fed natural soy. GM-fed babies were smaller, and possibly infertile. Testicles of rats fed GM soy changed from the normal pink to dark blue. Mice fed GM soy also had altered young sperm. Embryos of GM soy-fed parent mice had changed DNA, and mice fed GM corn had fewer, and smaller, babies. In India, most buffalo that ate GM cottonseed had reproductive complications such as premature deliveries, abortions, and infertility; many calves died.*

247

About two dozen US farmers said thousands of pigs became sterile from certain GM corn varieties. Some had false pregnancies; others gave birth to bags of water. Cows and bulls also became infertile. In the US, incidence of low birth weight babies, infertility, and infant mortality are all escalating..."

According to Dr. Joseph Mercola, *"Just about EVERY species of animal that is offered a GMO food versus a non-GMO food will avoid the GMO one. Many times they will do this to the point of starvation, as they have an intuitive sense of the danger of this food."*

The dangers of GMO are far-reaching. A study published in *Nature Biotechnology* stated, *"After we eat GMO soy, some of the GMO genes are transferred to the microflora of our intestines and those GMO genes are still active."* Another study, published in the journal *Reproductive Toxicology, "found Bt-toxin (used in genetically modified Bt corn) in the blood of 93% of the pregnant women studied and their babies."* In one independent study, the gene inserted into soy transferred into the DNA of the subjects' intestinal bacteria, and continued to function long after they stopped eating the GMO soy!

The American Academy of Environmental Medicine (AAEM) called on *"Physicians to educate their patients, the medical community, and the public to avoid GM (genetically modified) foods, [as] several animal studies indicate serious health risks associated with GM food,"* including infertility, immune problems, accelerated aging, insulin regulation, and changes in major organs and the gastrointestinal system. They concluded, *"There is more than a casual association between GM foods and adverse health effects. There is causation."*

Why is a *poison-producing company* pushing so hard to control the global food supply? Monsanto is the company that created Agent Orange (millions are still suffering from its effects in Vietnam), cancer-causing dioxin, DDT, and PCBs, the rBGH bovine growth hormone, and the cancer-causing Roundup® pesticide. They are the company responsible for introducing the poisonous and sterilizing GMO into our food supply. Their transgenic seeds are responsible for 93% of the US soy crops, 86% of corn crops, and US wheat production is next in their sights.

The world's leading producers of GM crops are the United States, Argentina, Brazil, Canada, India and China. GM crop production also reached noteworthy levels in Pakistan, Paraguay, Uruguay, Bolivia, Australia, and South Africa. In Portugal, Spain, Germany, France and the Czech Republic, transgenic crops are primarily grown for small-scale field trials. As of 2015, 28 countries grow GM crops and 38 countries have *banned* GM crops. Many food manufacturers in Europe and other countries have banned GMO food, but Monsanto is lobbying to get access to those markets…

To this day, GMO are still present in the **vast majority of processed foods** in the USA and Canada, despite the considerable health hazard they pose. If you consume processed foods, bread, pasta, crackers, cake mixes, canola oil, mayonnaise, soymilk, veggie burgers, corn tortillas, corn chips, corn oil, corn syrup, or anything else made from corn, soy, or cotton, you are usually consuming GMO.

It is estimated that the average person in the USA consumes 200 pounds of GMO foods per year! As a general rule, you should buy organic, and avoid products made with any GMO crops, such as corn, soy, canola, cotton, papaya, sugar. Check out www.NonGMOshoppingGuide.com.

Recently, many countries around the world have BANNED Roundup®, as have supermarkets and garden centers. The main ingredient of its highly profitable weedkiller, glyphosate, often used in conjunction with GM crops, has been declared a "probable carcinogenic". It has also been strongly suspected of contributing to the autism epidemic. In a surprising decision, California's Environmental Protection Agency dealt a blow to Monsanto recently, listing glyphosate as *"known to cause cancer"*.

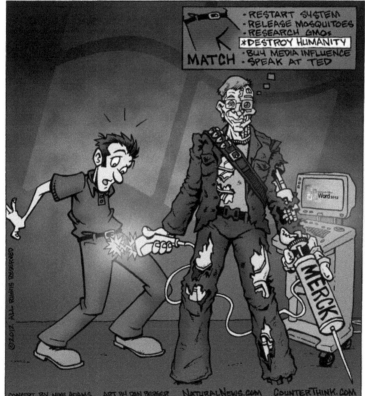

Thanks to Mike Adams and *www.NaturalNews.com* for the cartoon above.

In May 2015, world citizens staged <u>massive protests against Monsanto across 38 countries and 428 cities</u>, raging against the genocidal practices of the "world's most evil" corporation. The mainstream media did not report on this at all. Mike Adams wrote: *"Protesters from New York, London, Berlin, Paris, and even across South America, Asia and India rallied against the toxic agricultural practices of Monsanto, a corporation whose business model depends on poisoning the citizens of the planet, destroying the agricultural ecosystem, monopolizing the seed supply and hiring online character assassins to attack anyone who opposes its agenda."*

Despite research that shows that GMO crops produce **less** rather than more food, Bill Gates bought 500,000 shares of Monsanto and is actively pushing GMO crops on the developing world, in partnership with the infamous Rockefeller Foundation and Monsanto.

Toxic Food #3 – Soy Consumption Leads To Infertility and Cancer

More than 93% of soy in the US is now genetically modified and it also has one of the highest percentages of contamination by pesticides of any of our foods. For many decades, scientific studies have linked soy consumption to an increase in incidence of Breast cancer, Heart disease, Allergies, Hypothyroidism, Multiple Sclerosis, Brain damage, Immune system dysfunction, Endometriosis, and reproductive problems – Russian researchers recently found that GMO soy caused sterility in hamsters, as mentioned earlier – but **food corporations have suppressed the evidence**.

If that wasn't bad enough, soy also contains phytic acid, which blocks the uptake of essential minerals such as calcium, magnesium, copper, iron, and zinc in the intestinal tract. Soy literally sucks the nutrients right out of your body, and is known to contribute to widespread mineral deficiencies in third world countries.

A recent study of Japanese men living in Hawaii found that consuming two or more weekly servings of tofu was linked to the development of dementia. As far back as the 1950s, phytoestrogens were being linked to increased cases of cancer, infertility, and leukaemia. According to Dr. William Wong, *"Soy is poison, period!"*

Whatever you do, *don't* feed your children with soy-based infant formulas. In July of 1996, the *British Department of Health* issued a warning that the phytoestrogens found in soy-based infant formulas could adversely affect infant health.

Some "natural" food manufacturers are now using a toxic chemical called **hexane** to process soy in their products. The fumes from hexane go straight to your brain and cause damage almost instantaneously. Hexane is so toxic that the EPA has it listed as a hazardous chemical that causes cancer and birth defects and even Parkinson's disease.

In 2009, an independent lab found levels of hexane residue as high as 21 parts per million in soy oil and soy meal which is used in soy infant formula and protein bars.

Soy formula is one of the worst foods that you could feed your child. Apart from the hormonal effects, it also has over 1,000% more aluminium than conventional milk based formulas.

Soy causes cancer, destroys bones, and creates havoc with our hormonal systems. Stay away from it.

Toxic Food #4 – Unhealthy Fats and Oils

Refined oils **are produced and refined in such a way that they contain toxins and poison your immune system,** and make you exceedingly vulnerable to cancer.

Canola oil, for example, is actually made from a genetically modified hybrid version of rapeseed that has been heavily treated with pesticides. The rapeseeds are heated at high temperatures so that they oxidize, they are then processed with a petroleum solvent to extract the oils, acid is used to remove any nasty wax solids that formed during the first processing, the rancid brown oil is then treated with more chemicals to improve the colour, and then *even more* chemicals are used to deodorize the oil to mask the horrific smell from the chemical processing. Mmm… tasty!

Vegetable oils also contain very high levels of polyunsaturated fats (PUFAs) that are highly unstable, oxidize easily, and cause inflammation and mutation in cells. That oxidation is linked to all sorts of issues from cancer, heart disease, endometriosis, to Polycystic Ovarian Syndrome (PCOS), and more.

Many vegetable oils contain BHA and BHT (Butylated Hydroxyanisole and Butylated Hydroxytoluene), artificial antioxidants that keep the food from spoiling too quickly. They have been shown to produce potential cancer compounds in the body, and have been linked to things like immune system issues, hormonal issues, infertility, behavioural problems, mental decline, and liver and kidney damage.

People with fatty, unhealthy diets are often tired and sick, because <u>an excess of unhealthy fat makes your red blood cells stick together and move more slowly, resulting in far less oxygen</u> reaching your cells. Your cells become weaker and may even mutate and die. *That's* why so many studies show high fat intake related to cancer.

David Gillespie, author of *Toxic Oil*, reveals that an excess of seed oils not only causes cancer and heart disease but also damages our eyes and immune systems! Avoid entirely Canola Oil, Corn Oil, Soybean Oil, "Vegetable" oil, Peanut Oil, Sunflower Oil, Safflower Oil, Cottonseed Oil, Grapeseed Oil, Margarine and any fake butter substitutes.

Furthermore, when hydrogen is added to vegetable oil, you get "Trans-fats". Trans-fat is considered by many doctors to be the worst type of fat you can eat. Trans-fats and hydrogenated oils are used in food processing (packaged baked goods, snacks, margarine, French fries, crisps, donuts…) to prolong the shelf life of processed foods. They have been implicated in increased cardiac disease, cholesterol levels, and cancer. Once again, <u>it is advisable to stay away from all processed foods</u>.

In 1900 the amount of vegetable oils consumed was practically zero. Today the average person in the US consumes 70 pounds (31 kg) of vegetable oil a year.

WARNING: Avoid processed foods of any kind, and any foods that contain chemical additives!

Most processed foods contain hidden GMO, unhealthy oils, and chemical substances that aren't even listed on the labels. Processed foods in boxes, tins, cartons, etc. sit on supermarket shelves for months, or even *years!* That should tell you just how inert and 'chemicalized' they are. Almost all processed food is *dead* food that gives your body zero nutrition. You might as well be eating a bowl of cement. A friend of ours is a food scientist. He told us that **the Food Industry pays scientists *to hide certain chemicals in their foods***. *"We want to put this chemical in our product. Tell us how we can do it so that it is untraceable."* You should only eat organic produce, and *avoid processed foods!*

Toxic Food #5 – Milk Is a Poison That Causes Multiple Sclerosis and Cancer

Do you remember when milk used to go bad in your fridge after a few days? That rarely happens anymore, because of the chemical processing it undergoes. Processed milk is heated to the point of destroying any natural nutrition it contains. This turns the milk *brown*, so it has to be chemically processed to appear white again. Processed milk found in supermarkets gives your body nothing it needs, and actually **contains growth hormones, sex hormones, pus, pesticide residues, antibiotics, and artificially modified fats**. One study revealed that children with premature sexual development returned to normal when taken off cow milk! If that wasn't bad enough, milk covers your intestinal walls, where it hardens like concrete, preventing you from absorbing vital nutrients.

A study in Sweden found that women consuming more than three glasses of milk a day had <u>almost twice the mortality over 20 years</u> compared to those women consuming less than one glass a day, and they also had more fractures, particularly hip fractures. According to Dr. Robert Ellis – the world's foremost expert on calcium metabolism, who has conducted more than 50,000 blood tests on people – people who consume more than 2-3 glasses of milk a day have the lowest levels of blood calcium of any group tested! So here is the irony of the matter: <u>drinking milk actually *depletes* your calcium reserves and can *cause* Multiple Sclerosis</u>! This happens because milk sugars (lactose) metabolise into acid. To buffer this acidity your body leaches the alkaline calcium from your bones and attaches it to the acid so that it may eliminate it.

In 1994 Monsanto introduced rBGH (recombinant bovine growth hormone), a powerful genetically engineered drug which is injected into dairy cows to increase their milk production. In 1997 two Fox TV news reporters investigated how **consuming milk from rBGH cows promotes cancer** in humans. Monsanto pressured Fox and offered to pay off the two reporters if they kept silent about their report. After they refused to water down their report, they were promptly fired by Fox.

In 1998, Canadian scientists managed to acquire the full Monsanto studies that the FDA had kept secret due to their potential to *"irreparably harm"* Monsanto. The scientists learned that Monsanto's studies showed that <u>rBGH caused prostate cancer and thyroid cancer</u> in laboratory rats!

Since the emergence of rBGH, every industrialised country in the world has banned it – except the USA. American milk and milk products have been banned in over 100 countries as a result.

In his book ***Milk: The Deadly Poison***, Robert Cohen states *"The single most disturbing aspect of rBGH from a human safety standpoint, concerns Insulin-like Growth Factor (IGF), which is linked to breast cancer."* According to Dr. Samuel Epstein, *"IGF is not destroyed by pasteurization, survives the digestive process, is absorbed into the blood and produces potent growth promoting effects."* Epstein says it is highly likely that IGF helps transform normal breast tissue to cancerous cells, and enables malignant human breast cancer cells to invade and spread to distant organs.

Higher dairy intake has been linked to acne, food allergies, increased risk of prostate cancer, higher ovarian cancer risk, type 1 diabetes, higher rates of Multiple Sclerosis, and an increase in IGF-1 (Insulin-like Growth Factor-1) levels which have been implicated in several cancers.

Fun Fact: Did you know that cheese in many processed foods and pizzas *is not cheese at all*, but a cheaper chemical man-made substitute called 'analogue cheese'? In the UK, one raid on takeaway joints revealed that 19 out of 20 pizza places used fake cheese and fake ham!

Toxic Food #6 – Toxic "Factory" Meat

I eat meat two times a week, making sure that it is 'clean' and that my diet is 70 to 80% fresh organic "greens", since meat, fish, and eggs are acid-forming (as opposed to being "alkalizing" for our body). If you are going to eat meat, I recommend you source it from local, organic farms, rather than buy it at the supermarket. I prefer to **buy organic, locally-raised chicken, duck, goose, and rabbit** meat, which is plentiful where I live, as well as organic eggs. We buy local river trout, or locally caught fish when we are staying by the sea. Sourcing organic beef has proven more difficult.

Feeding animals a *species-appropriate diet* (cows grazing on grass, for example) significantly improves the nutritional quality of their meat, as one would expect. It also goes a long way towards eliminating toxins such as glyphosate and other pesticides. It is recommended that you choose *'grass-fed organic beef'* whenever you can. Look for the *100% USDA Organic* label and the *"Grass-fed"* label when buying beef in the US.

Truth be told, raising cattle is not the best idea from an environmental point of view.

- For each 16 pounds of grain and soybeans we give to cattle, we get just 1 pound of beef.

- 1 acre of land can produce 20,000 pounds of potatoes, but only 165 pounds of beef.

- US livestock consume enough grain and soy to feed the entire US population 5 times over.

In my twenties, **I was a vegetarian for four years**, mainly for ethical reasons relating to the treatment of slaughterhouse animals. Unfortunately, it did not do my health any favours. I lost a lot of weight and got very, very skinny. I looked pale and haggard, and my energy levels were low. After a while I began craving meat, and my health, energy, and strength returned when I started eating meat again.

It is not fashionable to talk about, but meat is an excellent source of a variety of nutrients, like vitamins A, D, several of the B-complex, essential fatty acids, magnesium, zinc, phosphorous, potassium, iron, taurine, selenium, carnitine, and coenzyme Q10. A plant-based diet does not adequately provide for some of these nutrients, typically.

Do Vegetarians Live Longer?

Some studies indicate that vegetarians live longer than meat-eaters. But this data needs to be viewed in its correct context. Vegetarians are also more likely to exercise, be married, smoke less and drink less alcohol—all factors that also contribute to a longer life. Furthermore, you need to differentiate between the effects of eating meat and those of eating chemicalized factory-produced *processed* meat. The causal relationship between becoming vegetarian and living longer is not straightforward.

It is worth noting that all of the longest-living cultures – such as the Hunza, Vilcabamban, Caucasus Georgians, etc. – *do* eat some meat, but they eat meat from clean sources.

A 2014 study conducted by the Medical University of Graz in Austria found that vegetarians had more doctor visits and a higher need for health care, and suffered more from Multiple Sclerosis, anxiety, depression, and asthma (though this was based on a sample of only 330 vegetarians, hardly enough to make sweeping generalizations).

Are The Ruling Class Vegetarians?

There might be another reason why eating meat is important. In 2009 I got to spend a week with a former employee of a secret US underground military facility. He had worked for the CIA and the US shadow government for over 13 years, and he explained that most of the information the public receives is merely disinformation, distraction, and propaganda – in effect, the *opposite* of the truth. This "mind control" process – controlling what American citizens think – is deemed by the ruling class as *vital for maintaining the status quo* in a large and diverse country such as the US. The Russians and Chinese killed tens of millions of "dissidents" in concentration camps instead, to maintain their *status quo*, so mind control and mass media propaganda is seen as a preferable more 'humane' option.

He told me what the ruling class know to be true: **the human body needs to consume animal flesh *for energetic reasons*** – the flesh of animals sustains our flesh <u>on an energetic level</u>. This is why vegetarians weaken past a certain age. He also informed me that the vegetarian lifestyle was introduced in the American culture by the CIA via their mass media lackeys (newspaper and magazine articles, TV interviews, book publishing), as a means of weakening the population. It would make them more docile, and less likely to revolt. A fascinating topic, certainly, but one that is outside the scope of this book.

While I recommend eating meat in moderation (duck, goose, rabbit, and fish from clean sources, for example), please note though, if you have a serious health issue you should start by doing a 30 day cleanse which would include <u>not consuming meat or animal products for that period</u>. They are acid-forming and meat is hard for your body to break down and digest. A 30-day detox is designed to give your body *a break* and help build up enough energy to cleanse and heal itself.

The Real Problem: Mass-Produced Meat Is Dangerous To Your Health

Here's the major problem when it comes to eating meat: mass-produced "factory" meat – aside from the ethical considerations of unspeakable mass animal cruelty – is filled with the most toxic products imaginable. **Chickens** are routinely found to contain banned antibiotics, antidepressants like Prozac, allergy medications, arsenic, Tylenol and Benadryl, caffeine, and other prescription drugs. Toxic chemicals such as *chlorine* are commonly used to treat chicken for contaminants in poultry plants. 8 billion chickens are slaughtered in the US every year, and the mechanized disembowelling process has the chicken carcasses soak in "faecal soup" for up to an hour, before being packaged for consumers. The soaked chicken meat is imbibed with faecal bacteria by the time it reaches our supermarket shelves, making it extremely toxic to the human body.

But what about **beef?** Cattle is fed ground-up parts of animals, such as **deceased horses, chickens, pigs, and chicken faeces** and feathers (chicken litter scraped off the floors of chicken houses are recycled as cattle feed). Apparently giving cattle natural, healthy feeds would be far too costly and unnecessary, because the consumer does not really care what the meat is made of as long as it looks like meat and it is *cheap.* Cattle is also fed **cement dust, radioactive materials, and GMO** soy and grains. French cows are fed **human sewage**. A few years ago a scandal broke because it was discovered that cows were fed the dead carcasses of *other cows,* causing "mad cow disease".

Of course, this unnatural diet makes the cows sick – they suffer from heartburn, liver disease, ulcers, pneumonia and other infections – so to keep them alive they are fed enormous doses of **antibiotics**.

Cattle are also pumped full of **growth hormones** to fatten them up and get them ready for market at just 16 months instead of 4-5 years. Growth hormones are finding their way into our meat and dairy products, with dreadful impact on our children. Consuming meat and dairy products may be to blame for the early sexual development of young girls: in the US nearly half of all African-American girls and about 15 percent of Caucasian girls now enter puberty when they are just 8 years old.

And that's just for starters. Cattle are also fed **anti-parasitic drugs**, and many of these drugs remain in the beef through the processes of cooking and consumption. The drugs *oxyclozanide, clorsulon, albendazole, closantel, ivermectin, mebendazole* and *fenbendazole* all remained in beef throughout a roasting or frying cooking process. The drugs *nitroxynil, levamisol, rafoxanide* and *triclabendazole* are reduced, though not eliminated, by conventional cooking.

And then it gets *much worse.* The Environmental Protection Agency reports that **meat is contaminated with higher levels of pesticides than any plant food**. Many chemical pesticides accumulate in the fatty tissue of animals. Animal feed that contains animal products compounds the accumulation, which is directly passed to the human consumer.

Worse still… *Dioxins* are a highly toxic group of hundreds of chemical compounds, that are a by-product of industrial processes that use chlorine – pesticide manufacturing, namely. Dioxins were a key toxic component of Monsanto's *Agent Orange*, used as herbicidal warfare. They are known to disrupt the immune system, endocrine system, nervous system, respiratory system; cause liver damage; cause hormonal imbalances; lower cognitive ability; slow neurodevelopment; induce depression; incite behavioural problems; cause low birth weight; and have damaging effects on reproduction. In men, dioxin exposure can cause low testosterone and low sperm count. In women, it has been linked with endometriosis. Dioxin is now recognized as a Group 1 carcinogen, and a typical American will receive 93% of their dioxin exposure from meat and dairy products.

And it doesn't stop there. **Sodium nitrate** and **sodium nitrite** are preservatives that are present in processed meats like salami, hot dogs, ham, bacon, livestock feed, etc. They make meats appear "fresh" rather than their natural rotten grey colour. A large amount of evidence indicates that these nitrosamines are human carcinogens. Research done at the University of California showed that children who eat as few as three hotdogs a week were 10 times as likely to develop leukaemia and brain tumours.

Mass-produced beef is *also* **contaminated with disease-causing faecal bacteria**. A large percentage of meat products become contaminated when the animals' intestines are punctured and their stool spills onto the meat being processed. Think 'liquid poo' smeared all over your steak... Ground beef is particularly problematic, as those bacteria get mixed throughout the meat, contaminating all of it. When meat from a number of cows is mixed together, one animal can contaminate the whole batch.

According to Mercola.com, in one test, *Consumer Reports* purchased 300 packages of ground beef from 103 stores in 26 cities across the US. This included 181 "conventionally raised" ground beef and 116 that were more sustainably produced. At a minimum, sustainably produced beef was raised without antibiotics (even better are organic and grass-fed methods). These 300 beef samples were then analysed for the presence of five types of disease-causing bacteria: *Clostridium perfringens, E. coli, Enterococcus, Salmonella,* and *Staphylococcus aureus*. The samples were also put through secondary testing to ascertain whether the bacteria were resistant to antibiotics used in human medicine.

Their results showed that:

- 100% of all ground beef samples contained bacteria associated with faecal contamination (*enterococcus* or *E. coli*), which can cause blood or urinary tract infections.

- Nearly 20% contained *Clostridium perfringens,* a bacteria responsible for an estimated **one million cases of food poisoning** each year in the US.

- 10% contained a toxin-producing strain of *Staphylococcus aureus,* which cannot be destroyed even with thorough cooking.

- 1% contained *salmonella,* which is **responsible for an estimated 1.2 million illnesses** and 450 deaths in the US each year.

- 1.7% of the conventional samples (3 out of 181) had *Methicillin-Resistant Staphylococcus aureus* (MRSA), which is **responsible for nearly 19,000 deaths each year**. None of the sustainably raised beef samples contained MRSA.

To combat foodborne pathogens the food industry uses **sterilization methods** that makes things even worse: high heat, chemicals (chlorine-based or lactic acid washes, for example), and **radiation**.

And finally, I believe that the utter terror that cattle experience prior to being butchered in a slaughterhouse and the *adrenaline* that their body produces in that moment acts as a poison for the human body, on an energetic level, when we ingest their meat.

Considering how toxic "factory farming" meat is, and how many bacteria and cancer-causing chemicals it contains, it is little surprise that consuming it creates serious health problems:

- ❏ The University of Hawaii conducted a 7-year study that included 200,000 people. They found that people who consumed processed meats (such as hot dogs and sausages) had a **67% increased risk of pancreatic cancer**.

- ❏ According to a federal study conducted by the National Cancer Institute, heavy meat consumption increases your risk of dying from *all* causes, including heart disease and cancer.

- ❏ Women who ate large amounts of red meat had a 20% higher risk of dying of cancer and a **50% higher risk of dying of heart disease** than women who ate less. Men had a **22% higher risk of dying of cancer** and a 27% higher risk of dying of heart disease.

- ❏ A 2009 study published in the Annals of Internal Medicine showed that eating meat **increases risk of prostate cancer by 40%**. Children have a **60% increased risk of developing leukaemia** if they consume meat products such as ham, sausages and hamburgers.

- ❏ *"I have found of 25 nations eating flesh largely,* **19 had a high cancer rate** *and only one had a low rate, and that of 35 nations eating little or no flesh, none of these had a high rate."* – Rollo Russell, *Notes on the Causation of Cancer*

- ❏ Most **food poisonings** today are related to eating meat. More than 500,000 Americans, most of them children, have been sickened by mutant faecal bacteria (E. coli) found in meat. This is the leading cause of kidney failure among children in the US.

- ❏ Children are especially vulnerable to antibiotic and hormone residues in meat. If you're serving tuna, salmon, or fish sticks to your family, you could be feeding them **mercury, PCBs, lead, arsenic, pesticides, or industrial-strength fire retardants**. Research done at the University of California at Irvine showed that <u>children who eat as few as three hotdogs a week were 10 to 12 times as likely to develop leukaemia and brain tumours</u>.

Recap – Toxic Foods and Acid Addictions

❑ Cigarettes contain over 4,000 chemicals, including 43 known cancer-causing compounds. Smoking killed 100 million people in the 20th century. You can't smoke *and* be healthy.

❑ Sugar consumption destroys your health in over 100 different ways; Sugar feeds cancer.

❑ Coffee is *pure acid*; it turns your bloodstream to *sludge* and robs you of energy.

❑ Genetically modified crops are designed to absorb considerably more toxic pesticides.

❑ <u>Several animal studies indicate serious health risks associated with GM food, including infertility, immune problems, accelerated ageing</u>, insulin regulation, and changes in major organs and the gastrointestinal system. Childhood cancer increased by 300% and babies with birth defects by 400% during the past decade in parts of Argentina where GMO soy is grown.

❑ US farmers revealed that thousands of pigs became sterile from eating GM corn.

❑ Genetically modified corn has adverse impacts on kidneys, liver, and detoxifying organs, as well as different levels of damages to heart, adrenal glands, spleen and haematopoietic system.

❑ Soy consumption can lead to infertility and cancer.

❑ Refined oils contain toxins that poison your immune system and that make you exceedingly vulnerable to cancer. They have been linked to cancer, heart disease, endometriosis, Polycystic Ovarian Syndrome (PCOS), immune system issues, hormonal issues, infertility, behavioural problems, mental decline, and liver and kidney damage.

❑ An excess of unhealthy fat makes your red blood cells stick together, resulting in far less oxygen reaching your cells. That's why so many studies show high fat intake related to cancer.

❑ Processed milk may contain hormones, pus, pesticide residues, and artificially modified fats.

❑ Milk covers your intestinal walls, preventing you from absorbing vital nutrients.

❑ Drinking milk actually *depletes* your calcium reserves and can cause Multiple Sclerosis.

❑ Higher dairy intake has been linked to acne, food allergies, increased risk of prostate cancer, higher ovarian cancer risk, type 1 diabetes, higher rates of Multiple Sclerosis, and cancer.

❑ Consuming milk from rBGH cows may promote cancer in humans. Monsanto's studies showed that rBGH caused prostate cancer and thyroid cancer in laboratory rats.

❑ Sex hormones given to cows to control their birth rates are passed on to humans.

❑ The human body needs to consume meat and animal protein, <u>from clean sources</u>, in moderation. The flesh of animals sustains our flesh *on an energetic level*.

❑ Buy organic, locally-raised chicken, duck, goose, rabbit meat, organic eggs, and fish.

❑ Chickens are routinely found to contain banned antibiotics, antidepressants like Prozac, allergy medications, arsenic, caffeine, and other prescription drugs. The chicken carcasses soak in "faecal soup" for up to an hour, imbibing the meat with faecal bacteria.

❑ Cows should be fed grass, but instead are fed chicken faeces, *human sewage*, deceased chickens, pigs, horses, *the carcasses of other dead cows*, cement dust, radioactive materials…

❑ Cows are pumped up full of growth hormones, which is affecting human hormonal development. Cows are also fed anti-parasitic drugs and enormous doses of antibiotics.

❑ Beef and chicken meat is contaminated with higher levels of pesticides than any plant food.

❑ Americans receive 93% of their dioxin exposure – a Group 1 human carcinogen – from meat and dairy products. Mass-produced beef is also contaminated with disease-causing faecal bacteria. More than 500,000 Americans, have been sickened by faecal bacteria found in meat.

❑ The food industry uses highly toxic chlorine and radiation to "sterilize" meat, and also cancer-causing preservatives to make the meat look "fresh"!

❑ <u>Avoid any and all processed or packaged foods, and any foods that contains chemical additives</u>! Eat fresh, organic, locally-grown produce and meat.

PART IV

17 Things In Your House That May Be Killing You

CHAPTER 22

Fluoride: A Crime Against Humanity

There is no scientific evidence that fluoride is a beneficial additive to water, and in fact there is overwhelming scientific evidence that proves that **fluoride is an extremely harmful poison**. Fluoride is a neurotoxic industrial waste of the Aluminium industry, which <u>has been proven to</u> <u>damage the immune, digestive, and respiratory systems</u>, as well as the kidneys, liver, brain, and thyroid. Fluoride has also been <u>linked to infertility, Alzheimer's, osteosarcoma, and even cancer</u>. It also accelerates ageing, and causes genetic damage at concentrations as low as one part per million – the exact level of fluoridation in the US water supply. Fluoride also prevents iodine absorption.

Fluoride is also an attack on our pineal gland, in which it causes calcification. Yogi masters, mystics and psychics consider the pineal gland to be the portal to our higher self, a doorway to higher consciousness and inter-dimensional experiences. *Fluoride may be cutting us off from our Higher Self.*

The Nazis were the first to use sodium fluoride. Produced by the I.G. Farben chemical plants in Germany, the Nazis used it in their water supply for the purpose of sterilizing their concentration camp populations and making them more calm and submissive. Sodium fluoride happens to be one of the basic ingredients in both Prozac® and Sarin Nerve Gas.

According to the research scientist sent by the U.S. government to take charge of I.G. Farben, Charles Elliot Perkins: "<u>The real purpose behind water fluoridation is to reduce the resistance of the masses to domination, control and loss of liberty</u>. Repeated doses of infinitesimal amounts of fluoride will in time reduce an individual's power to resist domination, by slowly poisoning and narcotizing a certain area of the brain, thus making him submissive to the will of those who wish to govern him.

Albert Einstein's nephew, Dr. E.H. Bronner, was a chemist who had been a prisoner of war during World War II. He stated: *"Fluoridation of our community water systems can well become their most subtle weapon for our sure physical and mental deterioration. Let me warn: fluoridation of drinking water is criminal insanity, sure national suicide. Don't do it... Even in small quantities, sodium fluoride is a deadly poison to which no effective antidote has been found. Every exterminator knows that it is the most efficient rat-killer..."*

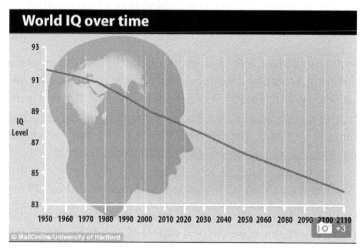

The IQ of the human population is being lowered (source: The Daily Mail)

Epidemiological studies by Dr. Dean Burk and Dr. Yiamouyiannis in 1977 showed that <u>fluoridation is linked to about 10,000 cancer deaths per year</u>. They stated: *"Fluoride causes more human cancer, and causes it faster, than any other chemical."*

A Harvard School of Dental Health study published in 2005 found that fluoride directly contributes to osteosarcoma (bone cancer) in young boys. *"Fluoridation is the greatest case of scientific fraud this century, if not of all time"*, concludes Dr. Robert Carton of the Environmental Protection Agency.

Fluoride causes dental fluorosis and **lowered IQ**. A dumbed-down population is easier to control, making fluoride one of the most effective weapons used by the ruling class.

Despite 90% of European countries having rejected, banned, or stopped fluoridation due to environmental, health, legal, or ethical concerns, 24 countries still use fluoride in their water supply, including the US, Canada, Australia, Ireland, and the UK. According to *Wikipedia*: *"Currently about 372 million people (5.7% of the world population) receive artificially-fluoridated water. Water fluoridation is rare in Continental Europe with 97-98% choosing not to fluoridate drinking water."*

There is no mention in that Wikipedia entry of *any* downsides of using this deadly poison in the water supply. A stunning example of propaganda and disinformation by omission.

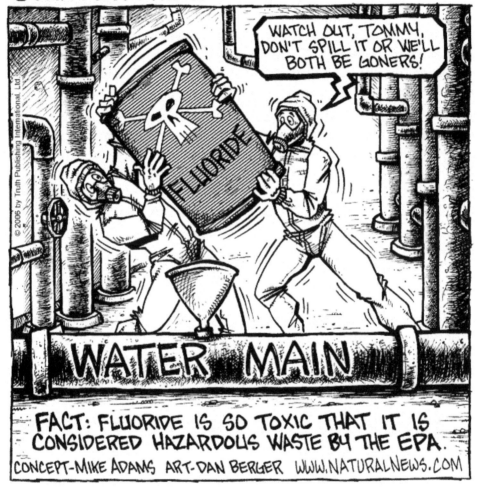

Thanks to Mike Adams and *www.NaturalNews.com* for the cartoon above.

The water supply in most American cities contains **chlorine**, sulphates, aluminium, nitrates, sex hormones, insecticides and herbicides, prescription medications such as antibiotics, anti-convulsants, and antidepressants, in the municipal water supplies. The U.S. Government does not require any testing for drugs in the water supplies; nor does it set safety limits for drug contamination. Unsurprisingly, **Salmon caught near Seattle was found to contain more than 80 drugs**, including cocaine, antidepressants, Flonase, Aleve, Tylenol, Paxil, Valium, Zoloft, Tagamet, OxyContin, Nicotine, Caffeine, Fungicides, antiseptics and anticoagulants, and numerous antibiotics. The presence of these drugs in the water appears to be related to the inability of the wastewater plants to fully remove the chemicals during treatment. Unless they're put in the water supply on purpose…

As if *fluoride* and *pharmaceutical drugs* is not bad enough, we are also faced with the chlorination of our water supplies. Organochlorines are chlorine by-products. Some types of Organochlorines are extremely deadly, such as Chlorine gas (a weapon used in both world wars), and the DDT pesticide. They are proven to cause cancer and they are endocrine disruptors. Organochlorines have been linked to breast cancer, endometriosis, prostate cancer, and testicular cancer.

According to the U.S. Council of Environmental Quality, ***"Cancer risk among people drinking chlorinated water is 93% higher than among those whose water does not contain chlorine."*** Another study found that 9% of all bladder cancers and 15% of rectal cancers in the USA are caused by chemical by-products of chlorinated water. Prolonged exposure has also been shown to produce birth defects, immune system problems, and reproductive disorders.

As biologist Joe Thornton explains, ***"There are no uses of chlorine which we regard as safe."***

From Paul Wittenberger and Chris Maple's documentary *The Great Culling: Our Water*:

❑ Fluoride inactivates 62 enzymes, it increases the ageing process, it increases the incidence of cancer and tumour growth, disrupts the immune system, causes genetic damage, increases arthritis, causes depression, and it is a systemic poison.

❑ Fluoride accumulates in calcium-rich tissues: bone, ligaments, cartilage, joints, and teeth. It gets stuck in your bones. Many arthritis cases are caused by FLUORIDE. Hip replacements, knee replacements… they weren't that common before fluoridation.

❑ Infant mortality is higher in counties with fluoridated water. A toxicologist in the U.K. recently found that perinatal deaths in a fluoridated area was 15% higher than in neighboring non-fluoridated areas. The fluoridated area also had a 30% higher rate of Down's Syndrome. Chile banned fluoridation because of research by Dr. Albert Schatz, which showed a link to infant deaths due to fluoridation.

❑ Fluoride leads to hypothyroidism – your thyroid needs iodine, and in the absence of it, it uptakes fluoride and chlorine instead.

- ❑ *"Fluoride is not being used to treat the water. It is being put specifically in the water supply to alter YOU, physically; to make a physical change in you."*

- ❑ It damages the neurones in the brain and causes memory problems. 24 IQ studies show even modest exposure to fluoride causes a decrease in IQ.

- ❑ In the US, fluoride is now in THOUSANDS of products… Coco Pops, Fruit Loops, dental fillings, baby water with fluoride, Lipton Ice Tea, milk, juice, mustard, ketchup… anything with water in it! And when you water your plants with fluoridated water, you ingest it in your produce.

- ❑ In the US, incredibly, most *bottled water* ALSO contains fluoride!

I recommend using a whole house water filter, drinking bottled water that is free of fluoride, and using toothpaste that is natural and fluoride-free (I use Aloe Dent® by Optima).

CHAPTER 23

From Pesticide To Genocide

More than one billion pounds of pesticides are used in the US each year, an amount that has increased five-fold since 1945. This includes 20,000 different products. The use of glyphosate alone increased 1500% from 1995 to 2005. Studies show that chemical contamination in our environment is growing at exponential rate. Could this be why **children today are sicker than a generation ago?**

According to the EPA, 60% of herbicides, 90% of fungicides and 30% of insecticides are known to be carcinogenic – **they cause cancer in humans**. There is no class of pesticide which is free of cancer causing potential, and most pesticides contain *multiple* dangerous toxins.

Pesticides Cause Cancer

In a recent study examining the toxicity of widely-used glyphosate-based herbicide formulations (such as Monsanto's Roundup®) on human placental cells, kidney cells, embryonic cells, and neonate umbilical cord cells, they found that it caused **total cell death** of each of these within 24 hours. Yet more than HALF of all foods sold in the US contain pesticide residues.

In 1983 the National Cancer Institute found that pesticide applicators that had been spraying for more than 20 years had nearly **three times the risk of developing lung cancer and two times the risk of developing brain cancer** than average.

Pesticides Cause Childhood Brain Cancers and Leukaemia

Brain cancer is the second most common childhood cancer, after leukaemia. According to a study published in the journal *Environmental Health Perspectives*, children living with parents who use pesticides around the home are significantly more likely to develop brain cancer than children who are not exposed to such chemicals. Manypesticides are known to exhibit hormone mimicking or immune-hampering effects that are especially dangerous for the developing bodies of foetuses.

269

A 1987 study by the NCI showed that children living in pesticide-treated homes had **nearly a four times greater risk of developing leukaemia**. If the children lived in homes where pesticides were sprayed on lawns and gardens, the risk of developing leukaemia was **6.5 times greater.** Indeed, multiple reports link pesticides to leukaemia in children.

Maternal Exposure To Pesticides Linked With Childhood Kidney Cancer

James and Nancy Chuda founded the *Healthy Child Healthy World* organization (healthychild.org) in 1992, after their young daughter Collette died of cancer (*Wilm's Tumor*, a type of cancer that starts in the kidneys). Doctors were at a loss to explain what could have possibly brought about this cancer. Until, that is, a 1995 study titled *"Parental Exposure to Pesticides and Risk of Wilm's Tumor in Brazil"* was published by the American Journal of Epidemiology. The study revealed that **maternal exposure to pesticides was most likely the cause of the disease** when the tumour was diagnosed 48 months after the child's birth. Colette was diagnosed when she was four years old — at exactly 48 months of age. The study also noted that *"the effects of pesticides could be brought about by exposure of the foetus in utero, or by exposure after birth from residues present in breast milk, in foods, in the home, or in the surrounding environment."*

Breast Cancer Risk Tripled For Women Exposed To Farm Pesticides

According to researchers from the University of Sterling in Scotland, women with breast cancer were nearly *three times more likely* to have been farm workers during adolescence. Developing breast tissue is especially vulnerable to exposure to toxic pesticides and other farm chemicals during teenage years, the researchers concluded.

Lawn Chemicals lead To Lymphatic Cancer, Non-Hodgkin's Lymphoma

The common lawn pesticide 2,4-D, produced by Dow Chemicals, is half of the recipe for Agent Orange. It is one of the top sources of dioxin in the USA. It has been shown to **increase the risk of lymphatic cancer in farmers six times the normal rate**, according to the National Cancer Institute. Exposure to 2,4-D has been shown to cause cancer, hormone disruption, genetic mutations and neurotoxicity. Lawn chemicals have been a significant factor in the 50% rise in non-Hodgkin's lymphoma over the past 20 years in the US, as well as being linked to **lymphoma in dogs** (pets are exposed to higher doses of pesticides because they are closer to the ground). Studies show that lymphomas are twice as prevalent in dogs whose owners treat their lawns four times a year.

270

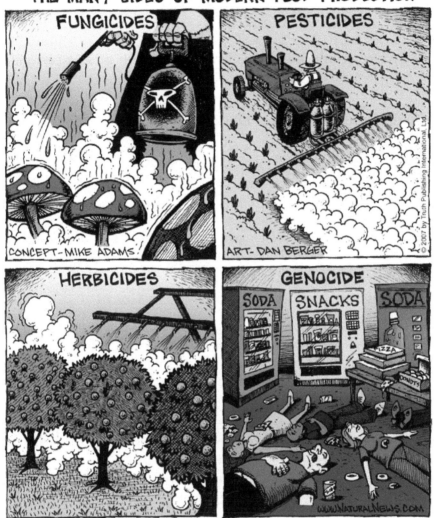

Thanks to Mike Adams and *www.NaturalNews.com* for the cartoon above.

Pesticides Linked To Autism, Alzheimer's, Parkinson's Disease

As I mentioned earlier, the Argentinian scientist Professor Andres Carrasco reported that glyphosate exposure can cause birth defects in the brain, intestines, and hearts of foetuses. Childhood cancer increased by 300% and birth defects by 400% in the past decade in parts of Argentina where GMO soy is grown to supply European farmers with cheap GM animal feed. Glyphosate has also been strongly linked to **Autism and Alzheimer's**. An acquaintance told me how his parents' farm had been contaminated

271

by heavy pesticide use in adjacent fields, causing Alzheimer's and Dementia in his mother and father respectively, and multiple neurological disorders in their neighbours!

In one study, a total of 17,429 hospital records were collected between 1998 and 2005. The risk of having **Alzheimer's disease, Parkinson's disease, Multiple Sclerosis and suicide were significantly higher in districts with greater pesticide use** as compared to those with lower pesticide use.

Pesticides Linked To Higher Depression Rates

Suicide for farmers in the U.S. is about twice the average of the general population. A 20-year study by researchers at the National Institute of Health established a connection between depression and conventional farming chemicals. After interviewing 84,000 farmers and their spouses over two decades, researchers confirmed that seven pesticides contribute to clinical depression in farmers. Organochlorine insecticides and fumigants increase the risk of depression by an astounding 90%!

Pesticides Cause Infertility and Low Sperm Count

Scientists found a substantial decrease in sperm count occurring among the regions of Aquitaine and Midi-Pyrenées in southwestern France, two large areas known for wine production. Vineyards apply more pesticides than any other agricultural process, and the chemicals used have been known to disrupt men's hormones and interrupt sperm production.

According to a recent study by Clemente Aguilar from the Medical Research Laboratory of the University Hospital San Cecilio, Granada, Spain, **even low-level exposure to common pesticides damages sperm and leads to fertility problems**. In total, researchers found 18 different pesticides in participants' blood, some of which are actually illegal in Spain. On average, participants had about 11 different pesticides circulating in their blood, and most of them had as many as 14 on average. Every participant had at least one detectable pesticide in his blood.

Another study in Europe proved that pesticides wreak havoc on reproductive health in men. They found that men with high levels of three common pesticides in their urine were **10 times as likely to have low sperm quality**. The study concluded that weed killers including alachlor, atrazine and diazinon had contaminated the water supplies and harmed the reproductive health of men.

Atrazine is a powerful herbicide used in 70% of US cornfields. This toxic chemical, which was recently banned by the European Union, is a suspected carcinogen and endocrine disruptor that has been **linked to low sperm counts among farmers**.

Traces of Atrazine routinely turn up in American streams and wells and even in the rain, and of course in the American food supply. Michael Pollan writes, in his article *The Way We Live Now:* *"Atrazine is often present in American waterways at much higher concentrations than 0.1 part per billion. But American regulators generally won't ban a pesticide until the bodies, or cancer cases, begin to pile up – until, that is, scientists can prove the link between the suspect molecule and illness in humans or ecological catastrophe. So Atrazine is, at least in the American food system, deemed innocent until proved guilty – a standard of proof extremely difficult to achieve, since it awaits the results of chemical testing on humans that we don't perform."*

Glyphosate and Roundup® Linked To Autism

Dr. Stephanie Seneff is a senior researcher from The Massachusetts Institute of Technology (MIT). She lists the following toxic effects of glyphosate, as identified by her research: Glyphosate kills beneficial gut bacteria and allows pathogens to overgrow; it interferes with function of cytochrome p450 (CYP enzymes); it chelates important minerals (iron, cobalt, manganese, etc.); it interferes with synthesis of aromatic amino acids and methionine, which leads to shortages in critical neurotransmitters and folate; it disrupts sulfate synthesis and sulfate transport.

Seneff remarks that a number of well-known "bio-markers of autism" such as low serum sulfate, disrupted gut bacteria, inflammatory bowel, serotonin and melatonin deficiency, mitochondrial disorder, zinc and iron deficiency and more *"can all be explained as potential effects of glyphosate on biological systems."*

Her research shows a remarkably consistent correlation between the rising use of Monsanto's glyphosate-based Roundup® herbicide on crops and the rising rates of autism:

273

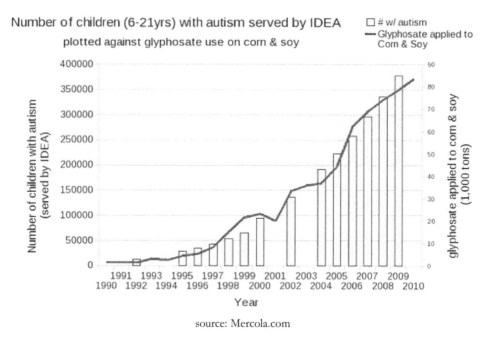

source: Mercola.com

Dr. Seneff believes that vaccines – especially those containing aluminium – may also be a culprit. (Pesticides contain aluminium and heavy metals).

Pesticides Are 1000 Times More Toxic Than You Are Told

Pesticide formulations may be up to 1000 times more toxic than what regulators commonly claim. Roundup® by Monsanto is in fact the most toxic of herbicides and insecticides used, and according to British researcher Robin Mesnage the safety evaluations of pesticides are incredibly flawed: "Adjuvants in pesticides are generally declared as inert and for this reason they are not tested in long-term regulatory experiments. It is thus very surprising that **they amplify up to 1000 times the toxicity of their Active Principles** in 100% of the cases where they are indicated to be present by the manufacturer."

He adds: "Our results challenge the relevance of the acceptable daily intake for pesticides because this norm is calculated from the toxicity of the active principle alone. Chronic tests on pesticides may not reflect relevant environmental exposures if only one ingredient of these mixtures is tested alone."

Monsanto's Glyphosate Causes Brain Cancer and Birth Defects

There is plenty of research confirming that mothers who are exposed to widely used pesticides give birth to children with lower intelligence, structural brain abnormalities, behavioural disorders, compromised motor skills, higher rates of brain cancer and small head size. It was revealed a few years ago that European regulators have known that Monsanto's glyphosate causes a number of birth and brain malformations *since at least 2002*. Regulators, in bed with the Agribusiness lobby, routinely mislead the public about glyphosate's safety.

Farmers in Argentina Sue Big Tobacco and Monsanto For Poisoning Them With Deadly Pesticides That Caused Devastating Birth Defects

A group of Argentinian farmers are suing Monsanto and Philip Morris after they were coerced into using dangerous amounts of Roundup® (glyphosate) and other pesticide and herbicide products on their tobacco crops, which eventually resulted in **a major spate of birth defects** throughout the local community. This new tobacco crop reportedly requires the use of much higher amounts of pesticides and herbicides, including Monsanto's herbicide, in order to grow, which suggests that the new crop may actually be a genetically-modified tobacco variety produced by Monsanto.

Microcephaly Birth Defects Caused By Monsanto Pesticide, NOT Zika Virus

You may remember seeing images of babies with shrunken heads on your television screen during the evening news. This television campaign went on for a couple of weeks. The dangerous "Zika virus" was blamed for this, and we were told that *genetically modified mosquitoes* were carriers of the virus. The Brazilian army was mobilized to spray pesticides and insecticides in some of the poorest areas of Brazil *to kill these dangerous mosquitoes*. Oh, and coincidentally, a couple of weeks after the outbreak, we were told on the news that a laboratory in Texas had magically *just* developed a Zika virus vaccine, that will ready for production soon. This media campaign was orchestrated so perfectly, all over the world, that it raised my suspicions.

Here's what you were *not* told, as revealed by Mike Adams of www.NaturalNews.com and John Rapaport of www.NoMoreFakeNews.com:

❑ The Zika virus has never been known to cause brain deformations in children. Previous Zika epidemics did *not* cause birth defects in newborns, despite infecting large parts of the population in those countries. Also, in other countries such as Colombia, despite plenty of Zika cases, there are no records of microcephaly. The cases of microcephaly being discovered in Brazil <u>have never been scientifically linked to the Zika virus</u>. The symptoms that are being attributed to the so-called "Zika virus" more likely resemble chemical toxicity, vaccine damage, and pesticide exposure.

❏ According to a study titled *"Urinary Biomarkers of Prenatal Atrazine Exposure"*, published in Environmental Health Perspectives on July 1, 2011: *"The presence of quantifiable levels of [the pesticide] atrazine or a specific atrazine metabolite was associated with foetal growth restriction… and small head circumference… Head circumference was also inversely associated with the presence of the herbicide metolachlor."* In other words, the pesticide compound *Atrazine* from Dow Chemicals is causing birth defects such as "shrunken heads."

❏ Brazil is <u>one of the largest global consumer of pesticides</u>. The Brazilian agriculture sector purchased more than 823,000 tons of pesticides in 2012, and 22 of the fifty main active ingredients used in pesticides in Brazil today have been *banned in most other countries.*

This amounts to chemical warfare on their own population.

❏ The Brazilian Ministry of Health failed to mention that in the area affected most, a chemical larvicide (pyroproxyfen) has been used in a sustained <u>18-month-long campaign of mass fumigation of low-income Brazilian people.</u> It was even added to their drinking water. This toxic poison is manufactured by Sumitomo Chemical, a subsidiary of Monsanto. As GM Watch reports, *"Pyriproxyfen is a growth inhibitor of mosquito larvae, which alters the development process from larva to pupa to adult, thus generating malformations in developing mosquitoes and killing or disabling them."* It is interesting to note that this chemical is *a growth inhibitor of developing organisms* (smaller baby heads, anyone?), and it was sprayed in the poorest areas of Brazil where women are told *"Don't have more children!"*

❏ In 2014, the Brazilian Minister of Health mandated that all expectant mothers receive the new Tdap vaccine (supposedly to protect the newborn babies from pertussis). This meant that, at 20 weeks' gestation, a vulnerable, developing young life would be exposed to aluminium adjuvant, mercury preservative, formaldehyde, antibiotics and a host of other chemicals that could damage a foetus's developing brain. It is no coincidence that birth defects have spiked in Brazil following this campaign, due to the toxic elements that pregnant women have been exposed to.

❏ In the U.S. approximately 25,000 infants are diagnosed with microcephaly each year. Brazil has had just over 400 cases, 17 of which tested positive for the Zika virus. In Colombia 3,177 pregnant women have tested positive for Zika virus, yet no cases of microcephaly have occurred. It is patently obvious that the "Zika virus" is not responsible for these birth defects.

❏ The so-called Zika virus didn't start spreading in Brazil until 2012, when the British biotech company Oxitec released genetically modified mosquitoes *en masse* in Brazil, supposedly to combat dengue. Oxitec is a company supplied with grant money from Bill Gates.

- The Indian company Bharat Biotech somehow got a head start on other pharmaceutical companies, and <u>began working on two Zika vaccines in November 2014</u>. This company just happens to be linked to Bill Gates as well. They received $50 million from the Bill and Melinda Gates Foundation *to research and conduct human trials on a malaria vaccine.*

- The mainstream media's false narrative is causing the public to fear a benign, asymptomatic viral infection, so that they rush and get *dangerous vaccinations,* while giving the governments the justification to push *even more* the use of toxic chemical fumigation and vaccinations on an unsuspecting population. President Obama has called for $1.8 billion in government handouts to vaccine companies and pharmaceutical corporations to combat Zika.

- A stunning report published in the June 2010 *British Medical Journal* revealed that top scientists who persuaded the World Health Organization (WHO) to declare the swine flu a global pandemic held close financial ties to the Big Pharma companies that profited from the sale of those vaccines.

  The WHO declared a pandemic, resulting in billions of dollars in profits for the Big Pharma vaccine manufacturers. The pharmaceutical industry seems to launch annual highly-mediatized 'virus outbreak scares' to frighten the public and governments into buying vaccines... Every year you see the same story playing out in the media... SARS... the bird flu... the swine flu... the West Nile virus... the Ebola virus... the Zika virus...

How To Reduce Your Exposure To Pesticides

According to the Environmental Working Group (EWA) "Dirty Dozen" list, apples you buy at the supermarket typically contain as many as 45 different pesticides, strawberries contain 40 pesticides, cucumbers are the worst, laced with as many as 86 pesticides, celery and spinach contain more than 50, more than 30 pesticides are found in potatoes... and 52 pesticide residues were found in blueberries by the USDA pesticide data program. Other fruits and vegetables that are heavily sprayed include cantaloupe, bell peppers, peaches, nectarines, pineapples, carrots, and grapes.

Fresh produce typically low in pesticide residue include: avocado, asparagus, mango, papaya, eggplant, cantaloupe, broccoli, cauliflower, kiwi, cabbage, watermelon, melons, sweet potatoes, grapefruit. But this is no guarantee.

In a 2010 article in The Guardian, Fernando Ramirez, the leading agronomist at the Costa Rica National University's toxic substances institute, explains the agrochemical cycle required to produce their top-selling fruit: *"Pineapples need very large amounts of pesticides, about 20kg of active ingredient per hectare per cycle. The soil is sterilised; biodiversity is eliminated. Fourteen to 16 different types of treatment are typically needed, and many have to be applied several times. They use chemicals that are dangerous for the environment and human health.*

The chemicals involved are legal in Costa Rica but include some of the most controversial in the world."

According to www.NaturalNews.com, Green tea from China was found to be contaminated with alarming levels of pesticides. And 96% of Indian-made tea contains pesticides, some of which have long been banned.

I *highly* recommend that you switch to buying organic whenever possible, even though it is more expensive. Eating an organic diet can reduce pesticide levels by 90%. Producing your own fruit and vegetables would be even better. If you can't find organic produce, here are some suggestions for eliminating a good amount of pesticide residue:

- ❑ Fruit and veggie wash recommended by Elena Ollick of DailyMom.com: "Fill up a large bowl or your kitchen sink with 1 part vinegar and 4 parts water. Let your fruits/vegetables soak in this mixture for up to an hour (non-organic apples can soak for an additional 30 minutes to an hour). Remove the produce from the mixture, give them another quick rinse with water.

  Alternatively, mix 1 tablespoon lemon juice, 2 tablespoons baking soda, and 1 cup water until the baking soda has dissolved, and pour into a clean spray bottle. Spritz the mixture onto your fruits and vegetables; let sit for 5-10 minutes. Rinse the mixture off, and enjoy your produce!"

- ❑ Fruit and veggie wash recommended by Becky Rapinchuk of www.CleanMama.net: Put ½ cup apple cider vinegar, ½ cup lemon juice, and ½ cup water in a spray bottle and shake. Spray liberally on fruits and vegetables then rinse in cold water.

- ❑ Fruit and veggie wash recommended by Ty Bollinger of www.CancerTruth.net: Mix twenty drops of grapefruit seed extract, one tablespoon of baking soda, one cup of vinegar, and one cup of water together in a spray bottle. Spray the produce, let it sit for about ten minutes, and then rinse thoroughly.

- ❑ Some produce wash products available include: Environne Fruit & Vegetable Wash, Biokleen Produce Wash, and Citrus Magic Veggie Wash.

CHAPTER 24

Toxic Mercury In Your Teeth Is Destroying Your Brain

Dr. Patrick Störtebecker, a world-renowned neurologist, states:

*"**Dental amalgam** is a highly unstable metal that easily gives off mercury vapour. The most dangerous route for transport of mercury vapour, being released from dental amalgams, is from the mucous membranes of the upper nasal cavity and directly upwards to the brain where mercury vapour easily penetrates the dura mater (i.e. the blood-brain barrier). Mercury (vapour) can act in a much stronger concentration straight on the brain cells."*

Dr. Dietrich Klinghardt, a mercury toxicity expert, adds: "As soon as anybody has any type of medical illness or symptom, whether medical or emotional, the amalgam fillings should be removed, and the mercury residues should be eliminated from the body, especially the brain.... Most, if not all, chronic infections diseases are not caused by a failure of the immune system, but are a conscious adaptation of the immune system to an otherwise lethal heavy metal environment."

Mercury poisoning has been linked to <u>depression, memory disorders, and chronic diseases such as cancer, Multiple Sclerosis, and even neurological disorders such as Alzheimer's, and Parkinson's</u>, among others. A patient may not notice its symptoms until 40 years later, when their immune system collapses entirely.

According to Ty Bollinger, mercury filling are acted upon by oral and intestinal bacteria to produce methyl mercury (an even more toxic form of mercury) which affects primarily the pituitary gland, thyroid gland, and the brain. He also notes that dentists have one of the highest rates of suicide of any profession, and they also suffer a high incidence of depression and memory disorders.

Well guess what. In my early teens my dentist gave me six mercury fillings. I started having acne on my nose and forehead shortly thereafter. Until recently, I regularly experienced painful inflammations of my jaw, and painful blisters inside my lower lip and gums, especially when I ate sugar. My gums bled for *years*. My concentration and my grades deteriorated rapidly in my teens. I suffered from intense depression from the ages of 13 to twenty-one. My thyroid swelled up, as mentioned earlier. It wouldn't surprise me if these symptoms were linked to the mercury fillings, which is why I recently got them removed.

Can You Reverse Alzheimer's By Getting Rid of Mercury?

It is looking increasingly likely that toxic mercury that has leached from amalgam dental fillings over a period of a few decades is the most common cause of Alzheimer's disease today. *"In large measure, those martyred by dementia are showing the results of toxicity from mercury, aluminium, lead, cadmium, arsenic and other heavy metals. Their neurons have been poisoned"*, writes Dr. H. Richard Casdorph, author of *Toxic Metal Syndrome: How Metal Poisoning Can Affect Your Brain.*

In his book, he claims that chelation therapy (to remove heavy metals from your body) has been shown to help at least 50% of elderly people with Alzheimer's who have tried it. They are documented as showing greater mental clarity, increased IQ, and improved memory.

Be careful when getting your amalgam fillings removed though, as this process – when not done properly – can release even more mercury into your system. A client of mine from Australia told me how her husband experienced acute renal failure and severe mental and neuro-motor disorders when he got his fillings removed. The emotional, physical, and financial effects were crippling and devastating for several years. They are currently attempting to cleanse his body of these heavy metals.

Some safety precautions:

- ❑ Seek out a "biological dentist" who understands the issues surrounding amalgam fillings.

- ❑ Request oxygen during the procedure – this will insure that you breathe clean oxygen rather than toxic mercury vapour when the fillings are drilled out.

- ❑ Request a rubber dam – this keeps pieces of the filling from falling down your throat.

- ❑ It is recommended that you do a heavy metals detox after the procedure. The quickest and most potent chelation method available today is intravenous EDTA chelation therapy. It requires twenty to fifty sessions, and costs $2,000 to $5,000. Oral EDTA costs significantly less – between $20 and $50 per month – but takes longer, since only 5 to 10% of an oral dose of EDTA is absorbed into the bloodstream (compared with 100% of an IV dose). High doses of chlorella (10 to 20 grams a day) have also been found to be effective for mercury elimination, and should be used together with coriander (also known as *cilantro*), since the latter removes toxic metals rapidly from the central nervous system. I personally use MSM and chlorella daily in my morning "Green Juice" (more on this later).

The Dangers of Root Canals

Root canals are another crime against our health notched up by dentists. Root canals is the term used to describe a procedure to replace infected pulp in a tooth root canal with an inert material.

Dentist Frank Jerome, author of *Tooth Truth*, states: *"The idea of keeping a dead, infected organ in the body is only thought to be a good idea by dentists. A root canal-treated tooth always negatively affects your immune system."*

According to Dr. James Howenstine, *"Many chronic diseases, perhaps most, are a result of root canal surgery."* Dr. Weston A. Price observed that when root-filled teeth were taken out of his patients then <u>a variety of health problems improved</u>, from arthritis to kidney problems to cancer.

Dr. Josef Issels in Germany treated terminal cancer patients for over 40 years. Despite the immune systems of his patients having been already destroyed by conventional treatments such as radiation and chemotherapy, Dr. Issels cured 24% of his 16,000 "terminally ill" patients. The first thing he always did: he got a dentist to take out their root canal teeth.

It is recommended that you remove your root canal teeth, and in any case, if you have root canals you should use an antiseptic mouthwash and supplement your meals daily with MSM, Co-Enzyme Q10, and Vitamin C.

CHAPTER 25

Cancer-Causing Chemicals Lurking In Your Bathroom

More than 13,000 chemicals are used in cosmetics, and according to the National Institute of Occupational Safety and Health nearly 900 of them are toxic to humans – though the true number is probably significantly higher. It is worth noting that the standard for testing most cosmetic and personal care products is very lax.

According to one study, the average adult in the Western world uses nine to 15 personal care products a day, exposing themselves to 126 different chemicals a day, on average. In another study, by the Environmental Working Group (EWG), the average woman in the US uses 12 personal care products and cosmetics a day, containing 168 different chemicals, while men in the US are exposed to about 85 such chemicals every day. Is it any wonder that hundreds of chemicals that didn't exist a century ago are now found in the human body?

Your personal care products are unfortunately putting your health at risk. Toxic chemicals are being absorbed through your skin and into your bloodstream, accumulating in your body over time. The problem here is not just *repeated* exposure to a single chemical – or even a number of chemicals – but *the combined effect* of thousands of chemical exposures and the interactions between them.

Here are some commonly-found chemicals you should avoid:

❑ **Parabens** – these chemical preservatives used in cosmetics have been linked to hormonal imbalance, breast cancer, and cancer in reproductive organs. These preservatives act like oestrogen in the body, throwing off your hormonal balance and disrupting your endocrine system. Parabens have been shown to accumulate in cancerous breast tumours. An estimated 13,200 cosmetic and skin care products contain parabens.

❑ **Phthalates** – also listed as Fragrance; used in personal care products to moisturize skin and as a solvent; also used in nail varnish and hair sprays. Phthalates are also found in detergents, packaging materials, PVC shower curtains, pharmaceuticals, food products, children's toys, paints, printing inks, lubricants, emulsifying agents, adhesives and glues, vinyl flooring, electronics, building materials, medical devices, food additives, textiles, pesticides, plastic wrap, plastic bottles, plastic food storage containers, nail polish, and cosmetics.

Phthalates have been shown to disrupt hormonal balance and lower testosterone levels, cause birth defects, reproductive impairments such as low sperm count, and liver damage. All 289 people in a recent test for body load of chemicals tested positive for phthalates. The CDC found most of the people they tested in the US had multiple phthalates in their urine. The data showed the "tolerable intake" of phthalates for children to be far exceeded, in some instances up to 20-fold. Women who are pregnant, nursing or thinking about getting pregnant should avoid all personal care products with the word phthalate on the label. Phthalates are recognized as toxic substances under environmental law, but companies are free to use unlimited amounts in cosmetics.

❑ **Fragrance or "Parfum"** – Many compounds in fragrance are carcinogenic or toxic. The term 'Fragrance' or 'Parfum' on a label may involve up to 4,000 different chemicals. Companies don't have to disclose the actual components of each fragrance, under the guise of being "trade secrets".

❑ **Sodium Lauryl Sulphate (SLS) and Sodium Laureth Sulphate (SLES)** Sodium Lauryl Sulfate is a chemical used in thousands of cosmetic products, as well as in industrial cleaners. It is present in nearly all shampoos, hair colour products, bleaching agents, toothpastes, body washes and cleansers, make-up foundations, liquid hand soaps, and laundry detergents. During the manufacturing process, ethoxylation results in SLES/SLS being contaminated with 1,4 dioxane, a carcinogenic by-product. SLS have been linked to organ toxicity, developmental and reproductive toxicity, neurotoxicity and endocrine disruption, cellular changes and cancer. It can also cause hair loss. Nearly 16,000 studies in the PubMed science library mention the toxicity of this chemical. It is toxic to the brain and central nervous system, kidneys, and liver. It is a leading groundwater contaminant. When SLS come into contact with any number of chemicals including TEA (triethanolamine), which is a commonly used ingredient in shampoos, it results in the cancer-causing nitrosamine NDELA. Avoid products with indications of ethoxylation, indicated by suffixes such as: "myreth," "oleth," "laureth," "ceteareth," "PEG," "polyethylene," "polyethylene glycol," "polyoxyethylene," or "oxynol". Also avoid polysorbate 60 and polysorbate 80. SLS may also be listed as sodium dodecyl sulfate, sulfuric acid, monododecyl ester, sodium salt, sodium salt sulfuric acid, sodium dodecyl sulfate, aquarex me or aquarex methyl. It is arguably the most dangerous of all ingredients in personal care products.

❑ **Tetrasodium EDTA** – chelating agent and penetration enhancer, made from formaldehyde and sodium cyanide. It helps the other chemicals get *deeper into* *the skin.* Tetrasodium EDTA has reproductive and foetal effects, albeit only at very high doses.

❑ **Diazolidinyl Urea** – readily breaks down in the product or on the skin and releases formaldehyde. It's an endocrine disruptor, a possible neurotoxin, a known immune system toxicant, and has a possible link to cancer.

❑ **Propylene Glycol** (PG) – This is <u>the active ingredient in antifreeze</u>. It is used as a penetration enhancer, meaning it's a carrier for other chemicals, bringing them into your skin and your bloodstream. It has been shown to cause cancer in lab tests, it is a possible endocrine disruptor, and a possible neurotoxin. It is found in more than 3000 personal care products, including lotions, deodorants, sunscreen, shampoo, conditioner and body washes.

❑ **Sodium benzoate** – this preservative is used because it is the cheapest mould inhibitor on the market. It promotes cancer and kills healthy cells. It deprives the cells of oxygen, breaks down the immune system and causes cancer. It has also been linked to premature ageing, Parkinson's, and other neuro-degenerative diseases. It is found in thousands of personal care products, even foods labelled as "all natural". It combines with vitamin C or E to form *benzene*, a highly dangerous known carcinogen.

❑ **Cocamide DEA, TEA & MEA** – used to thicken shampoo, body wash and facial cleansers. It offers no benefits to the skin, and disrupts hormonal balance. It has been linked to liver and kidney cancer, as well as miscarriages and inhibiting foetal brain development. Animal studies show damage to the immune system and organs. It can react with formaldehyde-releasing ingredients to form carcinogenic nitrosamines.

❑ **Linalool, Hexyl cinnamal, Benzyl alcohol, Limonene** – these synthetic fragrances are severe allergens, they can trigger asthma attacks, and cause central nervous system disruption.

These are just *a handful* of chemicals present in our day-to-day cosmetic and personal care products. There are *more than 13,200 chemicals* in personal care products today, and many are not even listed on the packaging. Just for fun, let's look at three commonly-used products and their ingredients…

Palmolive "Naturals" hand wash

Ingredients: Sodium C12-13 pareth sulfate, sodium laureth sulphate (SLS), Sodium Chloride, Cocamidopropyl Betaine, Cocamide MEA, Sodium Salicylate, Parfum, Sodium Benzoate, Styrene/Acrylates Copolymer, Polyquatemium-7, Tetrasodium EDTA, Citric Acid, Phalaenopsis Amabilis Extract, Benzyl Salicylate, Butulphenyl Methylpropional, Hexyl Cinnamal, Linalool.

Gillette shaving gel

Ingredients: Aqua, Palmitic Acid, Triethanolamine, Isopentane, Glyceryl Oleate, Stearic Acid, Isobutane, Sorbitol, Parfum, Glycerin, Hydroxyethylcellulose, Glyceryl Acrylate/Acrylic Acid Copolymer, PEG-90M, Ptfe, Menthol, PEG-23M, Propylene Glycol, Benzyl Salicylate, Hexyl Cinnamal, Limonene, Linalool, Sodium Nitrate, Glyoxal, Silica, Pvm/Ma, Copolymer, Polysorbate 60, CI 42053, Calcium Peroxide, Disodium Phosphate, Methylparaben, CI 42090, Propylparaben, BHT.

Head & Shoulders shampoo

Ingredients: Aqua, Sodium Laureth Sulfate, Sodium Lauryl Sulfate, Cocamide MEA, Zinc carbonate, Glycol distearate, Sodium chloride, Zinc pyrithione, Dimethicone, Cetyl alcohol, Guar hydroxypropyltrimonium chloride, Parfum, Sodium xylenesulfonate, Magnesium sulfate, Sodium benzoate, Ammonium laureth sulfate, Butylphenyl Mothoxypropional, Linalool, Sodium diethylenetriamine pentamethyl phosphonate, Magnesium carbonate hydroxide, Hexyl cinnamal, Benzyl alcohol, Eitdronic acid, Hydroxyisohexyl 3-cyclohexene carboxaldehyde, Limonene, Citronellol, Paraffi num liquidum, Sodium polynaphthalenesulfonate, Methylchloroisothiazolinone, DMDM hydantoin, Disodium EDTA, Tetrasodium EDTA, Methylisothiazolinone, CI 42090.

Next to pesticides, you couldn't create better *cancer-causing* and *infertility-causing* products if you tried. It is even more shocking to find out that many of these health-destroying chemicals are not needed in the product and confer no benefit whatsoever, but they put them in there anyway!

These products often contain toxic chemicals that are accumulatively dangerous to your health and your children's health:

- ❑ **Perfume** – perfume contains 250 chemicals on average. Most worrying: Benzaldehyde, Toluene. Possible side-effects: damage to sperm, linked to cancer, hormone disruption. And I'm not even talking about Lady Gaga's perfume that contains human sperm and blood.

- ❑ **Toothpaste** – most toothpastes contain fluoride, a deadly poison, as we've discussed already. They are loaded with other dangerous toxins and chemicals as well, such as Triclosan, Propylene Glycol, artificial sweeteners, Diethanolamine (DEA), sodium lauryl sulfate, and hydrated silica. All of these common ingredients have been found to be harmful to humans.

- ❑ **Shaving foam/gel** – Gillette shaving gel has parabens, PEG, laureth and propylene glycol. Neutrogena shaving cream has PEG and propylene glycol. Most shaving foams contain numerous toxic ingredients, including phthalates, parfum and triethanolamine — which also appear in many soaps, shampoos, detergents and toothpastes.

❑ **Deodorants** – contain 32 chemicals on average. Most worrying: Aluminium Zirconium, Isopropyl Myristate. Possible side-effects: breast cancer, hormone disruption. Scientists have established links between aluminium and breast cancer. It also blocks the pores of the skin, preventing the toxins we already have from being excreted through sweating. The toxins accumulate instead in the breasts or even the brain. It has also been linked with Alzheimer's. Aluminium compounds are known to be neurotoxic to humans.

❑ **Shampoo** – 15 chemicals on average. Most worrying: Sodium Lauryl Sulphate; Propylene Glycol, Methylisothiazoline. Possible side-effects: neurological damage to foetus, irritation, eye damage. <u>Hair follicles are significant transporters of harmful chemicals into your body</u>.

❑ **Sunscreen** – sunscreen lotions and creams *cause* cancer. One of the ingredients found in sunscreen products is Oxybenzone, which comes from benzophenone <u>that is shown to have oestrogenic activity and is known to attack DNA when illuminated by sunlight</u>! It is absorbed through the skin and wreaks havoc on the immune system, damage the liver and the heart, and even promotes systemic cancer. Another ingredient, octyl methoxycinnamate, has been shown to kill mouse cells even at low doses. It was also shown to be particularly toxic when exposed to sunshine. OMC is present in 90% of sunscreen brands!

❑ **Makeup** – The list of toxic chemicals in makeup is endless. Makeup also contains dangerous heavy metals. *Environmental Defense* tested 49 different makeup items, revealing serious heavy metal contamination in virtually all of the products: 96% contained lead, 90% contained beryllium, 61% contained thallium, 51% contained cadmium, and 20% contained arsenic.

❑ **Foundation** – 24 chemicals on average. Most worrying: Polymethyl methacrylate. Possible side-effects: disrupts immune system, linked to cancer.

❑ **Lipstick** – 33 chemicals on average. Most worrying: Polymenthyl Methacrylate. Possible side-effects: linked to cancer, allergies.

❑ **Eye Shadow** – 26 chemicals on average. Most worrying: Polythylene terephthalate. Possible side-effects: linked to cancer, infertility, hormonal disruption, and damage to your organs.

❑ **Blush** – 24 chemicals on average. Most worrying: Ethylparaben, Methylparaben, Propylparaben. Possible side-effects: hormone disruption.

❑ **Nail Varnish** – 31 chemicals on average. Most worrying: phthalates. Possible side-effects: linked to cancer, hormone disruption, fertility issues, and problems in developing babies.

❑ **Hair sprays** – 11 chemicals on average. Most worrying: Octinoxate, Isophthalates. Possible side-effects: allergies, hormone disruption, changes in cell structure.

❑ **Hair colouring** – contain PPD (Para-Phenylenediamine, a petroleum-derived chemical that includes benzene, naphthalene, phenols, aniline, and other chemicals. PPD in combination with Hydrogen Peroxide is very toxic and can lead to cancer. Ammonia may produce caustic burns and lung irritation. DMDM Hydantoin is a preservative that slowly releases the toxic formaldehyde chemical, which affects the immune system. They also contain Parabens, Lead Acetate with produces neurological problems, and other toxic chemicals that affect your endocrine system.

❑ **Tampons and sanitary towels** – 85% of tampons and feminine hygiene products are contaminated with Monsanto's cancer-causing glyphosate herbicide, due to the use of GMO cotton heavily sprayed with toxic pesticides. The rayon/viscose used in Tampax requires hundreds of chemicals and chlorine bleaching. The process creates chlorinated hydrocarbons, a hazardous group of chemicals with by-products that includes dioxins, some of the most toxic substances known.

❑ **Liquid soaps and Handwash** – these usually include a nasty cocktail of Triclosan, SLS and SLEs, Parabens, Ureas, Synthetic colours, Propylene Glycol, Fragrance, Diethanolamine (DEA), 1,4-Dioxane, Ethyl Alcohol, and many more chemicals linked to cancer, birth defects, developmental and reproductive toxicity, etc.

❑ **Diapers** – You wouldn't *believe* what disposable diapers are made from and the harmful chemicals they contain. Disposable diapers contain traces of Dioxin, an extremely toxic, cancer-causing chemical present because of the chlorine bleaching process used. Dioxins and sodium polyacrylate in diapers have been linked to cancer, reproductive and infertility problems, asthma and respiratory distress, hormonal problems, developmental and cognitive problems, suppressed immune system, diabetes, allergic reactions, chemical burns, Chloracne, and Toxic Shock Syndrome. Evidence suggests that increased exposure to dioxins is associated with increased incidence of endometriosis.

Diapers also contain chemicals such as Tributyltin (toxic to humans and causes irreversible damage to aquatic life), Xylene (toxic to the respiratory and central nervous systems), Ethylbenzene (damages organs, damages lungs, causes cancer and is toxic to the central nervous system), Styrene (cancer-causing and is toxic to the nervous system and upper respiratory tract, very hazardous to the eyes), Propylene (may cause central nervous system depression), Toluene (toxic to blood, kidneys, the nervous system, liver, brain, and central nervous system), Phthalates, and many more.

A study published in 1999 by Anderson Laboratories found that some types of disposable diapers release chemicals that are toxic to the respiratory tract, and that laboratory mice that were exposed to various brands of disposable diapers experienced asthma-like symptoms, as well as eye, nose and throat irritation.

This topic has become of particular interest to us since we became parents. Our babies are going to be using diapers for the first 2 to three years of their lives almost 24 hours a day, and we noticed already rashes on their skin from wearing diapers. After finding out what disposable diapers contain we have switched from Pampers to some more organic and chemical-free alternatives. These are not as effective in terms of "dryness" and practicality, and they are more expensive, but the alternative is too risky to consider.

Cleaning Products Are Dangerous Too

Cleaning products and detergents are extremely deleterious to your health as well, especially those that contain chlorine. Look for chemical-free alternatives to:

- ❑ Laundry detergents

- ❑ Bleaching products

- ❑ Dishwashing liquid and dishwashing tablets

- ❑ Window cleaning products

- ❑ Dry cleaning

The Dangers of Plastic Pollutants

BPA stands for bisphenol A. It is an industrial chemical that has been used to make certain plastics since the 1960s. It is found in containers that store food and beverages, such as Tupperware and plastic water bottles. As the plastic ages, the BPA leeches into the food and beverage contents. Low level exposure to BPA during foetal growth **causes breast cancer** in adults as well as insulin resistance. It is suspected of causing neurological and behavioural problems in foetuses and children. Researchers in Japan report that BPA levels are higher in women with a history of repeated **spontaneous miscarriages**, indicating that the BPA chemical may be an abortifacient.

Water is often bottled in #1 PET or PETE bottles (polyethylene terephthalate), which can leach DEHA, a known carcinogen, into the water, while plastics numbered 3, 6 and 7 contain BPA. BPA is only *one of a long list of plastic pollutants* (Phthalates are plastic pollutants, for example). Unfortunately, BPA and other plastic pollutants are extremely toxic and are everywhere around you, in your house, your car, your personal care products. I recommend you use safer alternatives to plastic and melamine dishware, such as glass or ceramics.

Women Are More At Risk

Women tend to use far more personal care products than men do. If you use commercially-produced cosmetics on a daily basis, you can absorb almost five pounds of chemicals and toxins into your body each year. Perhaps this explains why diseases such as thyroid disease, fibromyalgia, and Multiple Sclerosis are far more common in women. Dr. Theo Colborn dedicated herself to publicizing the dangers of endocrine disrupting chemicals to humans, animals, and the environment, for nearly 30 years. In her book *Our Stolen Future* she reveals that in many cases effects are not seen in the women exposed but *do* appear in her offspring.

I also recommend *Our Toxic World: A Wake Up Call* by Dr. Doris Rapp; she explains the many ways in which we are exposed to toxic chemicals and how they contribute to chronic disease.

The Dangers of Estrogen Dominance

No, this does not refer to a husband feeling overwhelmed by the presence of too many females in his household (ever felt like that? No? OK, only me, then). Actually, 'estrogen dominance' refers to a hormonal imbalance that can have serious repercussions for our health (especially women's health). According to David Wolfe, author of *Longevity Now*:

> "[Remove] bad estrogens from your system, in order to shut down hormonal signaling mechanisms **that damage and inhibit health and longevity**. Leveling the hormonal playing field not only improves metabolism, it rejuvenates us, and **improves overall immunity**. It is imperative to keep our sex hormones in a system of checks and balances throughout the years of our life. This becomes particularly important as we age. Hormone health is our key to a healthy future. [...] The correct amount of androgenic hormones improves internal levity and health within the body – meaning the correct balance of good hormones prevents and fights calcification, gravitation, and oxidation; and that **estrogen dominance (estrogen toxicity) as well as low hormone levels (in general) increase calcification, gravitation, and oxidation, thus accelerating age-related degeneration.** Ninety years of research and tens of thousands of studies indicate that low hormone levels, too many "bad" hormones and/or disruption in hormone production, absorption and detoxification **are at the root of chronic health challenges**, lead to calcification, and accelerate ageing." [...] "Hormones are secretions from our glands, and glandular health is a key indicator (along with levels of bad calcium and bad iron) or one's actual level of youthfulness. Hormones are cellular messengers that transmit information from one cell to another.

[...] **Due to ageing, birth control pills, estrogen replacement therapy, poor nutrition, stress, xenoestrogenic pollution, and/or lack of exercise, metabolic "bad" or nonmethylated estrogen builds up** along with the adrenal hormone cortisol and starts to swing the seesaw toward too much estrogenic metabolism and not enough androgenic metabolism. The latter is improved by building up testosterone (men), progesterone (women), DHEA, vitamin D3, and thyroid hormone while simultaneously lowering cortisol and bad estrogen levels (meaning the types of estrogen that are counterproductive to health)."

Dr. Igor Tabrizian writes, in his article *Strangers in the night: Xenoestrogens and health:*

"What is Estrogen dominance? This refers to the balance of Estrogen and progesterone [due to] Xenoestrogens: **Pesticides**; **Petroleum products** (car fumes, methlybenzene, toluene, benzene, styrene, pyrene); **Plastics** (PVC, PCB's, biphenyl, nonylphenyl, lunch wraps etc.); **Hormones** from doctors (oral contraceptive pill & Hormone Replacement Therapy) and from poultry industry and antibiotics in animal feed. These Xenoestrogens (especially the pesticides) over time have progressively been classed as carcinogens."

Here is a list of **symptoms associated with estrogen dominance**, compiled by Dr. Tabrizian: Autoimmune disorders, Lupus, Thyroiditis (Hashimoto's); Acceleration of ageing; Agitation or Anxiety; Allergy (asthma, hives, rashes, sinus congestion); Breast cancer (men and women); Breast tenderness with period; Cervical dysplasia (abnormal pap smear); Cold hands and feet; Copper excess; Decreased sex drive; Depression with anxiety or agitation; Dry eyes; Endometriosis; Fat gain around abdomen hips and thighs; Fatigue; Fibrocystic (lumpy breasts); Fibroids; Foggy thinking; Gall bladder disease; Hair loss; Headaches; Hypoglycemia (low blood sugar esp. 3-4 pm); Increased blood clotting; Infertility; Irregular menstrual periods; Irritability; Insomnia; Magnesium deficiency; Memory loss; Mood swings; Multiple Sclerosis; Ovarian cancer; Ovarian cysts; PMS/PMT; Polycystic ovaries; Pre-menopausal bone loss; Prostrate cancer (in men); Sluggish metabolism; Thyroid dysfunction; Uterine cancer; Water retention, bloating; Zinc deficiency.

Some Tips To Avoid Unnecessary Chemical Exposure

Here's what we've done in our home:

- ❑ We use PitRok® crystal deodorants – they last for ages, and are completely natural.

- ❑ We use Aloe Dent® natural toothpaste by Optima, that is free of fluoride.

291

❑ We use cleaning products from Ecover and Ecozone. We also create our own house cleaning products based on Tracy Rapinchuk's book *The Organically Clean Home.*

❑ We've replaced soaps and shampoos with Korres, Jāsön, and Kawar natural products.
Also: You can Google "homemade cosmetics" for thousands of recipes and instructions. Instead of mass-produced chemical shampoos, look for shampoos made with essential oils.

❑ We've replaced handwash liquid soap and dishwashing liquids with more natural products.

❑ We don't use sunscreen. Simply wear a T-shirt in the sun or don't stay in the sun too long!

❑ We use more natural diapers for our babies, such as Bambo® Nature.

❑ I've thrown out my Gillette shaving products (see picture above); I use a double-edged safety razor and Osma bloc soap with shaving brush instead. Back to basics! :)

❑ My wife has switched to more natural makeup and hair colour products. A healthy rule of thumb: don't put anything on your skin that you wouldn't *eat!*

❑ We buy products that come in glass bottles rather than plastic (chemicals can leach out of the plastic and into the contents; make sure your plastic containers and bottles are BPA-free).

❑ Twice a year we do a 10-day "detox" cleanse, to help our bodies flush out toxins.

❑ We've simplified our daily routine. Do you really need twenty different products to prepare for your day?

CHAPTER 26

Electro-Magnetic Radiation Causes Cancer

We are also exposed to another, more subtle form of pollution... I have mentioned earlier how in order to be healthy, we need to nurture *our cells*. One of the factors that can destroy our cells is <u>disturbances in the cell's electrical field</u>. If you disturb the electrical charges of the cell membrane (with a toxic substance or with EMF) you will damage this balance, and this can kill or mutate the cell. Electro-magnetic fields can cause such disturbances. We need to be wary of staying too long close to computers, cell phones, big electrical devices, and power lines, for example. Radiation is also emitted by our cell Wi-Fi routers, baby monitors, Bluetooth earpieces, antennas, smart boards, smart meters, cordless phones and other wireless devices.

According to Stewart Swerdlow, "Modern devices like cell phones, televisions, computers, all receive and transmit electromagnetic energy and microwaves. As these pass through your body, particularly your head, cells are disrupted and altered. This is why cancer and brain tumours are so prevalent these days."

Barbara Marciniak says: "A pregnant mother who is carrying cell phones, who is sitting in front of television, or who is going to movies and watching violent movies and having wireless signals all around... and every doodad in the house is electric... all of this is bombarding the foetus. It cannot survive it. It is not a nourishing environment. So you are going to see a huge increase in diseases. There is going to be an awakening. People are going to start realizing, 'we can't keep doing this to ourselves... We can't do this to our children and grandchildren anymore...'".

She also predicts that people who live in cities will increasingly become increasingly infertile. "*Look at the people who live the more natural lifestyle. They are going to be the most healthy*". I know of many couples that got pregnant almost soon after leaving the city and moving to the countryside.

Tim Ferriss, author of "The Four Hour Body", states that his own research has proven that as little as 1 hour of cell phone exposure severely reduces sperm count and affects sperm morphology and motility. He doubled his sperm count in three months, by avoiding exposure to his cell phone.

It is worth noting that sperm counts in industrialized countries are reducing by 1% a year. At this rate the human race will be extinct in four or five generations…

Dr. David Carpenter (School of Public Health), believes that <u>up to 30% of all childhood cancers may come from exposure to EMF</u>. Martin Halper, the EPA's Director of Analysis, says: *"I have never seen a set of epidemiological studies that remotely approached the weight of evidence that we're seeing with EMF. Clearly there's something here."*

It is estimated that we are now being exposed to a trillion times more EMF than our grandparents were. These unnatural energy fields are suspected of causing sleep disorders, chronic pain, chronic fatigue syndrome, depression anxiety, memory loss, tinnitus, respiratory problems, and a host of other health issues. EMF has been scientifically linked to breast cancer, prostate cancer, brain cancer, damage to the blood/brain barrier, Alzheimer's disease, miscarriages, ALS (Lou Gehrig's disease), Multiple Sclerosis, hypertension, diabetes, thyroid problems, and asthma.

Epidemiological studies conducted in Sweden showed that individuals exposed to high levels of EMF had a 3.7 times higher risk of developing leukaemia. Dr. George Carlo, a researcher from the Science and Public Policy Institute, conducted a study on cell phone radiation and cancer back in the 1980s. Dr. Carlo reported that the rate of death from brain cancer was higher among handheld phone users, and since then, ambient cell phone radiation has increased 500,000% in the average urban area…

The president of Environmental Health Trust, Devra Davis, says, **"Our grandchildren and children are being used as lab rats**. Even though we are well aware of the fact that EMF radiation damages DNA and impairs natural cellular repair processes, we continue to push it to the extremes. If radiation from Wi-Fi can cause diminished reaction time in children, decreased motor function, increased distraction, hyperactivity and inability to focus, what can it do to the fertility rates of adults?"

Camilla Rees of ElectromagneticHealth.org said: "Every 900 milliseconds, whether you are using the phone or not, your cell phone has a spike in radiation because it is looking for a signal from the tower…". She lists the following key impacts on children from cell phone and Wi-Fi radiation: Development of foetus in utero, Cognitive function, Attention, Memory, Perception, Learning Capacity, Low energy, fatigue, reduced motor function, Poor sleep, DNA mutations, Distraction and Hyperactivity, Inability to focus on long-term tasks, and Impaired Fertility.

Electromagnetic Frequencies and radiation (EMF) from mobile phones and wireless devices **weaken the immune system**. This is why, to protect ourselves and especially our children, we turn off the Wi-Fi in the evenings. We use *Q-Link* pendants, Q-Link diodes for our laptop and mobile phones (I keep the phone switched off throughout most of the day), and we use the *Aulterra* *Whole House Plug* that neutralizes the EMFs of every device that's plugged into a socket in our home.

Recap – Toxic Products You Should Remove From Your Life

❏ **Cigarettes** contain 43 known cancer-causing compounds.

❏ **Sugar** consumption destroys your health in over 100 different ways; Sugar feeds cancer.

❏ **Coffee** is *pure acid*; it turns your bloodstream to *sludge* and robs you of energy.

❏ Several animal studies indicate serious health risks associated with **genetically modified food**, including infertility, immune problems, and accelerated ageing.

❏ **Refined oils** contain toxins that poison your immune system and that make you exceedingly vulnerable to cancer. An excess of unhealthy fat makes your red blood cells stick together, resulting in far less oxygen reaching your cells.

❏ **Processed milk** contains hormones, pus, pesticide residues, and artificially modified fats.

❏ Higher dairy intake has been linked to acne, food allergies, increased risk of prostate cancer, higher ovarian cancer risk, type 1 diabetes, higher rates of Multiple Sclerosis, and cancer.

❏ **Chickens** are routinely found to contain banned antibiotics, antidepressants like Prozac, allergy medications, arsenic, caffeine, and other prescription drugs. The chicken carcasses soak in "faecal soup" for up to an hour, imbibing the meat with faecal bacteria.

❏ **Cows** are fed chicken faeces, *human sewage*, deceased chickens, pigs, horses, *the carcasses of other dead cows*, cement dust, radioactive materials… Cows are pumped full of growth hormones, anti-parasitic drugs and enormous doses of antibiotics.

❏ You should avoid any and all processed or **packaged foods**, and any foods that contains chemical additives! Eat fresh, organic, locally-grown produce and meat.

❏ **Fluoride** inactivates 62 enzymes, it causes a decrease in IQ, it increases the ageing process, it increases the incidence of cancer and tumour growth, disrupts the immune system, causes genetic damage, increases arthritis, causes depression, and it is a systemic poison. Infant mortality is higher in counties with fluoridated water.

❏ Cancer risk among people drinking chlorinated water is 93% higher than among those whose water does not contain **chlorine.** Prolonged exposure to chlorine has also been shown to produce birth defects, immune system problems, and reproductive disorders.

❑ **Pesticides** cause childhood brain cancers and leukaemia, birth defects, lymphatic cancer, Multiple Sclerosis; Alzheimer's, Parkinson's and other neurological diseases; autism, low sperm count, and depression. Some pesticides are 1000 times more toxic than you are told.

❑ Mercury poisoning from **dental amalgams** has been linked to depression, memory disorders, and chronic diseases such as cancer, Multiple Sclerosis, and even neurological disorders such as Alzheimer's, and Parkinson's, among others.

❑ **Deodorants** contain chemicals that can cause breast cancer and hormone disruption.

❑ **Sunscreen lotions** *cause* cancer. They even attack human DNA when illuminated by sunlight!

❑ **Makeup** contains a long list of highly toxic chemicals, including heavy metals like *lead*.

❑ Exposure to **plastic pollutants** such as BPA, phthalates, and dioxins leads to cancer, endocrine and hormonal disruption, and a range of neurological and behavioural problems.

❑ Cleaning products and **detergents** are extremely deleterious to your health as well, especially those that contain **chlorine**.

❑ Electromagnetic Frequencies and radiation (EMF) from mobile phones, Wi-Fi and wireless devices **weaken the immune system** and can impact children's cognitive function and energy.

PART V

How To Experience Vibrant Health, Superhuman Energy, and Live Longer

CHAPTER 27

Strengthen Your Immune System With Your Mind

Achieving great health is not just down to our environment and our nutrition, as important as these are. The mind has tremendous power over the body. Your mind can make you sick no matter how you eat, how you exercise, or how you breathe. Our habitual thought patterns – *our feelings, thoughts, and emotions* – produce a powerful effect on our physical health. For example, living in fear compromises your immune system. People who are fearful experience a drop in their T-cell count. Depression literally *depresses* your immune system. Fear, worry, anguish, anger, resentment, jealousy, stress, etc. are *mental poisons* for you body. They have a chemical effect. If you are in a state of anger or resentment, you literally create toxins and poisons in your system.

Conversely, happiness stimulates and strengthens your immune system. Positive emotions – *happiness, joy, laughter, enthusiasm, passion, excitement, etc.* – release endorphins, that reduce your perception of pain and trigger a positive feeling in the body, similar to that of morphine.

The Placebo Effect: How Our Thoughts Heal Our Physical Body

Take virtually any disease known to man, and usually 25-30% of patients treated with placebos will get well. This is quite astonishing. Our mind seems to be an incredibly powerful healing tool that can reverse practically any disease up to 30% of the time, with zero side-effects and at zero cost… and yet most doctors completely side-step this fact. Remember this important truth: you can use your mind to heal.

Countless studies have shown that a percentage of patients get healthy with nothing more than placebos and lifestyle instructions. Because they *believe* the pill will cure them, it does, when in fact the pills themselves have no effect on their bodies whatsoever. We are beginning to realize that our *consciousness* determines, to a large extent, what happens to our health.

A Baylor School of Medicine study published in the *New England Journal of Medicine* described an experiment conducted on patients with severe and debilitating knee pain. The patients were divided into three groups. In the first group, the surgeons actually shaved the damaged cartilage in the knee. For the second group they simply flushed out the knee joint, removing the material that was causing inflammation. These are the standard surgeries for people who suffer from severe arthritic knees. The third group received a "fake" surgery. The doctors merely made a small incision and splashed salt water on the knee. The results were astonishing: *the placebo group improved just as much as the other two groups who had surgery!*

In another example, the United States Department of Health and Human Services reported in 1999 that 50% of severely depressed patients taking drugs improved their mood, compared to 32% of those taking a placebo (and this second group didn't suffer any of the dreadful side-effects).

Psychology professor Irving Kirsch of University of Connecticut made some more shocking discoveries regarding antidepressants. He found that 80 percent of the effect of antidepressants, as measured in clinical trials, could be attributed to the placebo effect. Curiously, researchers have found that the placebo effect is somehow getting stronger, with drugs such as Prozac now proving less effective than placebos, a worrying trend for pharmaceutical companies.

Thoughts Alter The Physical Structure of Water

Experiments have been conducted over the past four decades on whether human intention affects the properties of water. Scientists have consistently found that positive intentions tend to produce symmetric, aesthetically pleasing crystals, and negative intentions tend to produce asymmetric, poorly formed crystals.

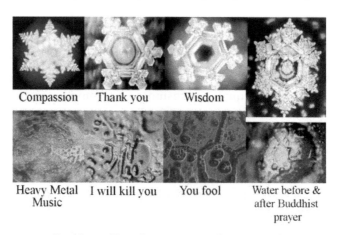

Compassion   Thank you   Wisdom

Heavy Metal   I will kill you   You fool   Water before &
Music   after Buddhist
                                             prayer

Dr. Masaru Emoto's experiments with water crystals.

Dr. Masaru Emoto in Japan photographed the crystals of frozen water after showing them certain words or pictures, playing certain music, and praying to water. The results were astonishing.

How come our thoughts and emotions can influence water's molecular structure? Is it the vibrational frequency of our thoughts that is being reflected by the water crystals? Since **the human body is 70% water**, one can imagine what negative emotions and thoughts do to our health. And *please* don't listen to Heavy Metal music or any loud music. Soothing classical music is better for your *health!*

Check out www.masaru-emoto.net/english to find out more, and I also highly recommend you watch the documentary '*What The Bleep!*'

The Power of Positive Thoughts

Start your day by setting the intention *"I'm having an AMAZING day today!"* Negative thoughts such as anger, hate, worry, and guilt weaken your immune system and are toxic to your body. Remember: Cancer is rooted in feelings of anger, unforgiveness, bitterness, and feelings such as *'I've been wronged', 'I've been screwed', 'I've been traumatized', 'I've been betrayed'*. All the poisons and toxicity in the world cannot really 'land' in you unless you create the emotional trauma to house it.

Your immune system is as strong as your *beliefs* are. If you think thoughts such as *"I am ill", or "I am tired", "I am a sickly being"*, etc. this weakens your immune system, and *attracts* those circumstances into your life. Monitor your mind-patterns. If you catch yourself having a negative or hateful thought, visualize a big brown "X" across that sentence or image, and replace it with a positive thought.

Learn to have a loving and forgiving spirit. Learn to relax and enjoy life. Program yourself daily with positive affirmations, such as:

- *I am healthy*
- *Every day in every way I am healthier and stronger*
- *I am calm and I am happy*
- *Every cell in my body vibrates with energy and health*
- *I take loving care of my body*
- *My body heals quickly and easily*
- *I have boundless energy*

I personally use **subliminal software** on my laptop to program my subconscious mind with positive affirmations such as the ones above. Learning how to use the power of your subconscious mind to achieve your outcomes is extremely powerful…

Learn To Love Yourself

Loving yourself is probably the #1 thing that will impact your life positively, more than anything else. Loving yourself means you are more likely to value your body and your health more, you are more likely to *earn* more (since you see the *value* in *you*), and you are more likely to be in a loving relationship. Only when you love yourself can you love someone else, now *they* see the value in you, and because you value yourself too much to accept anything less than a loving relationship, you don't punish yourself anymore by entering negative relationships, consciously or subconsciously.

Loving yourself strengthens everything in you. It strengthens your auric field around you, as well, which is your first line of defence. Conversely, doubting yourself, criticizing yourself, hating yourself, judging yourself, bad-mouthing yourself, and belittling yourself weakens you. Ground yourself in love, and ground yourself to the Earth. Visualize pale pink around you for unconditional love for yourself, and use the affirmation *"No matter what I have done or not done, I am worthy of love"*, and *"I love and accept myself"*. This is a powerful, transformative exercise: sit in front of a mirror and repeat *"I love you"* over and over again, until you can't hold back your tears…

The Importance of Love & Forgiveness

As I have mentioned previously, Barbara Marciniak states that *love is what returns people to a state of health*. She says: *"Understand that ill people are looking for love. There isn't enough love in their lives. It is LOVE that brings them back."* Dr. John Demartini confirms the healing power of *love* in his book *The Breakthrough Experience*: *"I've worked with terminal cancer patients who had spontaneous remissions, and in each case, some form of love and gratitude came into their lives and shifted them. A spiritual experience transformed their illness. Even watching a movie about love has been shown to increase the levels of immunoglobulin A in the saliva, the body's first line of immunological defence.* **We get ill to teach us to love.** *It's not a punishment or a mistake. It's a gift."*

He adds: *"Illness is your body's way of telling you that you're lying about life. Every symptom and sign in your physical body is designed to reveal to you what you're lying about."*

Live With Purpose and Integrity

Being true to yourself and living your life with passion and *purpose* strengthens your immune system. As does loving your partner with sincerity and integrity, and *working with integrity*, so that when you fall asleep at night you are pleased with your day and you are not hiding from yourself. Lying and being out of integrity weakens your body.

The centenarians from the world's Blue Zones have a strong sense of purpose in life, which propels them forward in life with energy and zest. What is *your* purpose? Why do you get up in the morning? What are you passionate about? What do you enjoy doing? What is truly important to you?

Research shows that the 2 most important factors in heart disease and predictions of fatal heart attack are: Job dissatisfaction – people who feel they have no meaning or purpose to their lives – and whether they answer *'yes'* to the question *'Are you happy?'* Pretty incredible, don't you think? If you're unhappy, or feel like your life lacks meaning… you become diseased and drop dead faster.

Having a Family and Being Part of a Community Makes You Live Longer

Did you know that single people die younger? Studies have shown that being married, or being in a permanent stable relationship, leads to living longer. Middle-aged people without a spouse or long-term partner were discovered to be at greater risk of premature death than those who were settled down with their other half. In fact, those who never married or settled down with a long-term companion were more than twice as likely to die in middle-age than those who had been in a stable relationship throughout their adult life. It makes sense, since having a family or community to contribute to gives you a sense a purpose.

In most cases, the centenarians from the Blue Zones built their entire lives around the core values of family and community. The social and emotional support that derives from that is probably one of the reasons why they lead such long, happy and healthy lives. It is important to learn to place our loved ones first and build ties with our friends and our local community. Rituals are important, so make sure you schedule family meals and prioritize things such as family vacations that help build the connection. Photo walls are wonderful. Make sure you have some sort of family shrine somewhere in the house where you can display family pictures.

Laughter Strengthens Your Energy Field

When you *laugh* you strengthen your energy field (your aura), and you strengthen your immune system. Remember: Truth, Love, and *Joy* are divine attitudes. Some people have laughed themselves into healing, and even cured themselves of cancer by watching funny movies. Norman Cousins claims to have cured himself of cancer by watching funny films for 8 hours a day!

Having great emotions running through your body releases completely natural 'happiness chemicals' into your bloodstream, and can bring about a positive change in your health with little change to your lifestyle. These natural chemicals in your body would cost you tens of thousands – even millions – of dollars to buy from a pharmaceutical company… and come without any of the side-effects!

The spiritual channeller Barbara Marciniak says: *"Laughter is a sign of an elevated spirit; laughter heals the body and opens up the chakras to take healing energy inside"*.

"Hope, purpose, and determination are not merely mental states. They have electro-chemical connections that play a large part in the workings of the immune system and, indeed, in the entire economy of the total human organism... The emotional state of the patient has specific effects on the mechanisms involved in illness and health. The modern physician, therefore.... Will prescribe not just out of the pharmacy or his little black bag, but out of the magnificent apothecary that is the human brain, which can activate and potentiate the healing system. The roster of emotions are hope, faith, love, will to live, festivity, playfulness, purpose, and determination. These are powerful biochemical prescriptions."

Norman Cousins, *Head First: The Biology of Hope*

Giving Thanks For Your Food Extends Your Longevity

Studies have shown that people who live the longest have this important thing in common: they bless their food. In *The Blue Zones*, Dan Buettner describes how people live longest in places where they are spiritually engaged, through prayer and giving thanks for their food. It would appear that <u>flowing your grateful intention and energy to *your food* brings about considerable health benefits</u>. This makes sense when you understand what Quantum Physics has shown us: everything in the entire Universe is just a singular unified *energy field*. We are "All One".

When I sit down for a meal, I say the following: *"I ask that this meal be blessed by God-Mind for the most effective and efficient use by all levels of my body. I ask that my body keep only what it needs while allowing what it does not need to be eliminated. Thank you for this abundance."* As you do this, create an image in your mind of your food nourishing you, with the nutrients reaching every cell in your body, replenishing you, and reenergizing you. Barbara Marciniak says: *"I always bless my food, put my hands together and do a 'Yummm' over it. What that's really doing is…. I'm thanking everything that's coming into my body and I'm asking that everything I add to my body to meet with my vibration or take me higher. A consciousness with food that most people don't have."*

Connect with Nature and Get Plenty of Sunshine

Barbara Marciniak also adds: "Nature will strengthen your immune system. If you don't feel well, or you want to get revitalized, go out and sit in nature, sit on the ground, connect to the earth."

She believes that exposure to sunshine is important for our immune system: "The sun is very important to keep the body healthy. Don't be afraid of the sun. You will keep your energy field strong with a good dose of sunlight."

Giving Your Attention To Plants Boosts Them

Many experiments have shown beyond the shadow of a doubt that the plants which get the most direct *positive* human attention, grow healthiest. Conversely, if you yell and scream abuse towards a plant, they wither, die, or simply fail to thrive. Our positive attention (and love) towards our plants is returned to us many-fold as they boost our strength when they are consumed.

Dr. Patrick MacManaway is the author of *"Energy Dowsing for Health"*. At a recent conference in Glastonbury, England, he revealed that his research showed that animals gravitated to the water that had been blessed, rather than water that had not, and the crops and seeds watered by that water grew considerably more. Through the use of subtle energies and 'extended sensory awareness techniques' he reports results such as a 20% increase in wheat and potato yields, 45% increase in sorghum yield, a 50% reduction in calf mortality, increased numbers of beneficial insects present, and many more astounding results.

"One of the greatest gifts we can give as humans is the gift of undivided, fully loving attention. When we give this to those around us, they and the space between us becomes filled with life and energy. We create an energy field within which things can thrive. The same applies when we extend our loving attention to the [plants and] animals in our life." – Dr. Patrick MacManaway

"The plant kingdom... it is essential that you focus on it. It will come into a much higher vibration, to help you. Not enough people say 'hello' to nature. You will eventually start talking to your plants, seeds, and flowers, to tell them what you need. Remember: nature supports you, so you should communicate with it." – Barbara Marciniak

Energy Work & Visualizing Health

If you focus on your disease, you will only experience *more* disease. Instead, you should focus on and visualize yourself being healthy and vibrant. **Visualize and focus on a mental picture of yourself being healthy, vibrant, and happy**. The Universe gives you more of who *you are*. What would you be doing if you were totally healthy? What would you believe? What would you say? How would you be around other people?

According to Stewart Swerdlow, everything we see around us in this Universe was created with 'the language of Hyperspace': <u>archetypes, tones, and colours</u>. We can use this esoteric language to create and manifest health, for example. To maintain a healthy body, he strongly recommends using daily visualization exercises such as:

- **T-bar balancing** – *this involves centering your consciousness at your pineal gland, and visualizing the letter* T *in its center.*

- **Chakra spinning** – *visualize your chakras spinning in harmony, like plates, along your chakra points.* Ill people tend to have their chakras spinning asynchronously.

- Visualize the **'Power Archetype'** in *red* in every cell of your body: ⋀

- Do your **affirmations** every day, 21 times for each one.

- **The Breathing Exercise** – *breathe in medium green colour in your heart chakra, and blowing out red (anger), blue (isolation), and grey (emotional confusion).*

- **The Child Within** exercise – *"there is a child within each person who has not developed into an adult. This little person causes you to emotionally react to difficult or unhappy interpersonal situations in your life. This visualization is designed to mature this child so that he/she reacts as an adult rather than as a child."*

- **The Golden Altar** exercise – this exercise is designed to release the images from the mind-pattern which perpetuate negative cycles that occur in your life, such as isolation, abandonment, and low self-worth issues. Visualize a Golden Altar, place upon it the person you need to forgive, and say: *"I forgive you and release you from all negative experiences between us, whether real or imagined, I forgive you and release you."* Then you place the next person on the altar. Finally, you place yourself there and say: *"I forgive and release myself from all negative experiences I have attracted to myself in this lifetime, whether real or imagined, I forgive and release myself."*

- **Communicating with your Oversoul** (e.g. daily meditation), visualizing a silver infinity symbol, and releasing all up to it.

These last three exercises are considered to be 'release work'. Stewart Swerdlow says: *"When you do the basics of chakra spinning, T-Bar balancing, breathing, and release work, the body responds with health, energy, and vitality."*

CHAPTER 28

Superfoods & Outstanding Nutrition

If you have removed the toxicity from your diet and your environment, you have a positive outlook and attitude and a strong sense of purpose, and you hydrate and oxygenate your body daily, the next thing on your agenda should be to optimize your nutrition. You need to **give your body the *fuel* it needs** to rebuild your cells, heal, create energy, and perform its myriad of functions.

I have found that the best way to integrate this information is to make it part of your daily routine. For example, I begin my day by preparing a 1.5 litre "Green Juice" smoothie for myself and my family. This consists of putting the flesh of an avocado and a handful of spinach in the blender, then juicing 5 apples, two cucumbers, and ⅓ of a celery (you'll need a good juicer and a blender). This "Green Juice" is extremely alkalizing and detoxifying to the body. I then add 20-30 supplements and **superfoods** into the blender, alternating the selection day by day. I find that when I drink this mineral-rich and vitamin-rich smoothie, I am not as hungry during the day, I eat less, I have more energy, my mood is brighter, and I don't crave sugar.

Let's take a look at some *awesome* superfoods you should consider making part of your diet! :)

Avocados

Avocados are one of the most nutrient-dense foods. They are high in fiber and contain very high levels of folate, potassium, vitamin E and magnesium. They also contain Vitamin K, Vitamin C, Potassium, Vitamin B5, Vitamin B6, and small amounts of manganese, copper, iron, zinc, phosphorous, Vitamin A, B1, B2, B3. Avocados contain essential Omega-3 oils needed by our cells. Eating avocado lowers chances of prostate cancer, helps lose weight, and lowers cholesterol. Avocadoes are a superb source of fats, specifically omega-3 and omega-9. According to the late Dr. Robert Atkins, *"Avocadoes are not only nourishing they are a heart promoting, cancer-fighting fruit that offers unequalled health benefits."*

Wheatgrass

Wheatgrass juice is *incredibly* healing. It contains all the minerals needed by your body (including calcium, phosphorus, magnesium, sodium and potassium in a balanced ratio), as well as vitamins A, B-complex, C, E, and K. It is claimed that two ounces of wheatgrass juice has **the nutritional equivalent of five pounds of the best raw organic vegetables.** Wheatgrass is a complete source of protein, supplying all of the essential amino acids. Wheatgrass juice is one of the best sources of living chlorophyll available (to get the full benefit, it is best to juice the living plant). It floods the body with therapeutic doses of vitamins, minerals, antioxidants, enzymes, and phytonutrients. It is also a powerful detoxifier, especially of the liver and blood, and cleanses your body of heavy metals, pollutants and other toxins.

According to health advocate Webster Kehr, "The number of ways Wheatgrass deals with cancer is incredible. It contains chlorophyll, which increases haemoglobin production, meaning more oxygen gets to the cancer. Selenium and laetrile are also in wheatgrass, and both are anticancer. Chlorophyll and selenium also help build the immunity system. In addition, wheatgrass is one of the most alkaline foods known to mankind. And the list goes on."

At the Hippocrates alternative health center in the US, their healing programs include drinking two ounces of wheatgrass juice twice a day. They recommend consuming it fresh, within fifteen minutes of juicing, undiluted and on an empty stomach, so that the nutrients are absorbed more efficiently. Studies have shown that wheatgrass powders and supplements are only 2% as effective as freshly juiced wheatgrass. They state on their website: "When it is consumed fresh it is a living food and has bio-electricity. This high vibration energy is literally the life force within the living juice. This resource of life-force energy can potentially unleash powerful renewing vibrations and greater connectivity to one's inner being. These powerful nutrients can also prevent DNA destruction and help protect us from the ongoing effects of pre-mature aging and cellular breakdown. Recent research shows that only living foods and juices can restore the electrical charge between the capillaries and the cell walls which boosts the immune system. When it is fresh, wheatgrass juice is the king of living juices. Wheatgrass cleanses and builds the blood due to its high content of chlorophyll. The high content of oxygen in chlorophyll helps deliver more oxygen to the blood. Chlorophyll is the first product of light and therefore contains more healing properties than any other element. All life on this planet comes from the sun. Only green plants can transform the sun's energy into chlorophyll, via photosynthesis. Chlorophyll is known as the 'life-blood' of the plants. This important phytonutrient is what your cells need to heal and to thrive. Drinking wheatgrass juice is like drinking liquid sunshine."

You can buy wheatgrass-growing kits online, which includes organic compost, seeds, growing trays, a wheatgrass juicer, and a set of instructions. It's super-healthy and fun for the whole family!

Aloe Vera

Aloe Vera has been used therapeutically for over 5000 years, and is mentioned eight times in the Bible, for its powerful therapeutic properities. It contains more than 200 active components including vitamins (A, C, E, folic acid, choline, B1, B2, niacin, B6, and even the rare vitamin B12), minerals (calcium, magnesium, zinc, chromium, selenium, sodium, iron, potassium, copper, manganese, and many more), amino acids (the building blocks of protein), enzymes, polysaccharides, and fatty acids (campesterol, and B-sitosterol, linoleic, linolenic, myristic, caprylic, oleic, palmitic, and stearic). Aloe Vera contains at least 18 of the 22 amino acids necessary for the human body.

Researchers have identified eight essential "glyconutrients" which are crucial to the proper structure and function of the 60 trillion cells in the human body. Unfortunately, six of those are missing from our modern diet. This is why it is important to supplement your diet with a product that contains all eight. Aloe Vera contains all eight **glyconutrients**, which have been shown to help people overcome a very wide range of diseases.

It is thought that Aloe Vera is a powerful adaptogen, which balances the body's system, stimulating the defense and adaptive mechanisms of the body. This allows you an increased ability to cope with stress and resist illness. Aloe also helps with digestion, it promotes weight loss, and it soothes and cleanses the digestive tract. It has been a great remedy for people with problems such as irritable bowel syndrome as well as acid reflux. Aloe also helps to decrease the amount of unfriendly bacteria in your gut, keeping your intestinal flora in balance. Aloe is also a vermifuge, which means it helps to rid the body of intestinal worms.

Aloe Vera also helps detoxify and alkalize your body, as well as boost your immune system. The polysaccharides in aloe vera juice stimulate macrophages, which are the white blood cells of your immune system that fight against viruses. Aloe is also an immune enhancer because of its high level of anti-oxidants. Aloe Vera is also great for the skin, and is known to help heal wounds, burns, abrasions, and psoriasis. It also helps reduce inflammation, as well as being a Disinfectant, Germicidal, Anti-bacterial, Anti-septic, Anti-fungal & Anti-viral! Next to wheatgrass, this is the best single plant to have around your home.

Dr. Robert Siegel cured himself of three different cancers (prostate, colon, and kidney) using the *Aloe Immune* available at www.aloeimmune.com. Precautions: Avoid taking Aloe internally during pregnancy, menstruation, if you have hemorrhoids or degeneration of the liver and gall bladder.

A note on the power of Glyconutrients

My friend Stephen had been in a terrible motorcycle accident in his twenties. This accident left him in a wheelchair, with more than 20 broken bones, no short-term memory, Asthma, a speech impediment, taking innumerable painkillers and anti-depressants. Doctors couldn't help him get better. And yet within 6 weeks of taking glyconutrients (the eight sugars contained in Aloe Vera) he could walk again, he no longer had Asthma, no longer required any drugs, his speech impediment was gone, and he had regained his memory. His body has kept growing stronger since then.

The results I have witnessed in people's health as a result of taking Glyconutrients have bordered on the miraculous. I have spoken to people who have overcome Cancer, Multiple Sclerosis, Arthritis, Lupus, Neurofibromatosis, type 1 Diabetes, and even reversed symptoms of Down Syndrome, blindness, paralysis, Parkinson's and Alzheimer's, thanks to supplementing their diet with glyconutrients.

Sprouts

Sprouting is the practice of germinating seeds. You can sprout alfalfa seeds, almonds, broccoli, cabbage, fenugreek, garbanzos, lentils, mung, peas, radish, red clover, and sunflower seeds. Sprouts are rich with vitamins, minerals, proteins, and enzymes and deliver them in a form which is easily assimilated and digested. Interesting, since sprouts are live foods, they will continue to grow slowly, and their vitamin content will actually increase after you harvest them, in contrast to store-bought vegetables and fruits which lose a lot of their vitamin content during shipping. Sprouts can be germinated at home, and it is a very effective way to add raw foods to your diet. Growing your own sprouts means having your own private supply of fresh organic vegetables every day from a couple square feet of counter space; and seeds can multiply up to fifteen times their original weight. Be sure to refrigerate your completed sprouts, though ideally you should eat them right after you pick them.

Nuts & Seeds

According to a number of studies, people who consume nuts five times a week have about a 50% reduction in risk of heart attack, and a 23% to 45% reduced mortality risk over the course of the study. In other words, **people who eat nuts regularly *live* longer.** People who eat nuts at least twice per week are 31% less likely to gain weight than people who seldom eat them. I add 10 different nuts and seeds to my daily "Green Juice", including:

Walnuts ($15.69 per kg)

Walnuts are high in unsaturated, Omega 3 fatty acids, iron, and B vitamins. They contain almost twice as many antioxidants as other nuts. Walnuts contain high amounts of alpha-linolenic acid, which is a major contributor to a healthy heart. In a study published in BMC Medicine it was shown that people who eat nuts more than three times a week have a reduced risk of dying from cancer or cardiovascular disease than those who do not. **Nut eaters had a 39% lower mortality risk** – a number that increased to 45 percent in the case of walnut eaters! Walnuts have a very high content of alpha-linoleic acid, phytochemicals, and minerals such as calcium, magnesium and potassium!

Brazil Nuts ($18.27 per kg)

Selenium is an essential component of a powerful antioxidant manufactured by the body: glutathione peroxidase. Sunflower seeds are very rich in Selenium (78mcg per 100 grams). But Brazil Nuts are the undisputed champions with a massive 1,917 mcg per 100 grams!

Selenium is <u>one of the most powerful anti-cancer nutrient there is</u>. Numerous studies have shown it to be an effective tool in warding off breast, oesophageal, stomach, prostate, liver, and bladder cancers. The number one nation in blood selenium level (Japan) had the lowest cancer level and consistently has rated highest in longevity, while the number two selenium level nation had the second lowest cancer rate, etc.

Simply put, <u>the more selenium available in the diet, the lower the levels of cancer</u>. A trial conducted by Dr. L.C. Clark at the University of Arizona found that the selenium-treated group developed 66% fewer prostate cancers, 50% fewer colorectal cancers, and 40% fewer lung cancers. Selenium is also an essential component of a powerful antioxidant manufactured by the body: glutathione peroxidase.

Pine nuts ($38.91 per kg)

Pine nuts are one of my personal favourites. I include them in many recipes, salads, and even smoothies. They are actually the seeds of pine trees, and they help suppress appetite and boost energy. They contain healthy fats and antioxidants.

They are a good source of protein, iron, and magnesium. Pine nuts contain monounsaturated fat, magnesium, vitamin E, vitamin K and manganese, which supports heart health. Pine nuts contain a wealth of anti-ageing antioxidants, including vitamins A, B, C, D, and E, and lutein, a carotenoid that may help you ward off eye diseases like age-related macular degeneration (AMD) and non-Hodgkin lymphoma.

Almonds (£21.76 per kg)

According to Ayurveda, almonds help increase high intellectual level and longevity. Almonds also reduce heart attack risk, they lower "bad" cholesterol, and protect artery walls from damage. They lower the rise in blood sugar and insulin after meals. Almonds help build strong bones and teeth, thanks to the phosphorus they contain.

They aid in weight loss. Almonds contain riboflavin and L-carnitine, which can boost brain activity and reduce the risk of Alzheimer's disease.

Chia Seeds ($20.36 per kg)

Chia Seeds are rich in antioxidants. They are typically organic, raw, Non-GMO, non-irradiated, and produced without pesticides. They contain so much fiber that they help you stay full for longer, and support your digestive system. Chia Seeds are 14% protein. A single ounce of Chia seeds provides 18% of your daily calcium needs, as well as containing phosphorus and magnesium. They also contain Zinc and Omega 3 fats, lowering your risk of cardiovascular disease, cholesterol, and colon cancer. Chia Seeds also help detoxify the body, repair your cells, and reduce inflammation.

Sunflower seeds ($4.08 per kg)

Sunflower seeds are rich in Selenium. One ounce of sunflower seeds contains 10 mg of vitamin E (35% of the recommended daily requirement), which helps protect cells against the effects of free radicals, and helps in the maintenance of blood circulation and production of red blood cells. Other health benefits are attributed to the seeds' content of Thiamine, a B-vitamin. This nutrient assists in obtaining energy from food. Humans require 1.2 mg of Vitamin B1 daily, with one ounce of sunflower seeds providing 33% of our daily requirements. Sunflower seeds also contain copper, which helps maintain the skin and hair, as well as supporting the mechanism of the body's metabolic processes to assist our cells in producing energy. One ounce contains 512 mg of copper, or more than 50% of our daily requirements.

Pumpkin Seeds ($12.80 per kg)

Pumpkin seeds contain magnesium, zinc, Omega 3 fats, antioxidants and fiber. These may provide benefits for heart and liver health. Research suggests that both pumpkin seed oil and pumpkin seeds may be particularly beneficial in supporting prostate health. They can help decrease blood pressure, hot flashes, headaches, joint pains and other menopausal symptoms in postmenopausal women. Pumpkin seed oil has been found to exhibit anti-inflammatory effects. Pumpkin seeds are a rich source of tryptophan, an amino acid that your body converts into serotonin, which in turn is converted into melatonin, the "sleep hormone", which helps promote a restful night's sleep.

Sesame seeds ($6.77 per kg, or $9.97 per kg of organic black sesame seeds)

Sesame seeds are packed with so many health benefits that they were worth their weight in gold during the Middle Ages. They are rich in vitamins, minerals, and fatty acids, including Manganese, Copper, Calcium (277 mg per ounce), Iron, Magnesium (99 mg per ounce), Tryptophan, Zinc, Thiamin, Vitamin B6, Phosphorous, fiber and protein. Sesame seeds can help prevent diabetes and lower blood pressure, due to their high magnesium content (it's in the Top 10 foods highest in magnesium). They help promote healthy skin and hair, due to their zinc content. They also improve bone health, as they are a great source of calcium. Sesame seeds contain higher phytosterol content – which is an important anti-cancer compound – than any other kinds of seeds and nuts. Sesame seed oil contains Omega 3, Omega 6 and Omega 9 fats which promote hair growth, as well as vitamins that feed your hair. Black sesame seeds are well known for darkening one's hair naturally. Sesame seeds contain nutrients that help relieve arthritis and reduce stress. Vitamin B1 has calming properties which have been used in treating depression.

Apricot Seeds ($42.50 per kg)

Apricot seeds are a rich source of Vitamin B17 (or 'laetrile'). Consuming apricot seeds is shown to strenghten your immune system and help your body combat infections. The anti-inflammatory qualities and natural analgesis properties of apricot seeds help reduce arthritis, as it relieves pain and swelling. They are used in Chinese medicine for the treatment of respiratory problems such as bronchitis, asthma, and emphysema. Apricot seeds are a superb source of unsaturated fats, and they help support heart function and lower cholesterol. And perhaps most importantly, <u>apricot seeds have been shown to kill cancer cells without side effects</u>.

Hemp Seeds ($8.50 per kg)

Hemp seeds are extremely nutritious. They are rich in healthy fats, protein and a range of minerals. They are exceptionally rich in two essential fatty acids, linoleic acid (omega-6) and alpha-linolenic acid (omega-3). They also contain gamma-linolenic acid and high amounts of the amino acid arginine, which have been linked with several health benefits. Hemp seeds are a great protein source, as more than 25% of their total calories are from high-quality protein. In fact, by weight, hemp seeds provide amounts of protein similar to beef and lamb. 30 grams of hemp seeds provide about 11 grams of protein. They are considered a complete protein source, which means that they provide all the essential amino acids. Quinoa is another example of a complete, plant-based protein source. Hemp seeds are also a great source of vitamin E and minerals such as phosphorus, potassium, sodium, magnesium, sulfur, calcium, iron and zinc. Hemp seed oil is also very healthy, and has been used as a food/medicine in China for at least 3,000 years. It may relieve eczema, dry skin, itchiness and reduce the need for skin medication. Hemp Seeds May Also Reduce Symptoms of PMS and Menopause. In a study of women with PMS, taking one gram of essential fatty acids (including 210 mg of Gamma-linolenic acid GLA) per day resulted in a significant decrease in symptoms. It decreased breast pain and tenderness, depression, irritability and fluid retention associated with PMS. It has been suggested that the GLA in hemp seeds may help to regulate the hormone imbalances and inflammation associated with menopause. Finally, whole hemp seeds contain high amounts of fiber, both soluble and insoluble, which benefits digestive health.

Cacao Powder ($19.31 per kg)

Raw cacao powder from the seeds of the Cacao tree contains more than 300 different compounds and nearly twenty times the antioxidant power of blueberries. Protein, calcium, carotene, thiamin, riboflavin, magnesium, sulfur, flavonoids, antioxidants, and essential fatty acids are also present. The precise blend of all these elements combined serve to kick in naturally occurring phytochemicals that have incredible benefits throughout the body, such as lowered LDL cholesterol, improved heart function, and reduced cancer risk.

Raw cacao powder contains Vitamin A, Vitamin B (1, 2, 3, 5 and 6), Vitamin C, Vitamin E, Magnesium (Cacao is the highest whole food source of magnesium), Copper, Calcium, Manganese, Zinc, Sulphur, Iron, Chromium, Phosphorus, Omega 6 Fatty Acids, Amino Acids, Soluble Fiber, Enzymes (including catalase, lipase and amylase), and other beneficial phytonutrients (such as the antioxidants oligomeric procynanidins, resveratrol and the polyphenols: catechin and epicatechin). Studies have shown that chocolate raises your serotonin levels and lifts your mood, releasing the compound anandamide, which produces euphoric feelings of relaxation and contentment.

The famous "Dutch study" followed over 200 Dutch men over the course of twenty years and found that <u>those who ate the most chocolate had lower rates of all major diseases compared to those who ate little to no chocolate</u>. Jeanne Louise Calment of France lived to be 122, and many say that one of her secrets to longevity was her consumption of 2.5 pounds of bitter dark chocolate a week. The third "official" oldest person ever to have lived was Sarah Knauss, who also regularly enjoyed the health benefits of chocolate, although not in as large quantities as Jeanne!

Herbs & Spices

Cat's Claw (Uña de Gato)   ($38.44 per kg)

In 1989 Austrian scientist Dr. Klause Keplinger isolated six oxindole alkaloids from the root of Cat's Claw, and discovered that four of these alkaloids have a pronounced enhancement effect on phagocytosis, which is the ability of the white blood cells and macrophage to attack, engulf and digest harmful micro-organisms, foreign matter, and debris.

According to Indian folklore, Cat's Claw has been used to treat digestive problems, arthritis, inflammation, ulcers, and even to cure cancer. In 1972, a 78-year-old Peruvian plantation owner named Don Luis was diagnosed with terminal lung cancer, and was sent home to die. An Indian medicine woman gave him tea made from Cat's Claw. After drinking the tea daily for six months, his cancer completely disappeared and he lived healthy and cancer-free until the age of ninety.

Cat's Claw possesses amazing healing abilities and benefits to the immune system with a plethora of therapeutic applications. Cat's Claw also seems to have the ability to break through severe intestinal disorders that no other available products can touch. It is known for its ability to cleanse the entire intestinal tract and its effectiveness in treating stomach and bowel disorders such as Crohn's disease, leaky bowel syndrome, ulcers, gastritis, diverticulitis, and other inflammatory conditions of the bowel, stomach, and intestines. Studies conducted in Peru, Austria, Germany, England, Hungary, and Italy suggest that Cat's Claw may be beneficial in the treatment of cancer, arthritis, bursitis, rheumatism, genital herpes and herpes zoster, allergies, ulcers, systematic candidiasis, diabetes, lupus, chronic fatigue syndrome, PMS, and irregularities of the female cycle, environmental toxic poisoning, numerous bowel and intestinal disorders, organic depression, and those infected with the HIV virus. Cat's Claw can be mixed with the Venus Flytrap extract (Carnivora™) for utmost results.

Echinacea ($32.76 per kg)

Echinacea is one of the herbs with the most beneficial effects upon human health. Its potency is derived from its impressive list of ingredients, including vitamins A, C, and E and a large number of nutritive minerals (copper, iron, potassium, and iodine). It is also rich in antioxidants and other beneficial elements (oils, akylamides, polysaccharides, phenols, and flavonoids). Echinacea stimulates and strengthens our immune system by activating white blood cells. Combining Echinacea and vitamin C reduced cold incidence by 86%, while Echinacea alone reduced colds by 65%.

Pau D'Arco ($15.91 per kg)

Pau d'Arco is a herb found in the rainforests of the Amazon and in South and Latin America. Pau d'Arco bark has been used by indigenous Latin populations for centuries to alleviate a range of health problems and today its strong resistance to harmful organisms is still appreciated. Pau d'Arco is commonly used to support indications of allergies, liver problems, and candida and yeast infections. Warning: people who are taking blood thinners should consult their healthcare provider. Pau d'arco should not be used during pregnancy.

Astragalus ($23.63 per kg)

This is an ancient Chinese herb. In China, astragalus is widely used in the treatment of Hepatitis, and there is strong scientific evidence that it indeed benefits liver function. In one study, astragalus was able to restore immune function in 90% of the cancer patients studied. In a 1994 Italian study, breast cancer patients were given a combination of ligustrum and astragalus. Patients showed a decline in mortality from 50% to 10%. In two other studies, cancer patients receiving astragalus had twice the survival rate of those who received chemotherapy or radiation treatments.

Dandelion Leaf ($16.29 per kg)

Dandelion promotes digestion, stimulates appetite, and balances the beneficial bacteria in the intestines. It can increase the release of stomach acid and bile to aid digestion, especially of fats. This superfood is a diuretic that helps the kidneys clear out waste and excess water by increasing urine production. Dandelion improves liver function by removing toxins and establishing electrolyte balance. Every part of the dandelion plant is rich in antioxidants that prevent free-radical damage to cells and DNA, slowing down the ageing process in our cells. It is rich in vitamin C and vitamin A and increases the liver's production of superoxide dismutase (which breaks down the superoxide O_2- radical into either ordinary molecular oxygen (O_2) or hydrogen peroxide H_2O_2). Dandelion may slow cancer's growth and prevent it from spreading. The leaves are especially rich in the antioxidants and phytonutrients that combat cancer. Recent animal studies show dandelion also helps regulate blood sugar and insulin levels. The fiber and potassium in dandelion also help regulate blood pressure. Dandelion reduces inflammation to help with gallbladder problems and blockages. Dandelion contains essential fatty acids, antioxidants, and phytonutrients that all reduce inflammation throughout the body. Studies also show that dandelion boosts immune function and fights off microbes and fungi. Warning: Anyone pregnant, nursing, or taking prescription drugs should talk to a healthcare professional before adding this to their diet.

Nettles ($12.73 per kg)

Nettle leaf alleviates arthritis, it is a herbal treatment for allergies, it relieves hair loss, treats Coeliac disease, bladder infections, skin complaints, neurological disorders and a long list of other conditions. It is often used as a spring tonic. It helps cleanse the body as it stimulates the lymph system and the kidneys. Patients with Lupus and other disorders suffering from joint pain experience relief from drinking a cup of nettle tea or eating stewed nettle leaves daily. Its diuretic action alkalizes and releases uric acid from the joints of gout patients eliminating pain. Nettle is high in iron making it excellent for combating anaemia and fatigue. It supports the liver and the female hormonal system. Pregnant women benefit from stinging nettle as it protects against bleeding and strengthens the foetus. Nettles can help increase milk production in nursing mothers. They also reduce PMS symptoms, help process estrogen to relieve menopausal symptoms and curb excess menstrual flow. It is often used in herbal tonics to remove fibroids and regulate the menstrual flow. Stinging nettles are helpful for bladder and urinary tract function in both sexes. The tea acts as a natural diuretic, increases urination and helps break down kidney stones. Nettles acts as a pelvic decongestant and reduces an enlarged prostate. Nettle tea relieves eczema and acne, and is applied as a warm compress to remove warts. It also helps regenerate both hair growth and restore original colour.

Nettle leaf is effective at reducing symptoms of the digestive tract ranging from acid reflux, nausea, colitis and Coeliac disease. Additionally, it is an effective herbal treatment for sore throats, swollen hemorrhoids, nose bleeds and mouth sores.

It supports the endocrine system including the thyroid, spleen and pancreas. It relieves chest congestion and coughing, bronchitis, and pulmonary disease. It relieves neurological disorders such as Alzheimer's, MS, ALS and sciatica.

Warning: Because stinging nettles can produce side effects and interact with other drugs and natural treatments, consult your healthcare practitioner before using it.

Ginger ($10.21 per kg)

Ginger is one of the world's healthiest foods. It can be consumed freshly grated, dried ground, or as a tea. Consuming ginger reduces the symptoms of osteoarthritis, contains powerful anti-diabetic properties, lowers the risk of heart disease, helps treat Chronic Indigestion, significantly reduces menstrual pain, lowers cholesterol levels, helps prevent cancer, improves brain function and protects against Alzheimer's disease. In his book *Cancer: Step Outside The Box*, Ty Bollinger shares the following story about the powerful healing properties of ginger: *"Bill is a former Stage IV cancer patient who cured his cancer with ginger. He says: 'When prostate cancer spread to and blocked my colon. I tried ginger. I took up to six capsules (500mg), four times a day. I was very lucky. It worked!'"*

Ginseng ($18.36 per kg, in powdered form)

Ginseng is effective in combating cancer, diabetes, stress, and fatigue. In a study conducted by Dr. Taik-Koo Yun published in 1998, consumption of ginseng resulted in a 67% decreased risk for stomach cancer and 70% for lung cancer. The ginsenosides in Ginseng fight cancer by preventing angiogenesis (creating of new blood vessels to the tumour), inducing normal cell death (apoptosis), and preventing metastasis (spreading).

Ashwagandha (or "Indian Ginseng"; $26.14 per kg)

Withania somnifera, better known as ashwagandha or "Indian ginseng," has been a staple of Ayurvedic medicine for over 3000 years. The herb has a wide range of activity that promotes physical and mental health, body rejuvenation, and longevity. It is known to inhibit anxiety and improve energy. In certain cases, ashwagandha may also promote healthy fertility.

The Department of Biochemistry at C.S.M. Medical University conducted a study involving sixty infertile men who, however, did have normal sperm production. Participants were given five grams of ashwagandha root powder every day for three months. At the study's conclusion, stress reductions and improvements in semen quality were observed in many of the participants and 14% of the participants' partners ended up becoming pregnant.

The Faculty of Sports Medicine and Physiotherapy at India's Guru Nanak Dev University conducted an eight week study in which forty elite cyclists took ashwagandha supplements. The study reported "significant enhancements in both cardiovascular and respiratory endurance".

The Department of Neuropsychiatry and Geriatric Psychiatry at India's Asha Hospital ran a placebo-controlled study involving 64 subjects with a history of chronic stress. They began supplementing with high-concentration, full-spectrum ashwagandha root extract. After two months, they reported significant improvements in all stress measurements and quality of life, compared to the control group.

Curcumin (Turmeric) ($20.64 per kg)

In a study on human breast cancer cells, curcumin reversed growth caused by a certain form of oestrogen by 98% and growth caused by DDT by 75%. It cleanses the skin, helps it maintain elasticity, nourishes the skin, and balances the effects of skin flora. Turmeric inhibits the growth of a variety of bacteria, parasites, and pathogenic fungi. If you combine curcumin with black pepper, **it multiples the effectiveness fo curcumin by 1,000 times**.

Cayenne pepper ($6.15 per kg)

According to Dr. Soren Lehmann, *"Capsaicin (Cayenne pepper) had a profound anti-proliferative effect on human prostate cancer cells in culture. It caused 80% of the prostate cancer cells growing in mice to commit suicide in a process known as apoptosis."*. Studies done at the Loma Linda University in California found that Cayenne pepper may help prevent lung cancer in smokers (Capsaicin might help stop the formation of tobacco-induced lung tumours, as well as liver tumours). If cancer-fighting capabilities weren't enough, its effects upon the heart are nothing short of miraculous. It has been known to stop heart attacks in 30 seconds. Dr. John R. Christopher states: *"In 35 years of practice I have never on house calls lost one heart attack patient, and the reason is, wherever I go if (if they are stilll breathing) I pour down them a cup of cayenne tea (a teaspoon of cayenne in a cup of hot water) and within minutes they are up and around."*

Rubbed on the skin, cayenne is a potent remedy for rheumatic pains and arthritis due to what is termed a "counterirritant effect." Cayenne is also a great metabolic-booster, aiding the body in burning excess amounts of fats. Scientists at the Laval University in Quebec found that participants who took cayenne pepper for breakfast were found to have less appetite. Cayenne is also an excellent agent against tooth and gum diseases, and as a topical remedy it has been used to treat snake bites, rheumatism, sores, wounds and lumbago. Dr. Richard Schulze states: *"If you master only one herb in your life, master cayenne pepper. It is more powerful than any other."*

Maca ($44.20 per kg)

Maca is rich in vitamins B, C, and E, calcium, zinc, iron, magnesium, phosphorous and amino acids. Maca is widely used to promote sexual function of both men and women. It serves as a boost to your libido and increases endurance. Maca balances your hormones and increases fertility. It relieves menstrual issues and menopause. It alleviates cramps, body pain, hot flashes, anxiety, mood swings, and depression. It is also known for increasing stamina and energy levels, which is why many athletes take maca for peak performance. Maca supplies iron and helps restore red blood cells, which aids anemia and cardiovascular diseases. Maca keeps your bones and teeth healthy and allows you to heal from wounds more quickly. When used in conjunction with a good workout regime you will notice an increase in muscle mass.

Many people take maca for skin issues, as for some people it helps to clear acne and blemishes. If you find yourself overcome with anxiety, stress, depression or mood swings, maca may help alleviate these symptoms. Some have reported an increase in mental energy and focus.

Warning: If you are pregnant or lactating you should avoid taking maca. Be cautious if you have liver issues, high blood pressure, or a cancer related to hormones like testicular and ovarian.

Brahmi ($23.56 per kg)

Brahmi (*Bacopa monnieri*) is a perennial, creeping herb native to the wetlands of southern India. Plants like brahmi and turmeric have been studied extensively for their ability to fight discomfort and systemic inflammation. A study evaluating brahmi supplementation reported significant mood improvement among participants, as well as decreased levels of cortisol, the stress hormone. This suggests that brahmi counteracts the effects of stress by regulating hormones involved with the stress response. A placebo-controlled study of 24 volunteers reported that brahmi improved cognitive performance. This could be helpful for people suffering from "cognitive issues, short attention span, foggy memory, and blurred focus", as the study reported.

Moringa Oleifera ($49.36 per kg)

Moringa Oleifera is a drought-resistant tree, native to the southern foothills of the Himalayas in northwestern India. It is said to treat over 300 diseases. It has the ability to retain high concentrations of electrolyte minerals. Moringa Oleifera also contains the vitamins, minerals, fatty acids, phytonutrients, and antioxidants necessary to sustain life. Moringa Oleifera is one of the most nutrient-dense plant known to man. It contains all 9 essential amino acids (thee building blocks of protein), properly sequenced and in the optimal ratios, as well as 90 nutrients, 46 antioxidants, 36 anti-inflammatories, and more.

319

Bee Products

Bee Pollen ($15.48 to $58 per 1kg)

Bee pollen is one of the most complete foods available. This "nature's perfect food" contains all the ingredients necessary for a balanced diet, including at least 22 amino acids (including all eight essential amino acids that the body cannot manufacture for itself), 18 vitamins (including all of the B-complex vitamins, vitamin C, D, E, K, and beta Carotene vitamin A), 25 minerals, enzymes and co-enzymes, and plant-source fatty acids. It is also very high in protein and carbohydrates.

According to researchers at the Institute of Apiculture, Taranov, Russia, *"Honeybee pollen is the richest source of vitamins found in Nature in a single food."*

Similarly, Propolis is a resinous mixture that honey bees collect from tree buds, sap flows, or other botanical sources. It is used as a sealant for unwanted open spaces in the hive. Propolis contains all the known vitamins except vitamin K, and all of the minerals required by the body, except sulphur.

Note: do not give bee pollen, propolis, or raw honey to infants under 18 months old.

Royal Jelly ($36.05 per 50g)

Royal jelly is the extremely nutritious, creamy liquid secreted by the hypopharyngeal glands of the nurse bees. It transforms an ordinary female been into a "Queen Bee", increases her life span of three months to over five years, and enables her to produce twice her own weight in eggs each day (over 3,000 eggs).

Royal jelly is rich in protein, the B-complex vitamins, vitamin C, vitamin E, and inositol. It's a great supplement to use for stress reduction. In fact, it contains 17 times as much pantothenic acid (vitamin B5), which reduces stress, as that found in dry pollen. Royal jelly contains gamma globulin, known to stimulate the immune system and fight off infections. It also supplies the minerals, calcium, copper, iron, phosphorous, potassium, silicon, and sulphur the body needs.

Berries

Goji berries ($20.57 per kg)

Goji Berries contain an extraordinary amount of unique nutrients and anti-oxidants. Goji berries contain 18 amino acids as well as huge doses of vitamin A (beta carotene), B1, B2, B6 and vitamin E. Goji berries contain more vitamin C per ounce than any other food on Earth. Goji berries also contain more iron than spinach as well as 21 other key trace minerals. Goji's are extremely rich in the phytonutrient antioxidants lutein and zeaxanthin, which are important nutrients for eyes and the nervous system. Goji berries are also rich in unique compounds that enhance your immune system.

Li Ching Yuen in China lived to be more than 160 years old. He gathered herbs in mountain ranges and learned of their potency for longevity. He lived on a diet of herbs such as lingzhi (reishi mushrooms), goji berry, wild ginseng, he shoo wu, gotu kola, and rice wine. According to one account, *his diet consisted mainly of goji berries.* His advice on living a long life: *"Keep a quiet heart, sit like a tortoise, walk sprightly like a pigeon, and sleep like a dog."*

Blueberries ($45.62 per kg of fresh blueberries; $12.9 per kg of frozen blueberries)

Blueberries – as well as raspberries, strawberries, blackberries, and Açai Berries – are packed with antioxidants and phytoflavinoids. They are also high in potassium and vitamin C. They boost brain power, fight Alzheimer's, lower your risk of heart disease and cancer, and are anti-inflammatory. They contain a variety of phytochemicals and antioxidants. Berries are also rich in many vitamins and minerals including zinc, calcium, and magnesium. They also contain ellagic acid, a compound that prevents cellular mutations and is an anticarcinogen. Ellagic acid is a naturally occurring substance found in almost 50 different fruits and nuts (like red raspberries, strawberries, blueberries, grapes, pomegranates, and walnuts).

The Hollings Cancer Institute at the University of South Carolina conducted a nine-year study on 500 cervical cancer patients. The study, published in 1999, showed that ellagic acid stops mitosis (cell division) within 48 hours and induces apoptosis (normal cell death) within 72 hours, for breast, pancreas, skin, colon, oesophageal, and prostate cancer cells. According to British researchers, red raspberries also prevent heart disease.

Schizandra Berries ($43.48 per kg)

Schizandra berries contain essential oils, amino acids and lignans, vitamins A and C, chromium, phosphorus, magnesium, silica and beneficial fats and antioxidants. They are a powerful adaptogen, which is used as an overall wellness tonic, exerting a normalizing effect on the entire body. In China, it is said to be the most protective of all herbs and plants. Schizandra was prized for thousands of years by Chinese emperors as an anti-ageing tonic and for its stress and fatigue reducing properties. The ladies of the court used the berries as a beauty aid for the skin. Schizandra increases energy at the cellular level. It is popular with athletes as it boosts nitric oxide levels in the body and fights fatigue. Schizandra berry can also raise the body's enzyme *glutathione*, a powerful antioxidant that detoxifies the body and improves mental clarity. It is widely taken by students in China for this reason.

Probably its best known property is as a protector of the liver, due to the lignans it contains. It helps maintain its proper functioning and regeneration and is also used to prevent liver damage. This amazing herb also contains antioxidants, and is often used in longevity formulas in Chinese medicine. This herb is popular with people who suffer from mental disorders such as anxiety, depression and mood swings. There is some preliminary evidence that Schizandra may inhibit cancer cell growth for some types of cancers, such as leukemia. This herb may be beneficial for lowering blood pressure, improving circulation and improving heart function, and helping impotence and erectile dysfunction since it has the ability to dilate the blood vessels.

Warning: Schizandra should not be taken by people who have gastroesophageal reflex disease (GERD), epilepsy, peptic ulcers or high brain (intracranial) pressure. Do not take Schizandra if you are pregnant or nursing.

Baobab Fruit ($46.78 per kg)

The Baobab has been used medicinally for centuries. It is high in nutritional value, providing as many nutrients as goji berries, and more calcium than milk (295 mg per 100g). It has more iron than red meat, more potassium than a banana and more magnesium than spinach. The baobab tree is a powerhouse of minerals, supplying your body with calcium (30% of your Daily Value), copper (1.6 mg or 80% of your DV), iron (9.3 mg or 52% of your DV), magnesium (90 mg or 23% of your DV), potassium (1240 mg or 35% of your DV) and zinc (1.8 mg or 12% of your DV).

The baobab fruit is considered one of the very best food sources of vitamin C, with only a handful of foods – including kakadu plums, camu camu, acerola, and rosehips – beating this fruit in terms of vitamin C content. A 100-gram serving of baobab fruit pulp has been reported to contain up to 500 milligrams of vitamin C, ten times more than oranges. The Baobab fruit has 12 times more antioxidant properties than Strawberries, 35 times more than Kiwi, and 110 times more than oranges. It is possibly a preventive treatment for Heart Disease and varicose veins, and a natural liver cleanser and detoxifier. Baobab extract was found to have significant protective effects against liver damage, possibly due to the presence of triterpenoids, beta-sitosterol, beta-amyrin palmitate and ursolic acid in baobab pulp.

Algae & Seaweed

Chlorella ($42.57 to $75.95 per kg)

Chlorella is a "miracle whole food". In a Japanese study, scientists placed lab mice on a chlorella regimen for ten days and then injected the mice with three types of cancer. Amazingly, over 70% of the mice injected with chlorella did **not** develop cancer, while 100% of the untreated mice **did** develop cancer and died within 20 days. In his book *Treating Cancer with Herbs*, Dr. Michael Terra states: *"I recommend Chlorella to all cancer patients. It acts as both a powerful nutrient and a detoxifying food."*

Chlorella also helps in balancing your body's pH level, helps remove toxic heavy metals, and contains a wide array of vitamins, minerals, and enzymes. It also stimulates the production of red blood cells, and it is safe for children. In a study conducted on identical twins, the one given chlorella grew much faster, healthier, and had fewer sicknesses than the twin who was not given chlorella.

Kelp ($10 per kg)

Kelp is a seaweed that is extremely rich in nutrients, including more than 70 minerals, trace elements, enzymes, iodine, potassium, magnesium, calcium, iron and 21 amino acids. This complex range of nutrients assists of glandular health, and it is also a natural antibiotic because of its iodine content, which helps the body fight bad bacteria and infections. The large concentration of iodine found in Kelp helps to stimulate the thyroid gland and control metabolism. Other health benefits include strengthening of the circulatory system, strenghtening bones and teeth, cancer fighting benefits, and reducing the risk of strokes and heart disease.

Spirulina ($41.97 per kg)

This blue-green algae is a freshwater plant from Hawaii, similar to Chlorella. It detoxes heavy metals from your body, eliminates candida, helps prevent cancer (*"spirulina increases production of antibodies, infection-fighting proteins, and other cells that improve immunity and help ward off infection and chronic illnesses such as cancer"*, according to The University of Maryland Medical Center), it lowers blood pressure, prevents atherosclerosis and reduces blood cholesterol levels, boosts energy levels, speeds up weight loss (because it is a nutrient-dense protein-rich food), and alleviates the inflammation that causes sinus issues.

Essential Oils & Fats

Our body needs certain fats and oils. The 'Essential Oils', known as Omegas 3 and 6 are absolutely essential for every aspect of our health, from energy and stamina, to weight loss, brain function, heart health, the immune system, the skin, detoxification, digestion, and fertility. Fats are an essential part of each and every cell and without them we would not be able to survive. Essential Fatty Acids that you absorb from avocados or nuts and seeds, for example, are very good for you.

Udo's Oil

I highly recommend the 'Udo's Oil' supplement for optimum cellular health. Udo's Oil contains a 2-to-1 ratio of Omega 3 and Omega 6 fatty acids which is crucial for good health. Diets high in omega-3 fatty acids and lower in omega-6 fatty acids can contribute to a decreased risk of heart disease, autoimmune diseases, breast cancer and colorectal cancer. Your body can't make essential fatty acids on its own, which makes them a crucial part of your daily diet. In addition to reducing the risk of certain health problems, **essential fatty acids also help repair your cell membranes, which enables them to absorb the nutrients from the foods you** eat. Healthy cell membranes also help remove toxins and waste from your body. In addition, fatty acids help your cells communicate with one another so each of your bodily systems works properly.

Coconut Oil

Coconut oil is extremely rich in lauric acid, which is found in nature in human breast milk. Lauric acid is used by humans to destroy viruses, and various pathogenic bacteria and microbes such as yeasts, fungi, bacteria, parasites, and moulds.

In the 1930s, Dr. Weston Price travelled throughout the South Pacific, examining traditional diets and their effect on dental and overall health. He found that those eating diets high in coconut products were healthy and trim, despite the high fat concentration in their diet. Mary Enig, the USA's leading expert on fats, writes: *"The health and nutritional benefits that can be derived from consuming coconut oil have been recognized in many parts of the world for centuries… coconut oil provides a source of antimicrobial lipids for individuals with compromised immune systems."* According to Dr. Bruce Fife, *"coconut oil is the healthiest oil on earth."*

Olive Oil

Olive oil is the only vegetable oil that can be consumed fresh pressed, and it is the most prominent source of omega-9 fats, also known as oleic acids. We use olive oil extensively in our food.

The Top 12 Superfoods That Can Heal Your Entire Body

We love Aloe Vera, Wheatgrass, Sprouts, Turmeric, Nettles, Limu juice, Maca, Goji berries, Chlorella, Garlic, Bee Pollen, and Coconut!

Supplements, Vitamins & Minerals

Due to modern farming techniques, food processing methods, and the effects of cooking, our food is often stripped of vitamins by the time it reaches our plates. Furthermore, the human body requires small amounts of about 25-30 minerals (14-16 of which are considered to be "essential") to maintain normal body function and good health, but due to modern dietary habits and soils eroded by intensive agricultural practices, most of us are mineral deficient; hence the need for supplements.

Most vitamins require the presence of other nutrients to be utilized properly by the body. For this reason, it may be best to obtain vitamins from a whole food supplement or a multiple vitamin-mineral formula, rather than taking supplement forms of individual nutrients. Here are some of the supplements, vitamins, and minerals that I use on a regular basis.

MSM (methylsulfonylmethane; $19.06 per kg)

MSM (a.k.a. 'The Miracle Supplement') is an organic sulfur compound that's naturally derived during the earth's rain cycle. Sulfur is present in many natural unprocessed foods, but it's quickly lost during the cooking process. MSM improves skin health and complexion. MSM is necessary for collagen production. Sagging skin and wrinkles, as well as dry, cracked skin are all developed through a loss of collagen. MSM works together with Vitamin C to build new, healthy tissues. MSM can normalize collagen formation and radically improve skin health. It improves joint flexibility, and it helps to produce flexible skin and muscle tissue. MSM detoxifies the body, by allowing toxins and metabolic waste products to easily be moved out of the cells, while essential nutrients and hydration can be moved in. It's a calcium phosphate dissolver, so it has a remarkable ability **to break up the bad calcium that's at the root of degenerative diseases.** MSM strengthens hair and nails. It is a bonafide "beauty mineral" that provides the sulfur needed to produce collagen and keratin.

It's also highly noted to contribute to exceptional strength and thickness of the hair and nails. MSM accelerates healing by increasing the ability of the body to eliminate waste products at the cellular level. It naturally increases energy and increases the absorption of nutrients. Finally, MSM is a powerful anti-inflammatory due to its ability to allow metabolic wastes to be removed from the cells. Sulfur needs to be present In order for these toxins and wastes to be removed from the body. When these byproducts can be removed from the system, then the cells can also dispose of excess fluids that were being stored as a buffer, resulting in natural weight loss.

Colloidal Silver ($27.02 per litre)

Colloidal silver is a suspension of extremely fine particles of pure silver suspended in water by a positive electric charge on each particle. A powerful germicidal, silver is an exceptional metal in that it is non-toxic to a healthy cell but <u>lethal to over 650 disease-causing bacteria, viruses, fungi, parasites, and moulds</u>. The daily ingestion of small quantities of colloidal silver is <u>like having a "second immune system."</u> Ancient Greeks realized that families who used silver utensils were rarely sick and had few infections. This knowledge passed on to kings, emperors, sultans, and their families and members of their royal courts. They ate from silver plates, drank from silver cups, used silver utensils, and stored their food in silver containers…

Himalayan Pink Salt ($6.41 per kg)

Rich in Iodine, Himalayan Pink Salt contains more than 80 minerals and elements including: sulphate, magnesium, calcium, potassium, bicarbonate, bromide, borate, and strontium. These minerals help your body increase hydration, regulate water content both inside and outside of cells, balance your pH levels (alkaline/acidity) and help to reduce acid reflux, prevent muscle cramping, aid in proper metabolism functioning, strengthen bones, lower blood pressure, help the intestines absorb nutrients, prevent goiter, improve circulation, dissolve and eliminate sediment to remove toxins. It is also reported to reduce the signs of aging, and detoxify the body from heavy metals.

Note: commercial refined salt is not only stripped of all its minerals, besides sodium and chloride, but is also chemically cleaned, bleached and heated at unnecessary high temperatures. In addition, it is treated with anti-caking agents which prevent salt from mixing with water in the salt container. These agents also prevent dissolving within our system leading to build up and then deposit in organs and tissue, causing severe health problems. Finally, the iodine that is added into salt is usually synthetic which is difficult for your body to process properly. Shockingly under U.S. law, up to 2% of table salt can be additives.

Vitamin C ($72.24 per kg in powder form)

Vitamin C is proven to cure over 30 major diseases, including pneumonia, herpes simplex, encephalitis, herpes zoster (shingles), mononucleosis, pancreatitis, hepatitis, bladder infections, alcoholism, arthritis, some cancers, leukemia, atherosclerosis, ruptured intervertebral disc, high cholesterol, corneal ulcers, diabetes, glaucoma, etc. Vitamin C kills cancer cells while leaving normal cells alone.

Dr Linus Pauling and Dr. Ewan Cameron in 1976 reported that cancer patients treated with high doses of vitamin C had survived three to four times longer than similar patients who did not receive vitamin C supplements.

Studies show that intravenous vitamin C is the best protocol for destroying cancerous cells (but must be performed under the supervision of a doctor). The key is to be consistent with large quantities of vitamin C, taken several times every day. Vitamin C is a viable treatment for skin cancer. When vitamin C comes into contact with skin cancer, it hardens the tumour and forms a crust, such that the scab falls off in a couple of weeks or so.

Scientists from India have demonstrated how the incidences of tumours of the breast in rats can be reduced 88% by a single application of magnesium chloride, vitamin C, vitamin A, and selenium.

Dr. Archie Kalokerinos in Australia found that that children experiencing adverse reactions to vaccinations would recover after receiving large doses of vitamin C and the numbers of children who suffered adverse reactions declined dramatically when only healthy children who had taken large doses of vitamin C received vaccinations.

Combining Echinacea and vitamin C reduced cold incidence by 86%, while Echinacea alone reduced colds by 65%. A team of scientists from Arizona State University discovered that people with low blood concentrations of vitamin C burned 25% less fat during a 60-minute walk, compared with those who had adequate levels of vitamin C in their blood. The potential weight loss effects of vitamin C may be linked to the fact that it is needed for the production of carnitine, a compound that encourages your body to turn fat into fuel, rather than store it as body fat.

Warning: Most commercially available Vitamin C today comes from GMO corn and is made in Chinese chemical plants. It's not Vitamin C at all. It is "ascorbic acid" synthesized from corn syrup. Make sure you source Vitamin C from reputable, organic companies, or absorb it from dietary sources such as: camu camu, Baobab, Avocado, Echinacea, Cacao, dandelion, bee pollen, blueberrie and Goji berries, organic strawberries, acerola cherries, grapefruits and lemons, black currant, dark leafy greens, fresh herbs such as corriander, chives, thyme, basil, and parsley.

Copper

According to Dr. Joel Wallach, a copper deficiency can cause aneurysms. Copper deficiency in human beings presents itself first as white, grey or silver hair, as it is required as a cofactor to manufacture hair pigment. Additional symptoms include crow's feet, skin wrinkles, varicose veins, haemorrhoids, liver cirrhosis, and iron resistant anaemia. When humans supplement with plant derived colloidal copper, their original hair colour can come back. Iodine and copper deficiencies caused Goiter in adults and miscarriages. Cerebral palsy could be due to a copper deficiency.

Zinc

Zinc is the most abundant trace element in cells, and increasing evidence emphasizes zinc's important role in both genetic stability and function. Zinc is found in over 300 enzymes, including copper/zinc superoxide dismutase, which is an important antioxidant enzyme, and in several proteins involved in DNA repair. Zinc also helps to protect cellular components from oxidation and damage. In addition, Zinc is the transportation system for the disbursement of laetrile (vitamin B17) in the body, thus building up the immune system against cancer. *(Men lose 420 mcg of zinc per ejaculation)*. A deficiency of zinc or folic acid can result in a cleft palate or spinal bifida in a farm animal. According to Dr. Joel Wallach: *"[We saw] lions, wolves, monkeys, and parrots with Multiple Sclerosis, a calcium and magnesium deficiency. Cerebral palsy in a llama, a copper deficiency; spina bifida in a monkey, a folic acid or zinc deficiency; cleft palate in arctic foxes, a vitamin A or zinc deficiency; ventricular septal heart defect in a kangaroo, a vitamin A or zinc deficiency."*

Magnesium

Magnesium has an incredible healing effect on a wide range of diseases as well as in its ability to rejuvenate the aging body. Magnesium is essential for over 300 enzyme reactions (especially in regard to cellular energy production), for the health of the nervous system and brain, and also for healthy bones and teeth. Regions with soil rich in magnesium have less cancer than those with low magnesium levels, according to epidemiological studies. Scientists from India have demonstrated how the incidences of tumours of the breast in rats can be reduced 88% by a single application of magnesium chloride, vitamin C, vitamin A, and selenium. Magnesium is also essential in the area of detoxification, especially heavy metals. Low levels of magnesium can lead to fatigue. Multiple Sclerosis is due to a deficiency of calcium and magnesium, and Asthma is due to a deficiency of magnesium, manganese, and essential fatty acids, according to Dr. Joel Wallach.

Calcium

No other mineral is capable of performing as many biological functions as is calcium. This remarkable mineral provides the electrical energy for the heart to beat and for all muscle movement. It is also the calcium ion that is responsible for feeding every cell, a feat accomplished by latching on to seven nutrient molecules and one water molecule, pulling them through the nutrient channel, detaching the load, and repeating the process. **One common denominator which links all people who live past 100 years is that they all get massive amounts (over 5 grams) of calcium daily.** As important as all these and hundreds of other biological functions of calcium are to human health, none is more important than the job of pH control. It has been said that *"Calcium is to acid, what water is to fire."* Calcium quickly destroys oxygen-robbing acid in the body fluids. We learned the many deficiency diseases that occur when single and multiple nutrients were missing from a ration. Calcium deficiency alone could result in as many as 147 different diseases ranging from Multiple Sclerosis, osteoarthritis, osteomalacia, kidney stones, etc. If you sweat out all of your calcium, magnesium, and sulphur and don't replace them by supplementation, you are at high risk of developing arthritis, Multiple Sclerosis, and kidney stones. In the wild, rhinoceroses, elephants, and other animals spent a great deal of time eating clay termite nests and crushed limestone road beds for calcium and trace minerals. Once the calcium has been broken down, its absorption into the body is totally dependent on the presence of vitamin D in the intestine, so be sure to get plenty of natural sunlight. Note: milk actually depletes your calcium reserves and drinking milk can actually *cause* Multiple Sclerosis.

Also, it is important to AVOID calcium supplements, and get your calcium from dietary sources instead, as "bad calcium" can calcify your arteries. Personally, I get my daily calcium from leafy green vegetables, wheatgrass, Aloe Vera, baobab powder, walnuts, maca, cacao, kelp, and Himalayan pink salt. Dr. Joseph Mercola states: "Bad calcium deposits are like concrete, "hardening" your arteries. Robert Thompson, M.D. wrote a book on this subject called The Calcium Lie, which explains that bone is comprised of at least a dozen minerals, and the exclusive focus on calcium supplementation is likely to worsen bone density In order for calcium to do your body good, it must be in a bioavailable form and balanced out with vitamins D and K and other important trace minerals, as part of a total nutritional plan. Good sources include raw milk and cheese from pasture-raised cows (who eat the plants), leafy green vegetables, the pith of citrus fruits, carob, sesame seeds and wheatgrass, to name a few. **Calcium from dietary sources is typically better absorbed and utilized than calcium from supplements**, which is why studies involving calcium from natural food sources have shown favorable results, including a 25 percent lower risk of dying from all causes."

Vitamin D

You produce Vitamin D in your body naturally, by staying 15 to 30 minutes a day in the sun. Sunlight is actually *good* for you! But you can also supplement your Vitamin D intake. Vitamin D has been shown to cut cancer risk by 77%! It enhances calcium absorption, and reduces metastasis and proliferation. Researchers have found that complications of pregnancy, such as preterm labour, preterm birth, and infection were lowest in women with the highest vitamin D levels. Many people are reporting healing from Arthritis, Crohn's disease, fatigue, and a host of other conditions by taking extremely high doses of Vitamin D3 (from 5,000 to 30,000 IU per day or more). In Jeff Bowles' book *"The Miraculous Results Of Extremely High Doses Of The Sunshine Hormone Vitamin D3 – My Experiment With Huge Doses Of D3 From 25,000 To 50,000 To 100,000 IU A Day"*, he states that "Appropriate vitamin D supplementation makes most conventional drugs and treatments obsolete (e.g. Multiple Sclerosis, fibromyalgia, cancer, schizophrenia, psoriasis, or arthritis). Sufficient vitamin D prevents all kinds of cancer and even depression. Vitamin D is antiestrogenic, anticortisol, and it promotes an adrogenic metabolism of healthy hormones. Vitamin D deficiency exacerbates types 2 diabetes and impairs insulin production in the pancreas. Infants who receive vitamin D supplementation (2000 units daily) have an 80% reduced risk of developing type 1 diabetes."

I recommend also using Vitamin K2, together with Vitamin D. Dr. Joseph Mercola writes: "Vitamin K2 is Crucial if You Take Vitamin D and Calcium: Vitamin K2 engages in a delicate dance with vitamin D; whereas vitamin D provides improved bone development by helping you absorb calcium, there is new evidence that vitamin K2 directs the calcium to your skeleton, while preventing it from being deposited where you don't want it -- i.e., your organs, joint spaces, and arteries."

Iodine

Iodine deficiency leads to cancers of the breast, prostate, ovaries, uterus, and thyroid. It can also lead to mental retardation and infertility.

Dr. Randall Tent states in his lectures that some people may experience a lot more energy if they help their thyroid through Iodine supplementation.

Coenzyme Q10 (400mg 60 capsules $42.31)

According to Wikipedia, Coenzyme Q10 is a substance which resembles a vitamin, and that is present in most eukaryotic cells, primarily in the mitochondria. "It is a component of the electron transport chain and participates in aerobic cellular respiration, which generates energy in the form of ATP. 95% percent of the human body's energy is generated this way. Therefore, those organs with the highest energy requirements—such as the heart, liver, and kidney—have the highest CoQ10 concentrations."

CoQ10 therapy has proven to be quite valuable in treating neurologic disorders such as Parkinson's disease, Multiple Sclerosis, amyotrophic lateral sclerosis (Lou Gehrig's disease), Alzheimer's disease, Huntington's disease, and strokes.

In the 1970s Dr. Karl Folkers of the University of Texas encouraged a cardiologist to use CoQ10 to treat congestive heart failure, with great success. According to Dr. Peter Langsjoen, "The clinical experience with CoQ10 is nothing short of dramatic. It is reasonable to believe that the entire field of medicine should be reevaluated in light of this growing knowledge. We have only scratched the surface of the biomedical and clinical applications of CoQ10 and the associated fields of bioenergetics and free radical chemistry."

Dr. Karl Folkers also followed the course of six cancer patients who were taking CoQ10 for congestive heart failure. Four of them had lung cancer and two had breast cancer. All six experienced remissions of cancer due to CoQ10 therapy. One patients had small cell carcinoma of the lung with widespread metastasis. He was given less a year to live by his oncologist. After one year of CoQ10 use, he had no sign of metastases, and he was still alive 15 years later! The only therapy he used was CoQ10.

Dr. Folkers who died in 1998, recommended the use of 500 miligrams of CoQ10 dialy in patients with malignancies. You can buy CoQ10 at www.mercola.com and www.lef.org.

It is recommended that if you're over 30 years old, you should be taking a CoQ10 supplement daily, since the body's production of CoQ10 diminishes with age as does the ability to convert it into ubiquinol. You'll feel the difference right away in your energy and stamina.

According to Ty Bollinger, an excellent way to improve the absorption of CoQ10 is to put the capsules in a cup of hot tea, and add a reaspoon of coconut oil to the tea.

Glutathione (30 capsules 500mg, $17.86)

Glutathione is an important antioxidant that prevents damage to important cellular components caused by free radicals, peroxides, lipid peroxides and heavy metals. Studies have shown that our body's supply of glutathione begins to decline by 10% to 15% per decade starting at the age of twenty. <u>Individuals who have low levels of glutathione are susceptible to chronic illness</u>.

According to Dr. Mark Hyman, "Glutathione is the most important molecule you need to stay healthy and prevent disease. It is the secret to prevent aging, cancer, heart disease, dementia, and more, and necessary to treat everything from autism to Alzheimer's disease. There are more than 89,000 medical articles about it – but your doctor doesn't know how to address the epidemic deficiency of this crucial life-giving molecule.... This is the mother of all antioxidants, the master detoxifier, and maestro for the immune system." The secret of glutathione's potency lies in the sulphur chemical groups it contains. Sulphur is a sticky molecule that acts like "fly paper". As a result, all the "bad guys" in your body (like heavy metals and free radicals) stick to glutathione which then carries them into the bile and the stool, then out of your body. Sulphur-rich foods (like garlic, onions, and cruciferous vegetables) support glutathione production.

Carnivora™ ($39.95 for 100 capsules)

Carnivora™ is the 100% pure extract from the Venus Flytrap plant and was developed by Dr. Helmut G. Keller in the late 1970's in Germany. In 1985, following the removal of malignant polyps from his colon, US President Ronald Reagan sent to Nordhalben, Germany for an herbal extract of the Venus Flytrap to take as a preventative against the spread of cancer. Thereafter, he drank thirty drops of the extract in a glass of water or tea four times a day, and continued to do so until 1995.

According to Dr. Morton Walker, *"Dr. Helmut G. Keller now has more than three decades of lab analysis, clinical investigation, and treatment of about 15,000 cancer patients to back him up. This plant is packed with 17 different substances that boost your immune system."*

Dr. Keller's terminally ill cancer patients would receive one three-hour intravenous injection a day, often making remarkable recoveries.

In addition to cancer and HIV, Carnivora™ has been successful in treating Arthritis, Lyme disease, hepatitis C, Crohn's disease, lupus, chronic fatigue syndrome, ulcerative colitis, and Multiple Sclerosis. According to Dr. Dan Kenner, *"If I could only choose a single plant medication to use, the answer would be simple: Venus flytrap. Its extract is the most versatile plant-based substance for the treatment of chronic infections and degenerative disease that I have ever experienced."*

In 1988, the active component of Carnivora®, "plumbagin," was isolated. It powerfully stimulates the immune system.

Warning: do not take Carnivora if you are pregnant.

New Chapter™ Every Man's One Daily Multi ($42.13, 48 count)

There are many excellent multivitamins available out there. I use New Chapter's organic multivitamin and mineral supplement, made from organic vegetables and herbs. It includes: Vitamin A, C, D3, E, K, Thiamin, Riboflavin, Niacin, Vitamin B6, Folate, Vitamin B12, Iodine, Zinc, Biotin, Selenium, Copper, Manganese, Chromium, Molybdenum, Organic Schizandra berry, Organic Maca, Organic Chamomile, Fenugreek seed, Oregano, Grapeseed Extract, Hawthorn berry and seed, Elderberry Extract, Eleuthero root, Astragalus root, Ginger extract, and Turmeric.

Living Fuel™ ($97 for for 910gr)

Living Fuel's *Superberry Ultimate* is a blend of organic, all natural foods that have been optimized with the most bio-available and usable nutrients. It contains concentrated sources of vitamins, minerals, proteins, essential fats, enzymes, co-enzymes, herbs, botanical extracts, and soluble and insoluble plant fibres from fresh, high-quality, organic, non-GMO, nutrient-rich foods and supplements. This includes: protein from brown rice, a strawberry, raspberry, blueberry, cranberry complex, chia seeds, dulse and kelp sea vegetables, enzymes, probiotics, amino acids; herbs: turmeric, ginger, dandelion root, astragalus, milk thistle, chlorella, Gingko Biloba; Antioxidants: green tea extract, grape seed extract, Glutathione, Coenzyme Q10; 17 different vitamins added, and more than 12 added minerals. Living Fuel provides you with high quality nutrition and has more potassium than bananas, more calcium than milk, more fiber than oatmeal, more friendly bacteria than yogurt, more protein that six eggs, and more vitamins, minerals, and antioxidants than a whole day's supply of fruits and vegetables.

Beyond Greens™ ($123 per kg)

Udo's Choice Beyond Greens contains greens from barley, alfalfa, oat and rye grasses, plus spirulina and chlorella. These provide calcium, magnesium, zinc, copper, selenium, B-vitamins, carotene and vitamins C and E. It also contasins soluble fibre from brown flax seed, sesame seed, sunflower seed, oat bran, rice bran, golden flax seed, and psyllium husk (without adequate fibre intake, food takes much longer to go through the digestive tract, and stagnates). It also contains antioxidant-rich whole food concentrates and phytonutrients such as carrots, soy sprouts, kale, bilberry, cinnamon bark, ginger root, peppermint leaf, licorice root, red clover blossom, lemongrass, artichoke leaf, dandelion root and leaf, rosemary leaf, thyme herb, and standardized grape seed extract.

Digestive enzymes are included to help the body absorb nutrients to build cells, tissues, organs, glands and entire body systems.

Vitamineral Green™ ($64.95 for 500 gr)

Created by Dr. Jameth Sheridan, one of the early pioneers of the organic, holistic, and raw foods movements, *Vitamineral Green* contains Nettle Leaf, Carob Pod, Alfalfa Grass, Barley Grass, Oat Grass, Dandelion Leaf, Horsetail/Shavegrass, Ginger Root, Parsley Leaf, Wheat Grass, American Basil, Chickweed, Holy Basil/Tulsi, Moringa Leaf, Yacon Leaf, Amla Berry, Shilajit, Spirulina, Chlorella, Kelp, Dulse, Bladderwrack, Alaria, Wild Atlantic Nori, VMG™ Enzyme Concentrate, Probiotics, and magnetic and vibrational Energenesis™ Energetic Enhancements.

Marine Phytoplankton (30ml; $35.65)

Marine Phytoplankton is a micro-algae single-celled organism that is rich in trace minerals, DHA, EPA, chlorophyll, essential amino acids, carotenoids, antioxidants, nucleic acids and necessary vitamins. It helps cell regeneration, liver health, brain & heart health, increase energy, and slows down ageing. Certain strains of marine phytoplankton can be hundreds of times more potent than chlorella and spirulina. It is responsible for creating over 90% of the earth's oxygen supply. In fact, NASA called Marine Phytoplankton the most important plant in the world, providing almost all of the Earth's oxygen and serving as a vital food supply for marine life. It makes up about 25% of all vegetation on the planet. The presence of hundreds of synergistic elements in phytoplankton have led scientists to call it the future of natural medicine.

pHMiracle PuripHy (2oz, $53.95)

PuripHy by Dr. Robert O. Young is a combination of liquid sodium bicarbonate, potassium bicarbonate and potassium hydroxide. Just a few drops of puripHy acts as an antioxidant and oxygen catalyst, helping your blood absorb more oxygen from the water you drink. It is water purification in a bottle, neutralizing algaes, bacteria, yeasts, moulds, parasites, exotoxins, and mycotoxins. It is designed to raise the alkalinity of your water.

Doc Broc Power Plants Green Drink

This nutrient-rich, chlorophyll-rich, alkalizing supplement by Dr. Robert O. Young is made from Avocado, Cucumber, Tomato, Lemon, Lime, Broccoli Sprouts, Spinach, Celery, Parsley, Cabbage, Collard Greens, Okra, Kale, Soy Sprouts, Lemon Grass, Wheat Grass, Barley Grass, Shave Grass, Oat Grass, and Couch Grass. Created by low-heat dehydration, it preserves the nutrients of these living foods. One scoop provides the same benefit as consuming 14 pounds of greens.

Other superfoods

Garlic

Recent studies on garlic have shown that it kills insects, parasites, bad bacteria, and fungi. It also eliminates various tumours, lowers blood sugar levels, lowers blood sugar levels, lowers harmful fats in the blood, and prevents clogging of the arteries. It also acts as a very potent antioxidant.

Cooking kills garlic's cancer-fighting properties. <u>There are cases on record where cancer was beaten with a good detox program and garlic alone</u>. Here's a powerful anti-cancer concoction: blend up some ginger, onions, raw broccoli, and garlic juice. If you can stand the taste, it's one of the most potent cancer-fighting concoctions available.

According to www.NaturalNews.com, garlic's healing properties are so intense that <u>it is 100 times more effective than antibiotic treatments</u>. Other natural antibiotics to survive infections include: Oregano and oil of oregano, Raw apple cider vinegar, Honey, Turmeric, Grapefruit seed extract, Echinacea, Extra virgin coconut oil, Fermented foods, Colloidal silver.

Asparagus

Asparagus is loaded with nutrients: it is a great source of fiber, antioxidants, folate, vitamins A, C, E and K, as well as chromium. This herbaceous plant—along with avocado, kale and Brussels sprouts—is a particularly rich source of the detoxifying compound glutathione. Eating asparagus may help protect against and fight certain forms of cancer, such as bone, breast, colon, and lung cancers.

Quinoa

Quinoa is a seed which is prepared and eaten similarly to a grain. It is loaded with protein, fiber and minerals, but doesn't contain any gluten. It also contains iron, lysine, magnesium, vitamins B1, B2, and B6, manganese, copper, phosphorus, and zinc.

Coconut Water

Coconut water is rich in nutrients, including: calcium, magnesium, phosphorous, potassium, sodium. It reduces blood pressure. It clears up and tones the skin, moisturizing the skin from within and eliminating large amounts of oil. Because of its high concentration of fiber, it aids digestion and reduces the occurrence of acid reflux.

There are many more superfoods out there, for you to discover. Amla, Pomegranates, Mangosteen, Kale, Limu juice, Reishi mushrooms, live sprouts, and cloves are just some of the extremely nourishing superfoods available today. Why not try adding one new superfood to your diet a month?

Fermented Foods

Eat organic fermented foods and live sprouts often. *"Cultured vegetables are the ultimate superfood"*, says Dr. Joseph Mercola. Fermented foods are potent chelators (detoxifiers) and contain much higher levels of probiotics than probiotic supplements.

David Wolfe writes the following about the benefits of eating fermented foods such as raw cultured vegetables (sauerkraut, kimchi, etc.), Kombucha, fermented cheeses, or cultured milk from cow, goat, or nuts and seeds: "Fermented or cultured foods have a very high enzymatic activity and thus have been used by natural health pioneers to accelerate healing and disease recovery. The process of fermentation in foods involves "friendly" bacteria (like acidophilus and bifidus) eating up compounds in the food, therefore helping it become more digestible. Once the fiber in the food has been broken down, it takes on a bit of an acidic quality, which helps our stomach produce more stomach acid for digestion. Digestive power is going to determine how much nutrition we actually absorb and are able to utilize from the food we are eating. Raw fermented foods help promote the growth of healthy bacteria in the digestive tract, including the colon. They are an integral part of our immune system.

It appears that the excretions (enzymes, antiviral/antifungal agents, fatty acids, amino acids, essential sugars, vitamins, trace minerals, etc.) of the great probiotic bacteria (Lactobacillus acidophilus, Bifidus infantis, Lactococcus thermophiles, L. salivarius, L. plantarum, Enteroccus faecium, etc.) play a pivotal role in keeping us healthy, modulating immunity, and rejuvenating our body. [...] Fermented foods may be eaten with green leafy vegetables to calm digestion. Fermented and/or cultured foods of one sort or another play a role in keeping the body young."

What David Wolfe Travels With…

David Wolfe is the author of *Superfoods: The Food and Medicine Of The Future*. I came across an interesting short video about what he travels with when he is on the road: a Magic Bullet blender, cacao powder, Coconut oil, Agave nectar, Vitaminerals by HealthForce, Goji berries, Maca powder, almond powder, blueberries, cordyceps mushrooms powder, Oceans Alive 2.0 Marine Phytoplankton, nuts, pumpkin seeds, Island Fire fermented noni (includes Tahitian Noni, turmeric, cayenne, ginger, Apple cider vinegar, and 140 enzymes), sprouted flax seeds, avocadoes, greens and lettuce, lemons, kimchi (fermented sauerkraut), cilantro, dandelion greens, almond butter, apples.

Foods That Fight Cancer

Ty Bollinger writes in *Cancer: Step Outside The Box:* "Foods that fuel cancer [include] mycotoxins, acidic foods, sodas, sugar, trans-fats, coffee, MSG, sodium nitrite, aspartame, processed foods, foods with pesticides, pasteurized milk and cheese, refined flours, fluoride, chlorine, etc. Foods that **fight** cancer include spring water, apples and their seeds, apricots and their seeds, purple grapes and their seeds, raspberries, blueberries, strawberries, cantaloupe, carrots, broccoli, peppers, tomatoes, avocadoes, garlic, lemons, limes, coconut oil, flax seeds, flax oil, raw walnuts, chlorella, spirulina, herbs, etc. [...] The typical American diet contains about 95% of the foods that fuel cancer."

Buy Organic Supplements and Grow Your Own Food!

According to Mike Adams' forensic food laboratory, many popular vitamins advertised on television have copper levels so high that they may cause mental instability and psychosis. *"They are pushing synthetic chemicals under the guise of all-natural, healthy vitamins. In most cases, the companies that manufacture these vitamins are owned in part or in full by Big Pharma. Popular children vitamins sold on supermarket shelves are designed to encumber neurological development. Common dietary herbs sourced from China contain extremely high levels of lead."* Personally, I recommend organic supplements from New Chapter, Premier Research Labs, Standard Process, and Udos Choice, among others, as well as growing your own food.

Secrets For Maximum Nourishment

Eat "Live" Foods

Anything you put into your body must be *assimilated* or *eliminated*. Most people eat food that *drains them* of their life force. Their body has to work overtime to eliminate it, wasting the energy they have, instead of being *replenished* with energy!

Do you want to feel *alive*? Then eat *living foods*, that are water-rich, that contain high electrical vibration levels, and that contain essential enzymes and minerals and vitamins (e.g. fruits, vegetables, grasses). Nature intended for us to eat enzyme-rich natural foods. People that are incredibly vibrant and healthy are so because they consume *live* foods. It takes a lot less energy when your food is 'live' because the body can use it immediately. And it is more cleansing to the system, too. Most food we eat nowadays is incredibly clogging!

The majority of people today eat "dead food" that contains little to no nutrition whatsoever. And as if that was not bad enough, you cannot ingest dead substances without your body requiring immense amounts of energy to eliminate them. That's why many people need more than 6 hours of sleep and still feel tired.

If you cook your food, that's *dead* food you've got on your plate. Microwaving, for example, destroys 97% of nutrients in vegetables. Cooking vegetables destroys their enzymes. Ed Douglas, director of the American Living Foods Institute, states, *"The source of most health problems is what we eat. Whoever started cooking food 40,000 years ago didn't realize that we are not designed to eat cooked food. We're designed like other species to eat food in the raw form."*

The more your foods are cooked or processed the more nutrition they lose. Any food that you buy that comes in a package, a box, or in a jar is basically <u>dead food</u>. Any stored food loses most of its nutritional value after a few days. To *truly* get the most out of your vegetables and fruit you should grow them yourself and eat them "fresh from the vine".

Also, buy yourself a juicer *today*. Fresh vegetable juices in the morning are delicious, easy, quick to make, and are an absolute *gift* for your body!

Good Vibrations – Your Body Needs High-Energy Food

Your body operates on a subtle electro-magnetic current. Nerve signals are actually tiny *electrical charges*. Your cells communicate with each other through pulses of electricity. Your brain, your heart (in fact, all the organs in your body) emit these fields of electrical current. Even the nutrients you ingest are carried to your cells via electrical charges.

Foods only provide value when they can be converted into the elements necessary for your inner chemistry to continue producing electrical charges. <u>Foods with higher electrical vibration levels help us stay at the right vibration levels ourselves</u>. Are all foods equal in their electrical vibration levels? Absolutely not! You must avoid foods that take away more energy than they provide.

Each of the organs in your body needs to function at a certain level of electrical vibration (measured in megahertz) for it to be functioning healthily. The average for your core organs (your brain, your heart, and your lungs) is 70 MHz. If we eat something that is lifeless (where its electrical energy is vibrating at a very low frequency) then you are not going to get the energy that your body deserves. It is actually taking away more energy than it is giving.

Only 1 to 3 megahertz are available in chocolate cake. A Big Mac has 5 megahertz. Think about it. If your body needs to operate at 70 MHz and your primary diet is made up of Big Macs and chocolate cakes, are you going to be in a state of energy deficit or abundance?

When you are in deficit, you lack energy. The organs of your body will not be working at their total functional peak efficiency, and as those systems start to shut down, you build up more toxic waste than your body can naturally get rid of. Consequently, your body no longer has enough energy to function properly, and you begin the slow decline most people call 'ageing'.

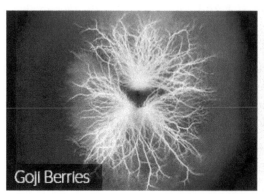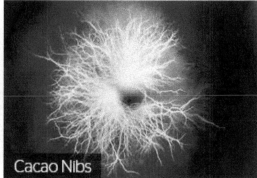

Kirlian photography of high vibrational frequency Goji berries and Cacao nibs

For total organ functional efficiency, you must cleanse your body, and provide your it with nutrients at high enough electrical frequency levels. Most supplements are in the 10-30 MHz range, and that's assuming your body can absorb them. Raw almonds have 40-50 MHz. Live fresh wheatgrass and green vegetables are in the 70-90 Mhz range. Cucumbers, too, are very high in vibrational energy. Furthermore, wheatgrass, cucumbers and green vegetables are extremely alkaline. Fruits provide a lot of energy too – they're 'alive'. But you want to eat them properly (on an empty stomach, and not combine them with protein, for example). Dr. Robert O. Young's "Supergreens" powder, made up of over 40 grasses, is extremely alkaline and is apparently in the 250 to 350 MHz range.

Bruce Tainio is a microbiologist who studied *vibrational therapy*. He claims that **a healthy person's body generates a frequency range of 62 to 78 MHz**. According to Tainio, disease starts at 58 MHz, the human body is receptive to Cancer at 42 MHz, and death begins at 25 MHz.

Dr. Royal Raymond Rife's research indicated that every single disease has a specific frequency. He claimed that if researchers could discover the specific frequency of a disease, vibration therapy could cure it. In the early 1900s he showed that by exposing microorganisms such as viruses and bacteria to certain frequencies he could destroy them without harming healthy cells and tissues. His 'Rife machine' is believed to have cured many diseases in his patients, including cancer. Dr. Hulda Clark seems to have continued Rife's and Tainio's research, and it appears she has had quite a bit of success in curing people. Change your frequency, and you can't have that disease anymore.

The takeaway point is this: if you want to be healthy, move away from things that lower your vibrational frequency, and **move towards things that *raise* your vibrational frequency**. As professor William Tiller stated: *"Future medicine will be based on controlling energy in the body."*

Invest In Some Quality Supplements

The better your nutrition, the better your self-healing ability, the better your mental function, your immune system, nervous system, cardiovascular system, and skeletal system; the function of every organ in your body will also improve – heart, kidney, brain, liver, pancreas, colon etc. Nutrition is a vital area to study if you choose to lead a healthy life.

I strongly urge you to invest in some quality nutritional supplements. *"But that's expensive"*, I hear some of you moan. Expensive? Compared to what? How much does it cost you to suffer from Cancer, heart disease, diabetes, arthritis, Multiple Sclerosis, fibromyalgia, gout, impotence, Alzheimer's, Parkinson's, Multiple Sclerosis…? Think of the pain involved. Think of the tens (hundreds) of thousands of dollars in medical bills incurred, lost productivity, years, decades of your life cut short…

What is your life worth? What are 20 years of life actually worth to you?

Prevention through proper nutrition is a bargain, trust me.

Food Combining: Don't Mix Protein With Carbohydrates

To really get *the most* out of your food, you need to properly combine your foods. The key lesson here is simply: do <u>not</u> mix carbohydrates with proteins. This comes down to fundamental bio-chemistry. Carbohydrates require *alkaline* digestive juices to break them down. Proteins are digested with the use of *acidic* digestive juices (Hydrochloric Acid). When you eat proteins and carbohydrates at the same time (say, potatoes + a steak) these different digestive juices **neutralise** each other but the food still needs to be digested. Your body uses immense amounts of nerve energy every time it does this – and your food is *still* not fully digested! As a result, the carbohydrate ferments, and the protein putrefies – drastically slowing down your digestion, and your body has used up huge amounts of energy in the process.

Forget how you've been taught to eat in your culture, this is how your body actually *works*. If you *don't* follow this guideline, you will have taken a 3-hour digestive process and extended it to 11-14 hours. All night long, instead of resting, your body will be working overtime to break down this food, usurping your energy. Use your common sense. Look at nature: animals eat just *one* concentrated food at a time. *Don't let food become recreation instead of nutrition!*

Also, only eat *comfortable* amounts of food. Don't force yourself if you are not hungry. And please, whatever you do, *don't eat while you are stressed*. Stress instantly stops the normal secretion of digestive enzymes. Whatever you eat will either ferment or putrefy (it will rot in your system).

Don't Drink While You Eat

Drink water *before* your meals, not during or after. Drinking water during or right after your meal will hamper your digestion as it dilutes your digestive fluids and your body then needs to produce extra digestive juices to get the same job done. So wait at least 20 minutes after a meal before drinking.

Check Your Levels Of Nutrition

Before embarking on this new *superfood* and supplementation lifestyle, I highly recommend you do some tests to find out what minerals and vitamins are lacking in your body. You can do a hair analysis, a food sensitivity analysis, a heavy metals test, a test to check out your hormone levels, and for more in-depth analysis contact Dr. George Georgiou at www.naturaltherapycenter.com, Dr. Raj at www.sainutrition.com, or Cliff Wilde at www.WildePerformance.com. In any case, considering the reduced levels of nutrition in our modern food, you should at the very minimum take an organic, natural multivitamin every day.

A food sensitivity test conducted by Dr. Georgiou revealed that my immune system reacted to All **Dairy**; **Potato**, Tomato, Aubergine, Red/Green Pepper, Mushrooms; **Sugar**; All **Gluten**: Wheat, Bread, pasta, oats, barley, rye; Yeast (it's a good thing that I cut out Sugar after watching the documentary *That Sugar Film* and I cut out bread and pasta shortly thereafter); **Avocado** (I had been eating an avocado a day for far too long!); Orange, **Lemon**, Grapefruit (I had been using lemon juice in my water for far too long!); **Chocolate**/Cocoa, Tea, Coffee; All Alcohol (I never drink alcohol nor tea or coffee, but chocolate was definitely a weakness!)

CHAPTER 29

Hydrate Your Way To Health

Water is only below oxygen in its value and importance, and can have a major impact on your health. It is absolutely critical to life. It is critical to your blood and to your cells as it helps transport nutrients and oxygen through your blood to every cell in your body. It is also the #1 way to cleanse the body. Without water, you *clog up*, and this creates major health problems. This is why *"Pee Your Way To Health"* is one of Dr. Robert O. Young's mottos.

Water is involved in every reaction in the body – most chemical reactions in the body can only be carried out if the reacting substances are dissolved in water. Water is also an actual ingredient in many bodily reactions. Water is essential for the blood to flow, and for messages to pass along our nerves. Our bodies *can* operate on a low ration of water, but this means that every function in the body is slowed and reduced in efficiency. Because we are losing water constantly when we sweat, breathe and eliminate waste, and we are too busy to take a sip of water throughout the day, most people are constantly in a state of dehydration.

A person is dehydrated long before they feel 'thirsty'. The body is programmed for survival at the minimum level of hydration, so it will start to shut down systems that are not absolutely and immediately essential to life. Mental clarity is the first thing that goes. Closely followed by your digestive process. It is not long before the body starts to overheat. Constantly depriving yourself of water is a certain recipe for disaster.

Are you constantly tired? Do you get headaches or just feel sluggish? Do you wonder why you are not as clearheaded as you used to be and can't seem to think straight? Are you dogged by constipation? Are you overweight? Chances are that you are dehydrated. Drinking enough water can clear up many of the above symptoms. You will have more energy, and more mental clarity, for starters.

Your Body's Many Cries For Water

Dr. Fereydoon Batmanghelidj was born in Iran. When the Iranian Revolution broke out in 1979, he was thrown into Evin Prison for two years. It was there he discovered

341

the healing powers of water. One night, he had to treat a fellow prisoner with crippling peptic ulcer pain. With no medications at his disposal, Dr. Batmanghelidj gave him two glasses of water. Within minutes, his pain disappeared. He was instructed to drink two glasses of water every three hours and became pain free.

He successfully treated 3,000 fellow prisoners suffering from stress-induced peptic ulcer disease with water alone. While in prison he conducted extensive research into the medicinal effects of water in preventing and relieving many degenerative diseases. In 1992, he stated in his book *Your Body's Many Cries for Water* that dehydration actually produces pain and many degenerative diseases, including asthma, arthritis, hypertension, angina, adult-onset diabetes, lupus and Multiple Sclerosis. His message to the world is, *"You are not sick, you are thirsty. Don't treat thirst with medication."* (Read more at www.watercure.com).

You should be drinking approximately 1.5 to 2 litres of water per day. And I am talking about *water*, here – not tea or coffee which actually *de*-hydrate you. I start my day with a glass of water with some lemon juice. This hydrates the body after many hours without water, and helps cleanse and alkalize my bloodstream. Keep yourself hydrated throughout the day. Drink only water, herbal teas, and juices you've made yourself from organic produce. Also, eat 70% water-content food (fresh vegetables and greens), as this facilitates your digestion.

Can Drinking A Gallon Of Water Every Day Make You Healthier?

The freelance writer Wil Fulton recently took on a 30-day challenge that involved drinking one gallon (3.8 litres) of water per day. He kept his expectations low when he started, but the results really surprised him.

Five days into the challenge, he found that – apart from having to urinate frequently – he was eating a lot less food and yet he felt full most of the time. By day 10, he noticed that his hair was shinier, his complexion had improved, and he felt 'handsomer'.

He also slept better, he felt more refreshed when he woke up, and didn't need to rely on coffee to get through the day. His thinking was clearer. He felt much more *energy*. He was even running a little *faster* during his evening jog. (Source: www.thrillist.com/drink/nation/i-drank-a-gallon-of-water-a-day-for-30-days-water-gallon-challenge).

While drinking 3.8 litres a day might be a bit extreme, perhaps doing this for 30 days is quite detoxifying. I personally drink 2.5 litres of water every day, with lemon juice added to alkalize it, and another litre of "Green Juice" (my daily avocado smoothie).

CHAPTER 30

Get Plenty of Rest and Avoid Stress

Your body needs rest. That much is obvious, of course, but you would be surprised at how many people burn the candle at both ends. The motto *"Work Hard, Play Harder"*, or *"Work Hard, Party Harder"* is a recipe for burnout and crippling health problems by the time you reach your forties.

It is important you go to sleep early, and **get quality rest,** with no electronics around you, and fresh air coming into your room. Do not eat after 6pm, as your body will actively be trying to digest your food throughout the night, rather than restoring you, and rejuvenating your cells. Also, avoid or **reduce stress to a minimum**.

Stress has your body in *fight or flight* mode, ready to run away or fight off a danger. Your blood flow is focused on your arms and legs, and adrenaline and cortisol floods your body. This shuts down your digestion, toxicity accumulates, and this impacts your general health in the ways we have described previously.

Stress has been linked to cancer, lung disease, fatal accidents, suicide and cirrhosis of the liver. Researchers at Johns Hopkins University have discovered that children exposed to chronic stress are more likely to develop a mental illness. Stress can affect a man's body weight, testosterone levels, sexual desire, and even lead to impotence. High levels of stress in pregnant women may also trigger changes in their children, specifically behavioural and developmental issues.

Stress damages your heart (stress hormones increase your heart rate and constrict your blood vessels). This forces your heart to work harder and increases your blood pressure. Stress **weakens your immune system**, and **is a major contributor to premature ageing** (wrinkles, weak muscles, poor eyesight and more).

Eat in a relaxed state. Turn the TV off, and eat slowly, chewing your food well. Chew your food properly and eat slower. Focus only on your food, this means turning off the TV and getting rid of all other distractions. When you eat, make sure you do JUST that. DO NOT eat on the run. Sit down and eat your food to help you notice how much of what you're actually eating. Have your smallest meal in the late afternoon or early evening, NOT the other way around.

How to reduce your stress levels:

☐ Find your purpose. Do what you truly love. What is your passion? What is your *unique ability?*

☐ Simplify your life; eliminate the clutter in your life.

☐ Meditate for 15-20 minutes twice a day.

☐ Adopt a spiritual understanding of life. Let go of the illusion that anything in the Universe is not exactly as it should be…

☐ Educate yourself about wealth creation and master your finances – keep a budget, spend less than you earn, and invest the difference. Financial abundance cuts out a lot of sources of stress, typically.

☐ Turn down the noise; minimize your time spent watching TV and using the Internet to help reduce aural and mental clutter in your life.

☐ Plan ahead and make sure you're always on time or at least 15 minutes early for appointment. This helps reduce stress that can arise from traffic or underestimating travel times. Ultimately, it allows you to slow down and focus before an event.

Meditate

Close to 600 scientific studies have shown that meditation brings **distinct improvements in health,** including a decrease in **Stress** and **anxiety** levels, sleep improves, vitality and **energy** levels increase, the **ageing** process slows down, blood pressure normalizes, chronic illnesses decrease, and creativity and the ability to **focus** and think clearly increases.

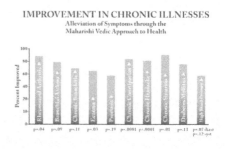

I rest my body twice a day, for 15-20 minutes at a time, with a quiet meditation. This allows me to slow down, take deep diaphragmatic breaths, visualize my perfect outcome, connect to nature, connect to my Oversoul and reminded myself of the spiritual nature of the world – and of *me* – and connect to what I feel *gratitude* for.

I started meditating after seeing an interview with Jerry Seinfeld, the comedian. I thought to myself, "*He looks great for a guy in his forties…*". Imagine my surprise when I looked him up on Google and found out that he is *sixty years old!* I had the same reaction when a couple of days later I found out that the British singer *Sting* is also in his sixties (though he looks like he's in his forties as well). What do they have in common? They both meditate. :)

"More than money, more than love, more than just about anything, I love ENERGY. I love it and I pursue it, and I want more of it. Physical and mental energy to me is the greatest riches of human life. And transcendental meditation is like this free account of an endless amount of energy. It is like your body is a mobile phone, someone hands you a charger for the first time, and you go 'Oooh, so THAT'S how it's supposed to work!'"

Jerry Seinfeld, comedian

CHAPTER 31

Exercise and Oxygenate!

Your cells require oxygen, nutrients, and the ability to eliminate their own waste. How does your body eliminate that metabolic waste? As I explained in earlier chapters, your lymphatic system is the **'sewage system' of the body**, draining your body of waste and toxicity. Although you have 4 times more lymph than you have blood in your body, it has no 'pump' (the bloodstream has the *heart*). The only way your lymph system can *circulate* is through physical movement and deep diaphragmic breaths. This is why exercising and playing sports helps your body **detoxify** (it helps **oxygenate** your bloodstream, to boot). This is why studies show that sitting all day is one of the worse things you can do for your health, and why 1 in 3 Americans get cancer, but only 1 in 7 American *athletes* do.

I spend a lot of time at my laptop, but I make sure I use my **rebounder** and go for walks twice daily.

Rebounding increases lymph flow by up to 30 times, and helps keep your blood cells healthy (rather than slamming into each other, they bounce around more freely).

Studies have shown that <u>cancer cells cannot thrive in an oxygenated environment</u>. Dr. Otto Warburg, a cancer biochemist and the 1931 Nobel Laureate in Medicine, discovered that **cancer occurs whenever any cell is denied 60% of its oxygen requirements**. Exercising daily, and deep breathing, help to get more oxygen down to the cellular level. This is why it is vital that you have a physically active life. This is a *must* if you want to be healthy and avoid diseases.

Health basically comes down to *Energy*. Energy is created at a cellular level, and cells need a lot of OXYGEN in order to create the ATP (Adenosine TriPhosphate) that fuels the body. Without ATP our bodies would immediately shut down, and without oxygen, there would not be any ATP. Consequently, **optimal oxygenation of your cells**, through proper nutrition, exercise, and fluid intake is absolutely vital when it comes to experiencing vibrant levels of Health. And we can increase the amount of oxygen that gets to our cells through Movement and Deep Breathing. It is worth noting that the longest-living populations in the world (the "Blue Zones") **exercise moderately every day**.

Energizing Breathing

Oxygen is the number one thing that cells use and *must* have, and the major factor of how much oxygen we get is *the way we breathe*! Most of us are so stressed that we don't allow ourselves to have a full breath. Lymphologist Dr. Jack Shields discovered that **a deep diaphragmic breath** sucks the lymph up the thoracic tract and stimulates the lymph in your body (thus *cleansing* you) 10 times more than through any other normal activity! This is the equivalent – metaphorically speaking – to taking a vacuum cleaner to your bloodstream and sucking out all the poison. When you are tired your body makes you *yawn* in order to get much more oxygen into your body! If you breathe deeply 10 minutes every morning you will experience a huge shift in your energy levels, thanks to your lymph system being stimulated and the consequent cleansing effect for your body.

The cells that take in the most oxygen into your body are reached through deep diaphragmic breaths. It opens up the lower lungs, where the richest blood flow is. Shallow breathing can give you stomach upsets and heartburn, panic attacks, chronic or intermittent fatigue, chest pains and palpitations, tingling and numbness in the arms and legs, muscular cramps, hallucinations, nightmares, etc.

Aerobic Exercise

Aerobic Exercise is critical to your health. This is because Aerobic Exercise relates to your body's ability to carry **oxygen**. Training yourself aerobically does wonders for your heart, it helps you eat better, digest better, circulate nutrients better, eliminate waste better, it makes your lungs operate more efficiently, your blood vessels become enlarged, and your blood supply increases, and it helps you sleep better. In fact, exercising aerobically stimulates your entire system.

A diminished blood supply causes cells to weaken, because less oxygen flows to your cells. But if you train in a gentle, comfortable, aerobic fashion for a period of 6-9 weeks, you can increase our blood supply considerably. When you increase your aerobic capacity, **you will have a lot more energy**, because you will have a lot more oxygen available. You must exercise aerobically so that you have enough blood to keep every cell in your body completely vital and *alive*. Try it for 10 days.

The Benefits of Aerobic Training

According to Anthony Robbins' training course titled *Living Health,* daily aerobic exercise provides you with the following benefits:

❑ Your lungs operate more efficiently.

❑ Your blood vessels become enlarged, making them more pliable and reducing the resistance to blood flow. Your oxygen supply increases, especially the red blood cells and haemoglobin.

❑ It reduces your risk of dementia, Alzheimer's and Parkinson's. Aerobic exercise helps to encourage regular brain function, and can help keep the brain active.

❑ Beat cancer patients who walk or do other kinds of moderate exercise for three to 5 hours a week are about 50% less likely to die from breast cancer than sedentary women.

❑ Aerobic training creates healthier body tissues that can supply more oxygen.

❑ It develops the heart into a strong and healthy muscle that works more efficiently.

❑ It helps you eat, digest, and eliminate waste better.

❑ It helps you sleep better. People who exercise regularly tend to sleep better than those who don't. They usually fall asleep more quickly, sleep more deeply, and awake less often.

❑ It enhances your outward appearance. Aerobic exercising can help you look toned and fit, and keep your body at a healthy weight.

❑ It may even make you feel better mentally and emotionally! Researchers found that an hour of aerobics reduced tension, anger, and fatigue, especially among those who felt depressed.

❑ The human body is designed to develop and maintain itself *through motion!*

'Being Healthy', by the way, means having all the systems in our body (the muscular, nervous, circulatory, digestive, lymphatic, and hormonal systems) working *optimally*. It does *not* mean only 'Having Great Muscles'. So don't go out and 'murder' yourselves at the gym. If you are exercising with pain, and you do not have a solid aerobic base first, you are making a huge mistake.

Take Care of Your Spine

Nerve impingement is a further source of disease. Your nervous system sends messages across your entire body (e.g. *'There's a challenge here, send help!'*), through your spine and your nerve connections.

Very often certain aspects of our spine become 'mis-aligned', which puts pressure on some nerves. Our nerve flow of information and energy is then reduced. Go see a **chiropractor** for an adjustment a couple of times a year, and do **yoga** – the more flexible you are, the more energy and vitality you have. I practice Yoga, and I always feel much better and freer in my body when I do.

"You are only as old as your spine. if your spines are rigid, so are your bodies and minds."

Paul Bragg, father of the Natural Health Movement

CHAPTER 32

The Truth About Obesity and Weight Loss

Many obese people are actually *starving*. Their food is so lacking in essential minerals that they eat and eat and never feel full. They are starved of minerals and vitamins. Changing your diet to eating greens, whole foods, and consuming nutrient-dense superfoods goes a long way towards maintaining a healthy weight.

But that is just one factor. According to Dr. Robert O. Young (author of *Sick And Tired* and *The pH Miracle for Weight Loss*), when you are too toxic and too acidic **your body creates fat reserves to preserve the integrity of your organs and tissues.** The excess acidity would otherwise eat away at your tissues and even your *brain*, destroy your cells, and affect your body's ability to maintain an inner pH level of 7.36 (which is slightly alkaline). When you detoxify and alkalize, by eating a diet that is 70% to 80% greens and vegetables), your body naturally eliminates the excess fat reserves on your body, with no effort.

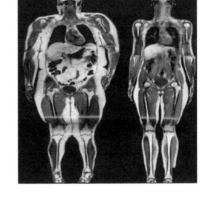

According to Dr. John Bergman, being obese is actually an **inflammatory response** to environmental stimuli: the poisons in vaccines, pesticides, our food, our water, our personal care products, cleaning products etc. are causing inflammation of the cells in your body – and your body responds by diluting this toxicity by withholding water and by **storing these toxins away in your fatty tissue** until it has enough energy to break them down and eliminate them from your system.

Forget about "calorie counting". You are NOT fat because you "eat too many calories". That is a falsehood of monumental proportions, designed to hide the truth. The truth is that most of what you eat is full of *sugar* AND completely devoid of nutrition.

I highly recommend Damon Gameau's documentary *That Sugar Film* where he reveals how food manufacturers <u>have put sugar into nearly 80% of all the products</u> at your grocery store. He states:

"After sugar enters the body, it splits into two parts... fructose and glucose. Both of which make their way to the liver. Now, once in the liver, the glucose is dealt with efficiently. It's either used immediately for energy or it's stored for later, like a spare battery. But the fructose half of sugar is very different. The liver doesn't have a system to regulate the fructose because it was so rare in nature, so it hoovers it out of the bloodstream whether it needs it or not. And if all our spare batteries are full, <u>then it rapidly turns it into fat</u>. Some of that fat is going to stay in the liver and you're going to have increased risk for insulin resistance and diabetes. [...] So when we're eating lots of sugar, we're putting fat into our bodies via the fatty liver. Plus, because of all the glucose, we maintain the level of insulin, which tells our fat cells to hold on to the fat. We can't burn off fat when insulin is around dealing with all the sugar! This is what may be happening to a huge number of the population."

Excess weight is actually due to *inflammation*. People are overly toxic, overly acidic, filled with chemical toxins from vaccines, they don't exercise so their lymphatic flow is stilted, they eat processed foods devoid of any nutrition and that are filled with **sugar** (which destroys your health in over 100 different ways, *and* is stored away as **fat**), they don't have the *energy* to get rid of all this gunk… and then we wonder why we have an obesity epidemic on our hands!

CHAPTER 33

How to Experience 300% More ENERGY

'Chronic Fatigue Syndrome' affects up to 4 million people in the US, and over 250,000 people in the UK. Tens of millions of people around the world feel "tired all the time". But if you do the things we recommend in this book, your energy levels will *take off* and you'll be bouncing off the walls in no time. Here are some specific recommendations to increase your energy levels:

Nutrition

❑ Cut out foods that *rob* you of energy: **cut out sugar; cut out coffee**; cut out sugary drinks (soft drinks, ice tea, coca cola, "energy drinks" etc.); **cut out dairy products** (milk, yoghurt, ice cream...); **cut out wheat products; cut out processed foods** (any food sold in a tin, box, etc.)

❑ **Eat healthy fats** like nuts, avocado, salmon; get plenty of Omega 3, 6, and 9 (I recommend 'Udos Oil'); Eat more vegetables and salads – especially green, leafy vegetables; Eat **fruit**, in moderation; **Eat nutrient-dense foods**… lentils, beans, quinoa, nuts, superfoods…; Consider making yourself a 'Green Juice' for breakfast; Consider going organic and eating *clean* meat;

❑ **Food combining**: do not eat *protein* and *carbohydrates* together. It makes for inefficient digestion, food rots in your stomach, it takes longer to digest, and drains your body of energy.

❑ Do **a 30-day DETOX** (eliminate the toxins that have built up in you over the years).

❑ Take an organic **MULTIVITAMIN** every day.

❑ Check your thyroid. Take an **Iodine** supplement daily and see your energy levels take off.

❑ Your cells require oxygen and nutrients to product the Adenosine Triphosphate that powers your body (i.e. to produce ENERGY). GIVE YOUR CELLS MUCH BETTER NUTRIENTS! Consume 5 to 10 times better *nutrition!*

Hydration

☐ **Keep hydrated**, with *water*, so that your bloodstream can bring oxygen and nutrients to your cells more efficiently and for your liver and kidneys to detoxify your body more easily. A survey of 300 GPs in the UK has found that **a fifth of all doctor's appointments are down to tiredness and fatigue**, a syndrome which is known as TATT (Tired All The Time). *"I see many people in my surgery who are feeling tired all the time. There are, of course, several reasons, but **a surprisingly common cause is that they are dehydrated**,"* writes Dr. Roger Henderson.

Mindset

☐ **Are you doing what you love?** Do you love *what you do?* Do you have an exciting, inspiring, motivating *purpose* in life right now? Do you have a burning desire that gets you excited about getting up in the morning? What would you *love* to be doing with your life instead?

☐ Anthony Robbins states: "Where does ENERGY come from? Sleep? Food? NO! It comes from being excited! Having a compelling vision for your future! Having compelling goals that get you excited about getting up in the morning!"

☐ According to Richard Moat, the **psychological and emotional *root causes* of fatigue** are: missing a sense of purpose; avoiding responsibility; feeling worn out from trying too hard; over-giving and under-taking.

☐ Are you feeling depressed? Are you sad about something? Aside from the fact that anti-depressants cause fatigue and a host of other negative side-effects, affecting the chemical balances in one's body (dopamine, endorphins, serotonin), a depressed state of mind can drain you of energy faster than anything.

☐ Stress and *fear* drain us of energy too. They depress our immune system. How can you move your life **from a vibration of *fear* to a vibration of LOVE and GRATITUDE?**

☐ Be more giving to yourself, take care of your own needs as well.

☐ Use daily **affirmations** such as: *I Am Amazing! I Am Inspiration! I Am Power! No Matter What I Have Done Or Not Done I Am Worthy Of Love! Every Day, In Every Way, I Am Healthier & Stronger! Every Day In Every Way I Am Better & Better! I Am Vital, Healthy, Energetic, and Productive! I Have Boundless Energy! I Love My Life!*

☐ **Visualize** yourself with boundless energy, happiness, and vitality. Also, visualize the 'Power Archetype' in *red* in every cell of your body: ⋀

Exercise & Oxygenation

- ❑ Exercise at least 20 minutes a day. Move your body. Your lymphatic system is responsible for eliminating toxins from your body, and it relies on you *moving your body* to operate effectively. *Sitting* all day long could be one of the biggest killers out there!

- ❑ Aerobic exercise increases the blood supply in your body, making more oxygen and nutrients available to your cells!

- ❑ Use a rebounder! Rebounding has been shown to increase lymph flow by up to 30 times.

- ❑ Get plenty of clean air into your lungs. Take deep diaphragmic breaths.

Remove "Energy-Vampires"

- ❑ Do you have 'energy-vampires' around you? Remove from your life negative people that drain your energy, put you down, put out 'negative vibes', make you sad, etc. Life is too short.

- ❑ Cut out TV watching. Instead, spend time playing sports or with people you love!

- ❑ Don't watch the news, don't read magazines or newspapers (cut out exposure to advertising).

- ❑ Take action and complete your tasks. Confront whatever or whoever you need to confront, even if you are afraid of conflicts. Procrastination and "incompletions" drain you of energy.

Detoxify Your Body To Get a Good Night's Sleep

- ❑ Cut out toxic chemicals from your environment and *food*; phase out pharmaceutical drugs.

- ❑ If you don't sleep well at night, I guarantee you that you are 'toxic'. One of the reasons people don't sleep well is because they've clogged themselves up with so much junk that their body is working overtime to carry oxygen through.

- ❑ Most people's diets require their body to work overtime during the night, to break down all the junk they have put in there. As a result, they wake up still feeling tired, because although they have *slept*, their body did not rest. And since there is no lymph flow when you're sleeping, your cells are 'screaming' from all the toxins inside of you! As a result, you toss and turn to try and move yourself, in order to help circulate the lymph.

355

❑ What you need to do is breathe properly and super-hydrate (to cleanse your body), and make sure you get some aerobic exercise (minimum 4 times a week).

❑ Whatever you do, do NOT eat late at night (especially animal products), and don't sleep with any electronic devices or TV set anywhere near your bedroom.

❑ Remove your **dental amalgams** and chelate the mercury out of your body. People report recovering "miraculously" of Chronic Fatigue when they remove the *mercury* (a deadly neurotoxin) from their body.

❑ Do a **parasite cleanse**. The burgdorferi borrelia parasite, linked with Lyme Disease, Multiple Sclerosis, Fibromyalgia, and Chronic Fatigue – as well as other parasites and viruses present in vaccines – could be a cause for persistent tiredness.

Alkalize! An Acidic Inner Terrain Destroys Your Energy Levels

❑ Your blood is your *'river of life'*, bringing oxygen and nutrients to every cell in your body. Your red blood cells carry the oxygen through your body, and the outside of each blood cell has a negative (-) electrical charge. This keeps the blood cells from sticking together (they constantly repel one another). An acidic environment *strips* these negative electrical charges from your red blood cells and as a result, **the blood cells start to slam into each other, clumping together**, moving slower and ripping apart. With the blood cells sticking together, they now go through the bloodstream more slowly and less oxygen and nutrients flow through your body. As a result, **your energy goes through the floor**.

CHAPTER 34

Health Advice from Stewart Swerdlow

This is the advice Stewart Swerdlow, author of *The Healer's Handbook* gave his clients recently, "for purging the body, mind and emotions of all old junk and toxins so that you may begin a new and better phase of life":

- Eat only **organic** foods and **stay away from all processed** and fat foods.

- Drink distilled water, herbal teas, organic fruit juices and red wine.

- Take **organic supplements** daily; do not skip days.

- **Exercise daily**, including weight-training every other day and **low-impact aerobics** daily.

- **Avoid wheat**, grain and any foods with additives.

- Do not eat **soy** or soy products.

- Do not eat foods that have corn syrup or any genetically altered components (GMO).

- Do your **release work** and grow up *the child within*.

- Take **sea salt baths** frequently.

- Spin your chakras every morning and balance your T-bar several times daily.

- Do breathing techniques and the green flush exercise.

- Take far infrared **saunas** as often as possible.

- Do a **colon cleanse** twice per year followed by a series of colonics.

- Communicate with Oversoul daily and release all up to it (the silver 'infinity' symbol).

- Use *Ultimate Protection* 24/7. Do *White Winged Lion* and *White Winged Dragon* often.

- Use the brown merger symbol at the pineal gland daily.

- Get **Rife treatments**/ foot baths frequently.

- Get deep tissue massage and **chiropractic adjustments** a couple of times per month.

- Eat organic **proteins** several times per week.

- Eat **organic fermented foods** and **live sprouts** often.

- Use organic castor oil and virgin organic coconut oil on the skin.

- Monitor your mind-patterns and only think positive, beneficial thoughts.

- Take plenty of **Vitamin D**.

- Consider taking a **course of MMS** to kill viruses and bacteria.

I highly recommend you get Stewart's books *Stewart Says* and *The Healer's Handbook* to further your understanding of how to use your mind for healing. You can also get a personal consultation with him at www.expansions.com.

CHAPTER 35

How I Integrated This Knowledge Into a "Daily Routine"

I have shared with you a lot of information in this book. The important thing now is for you to *integrate* this knowledge into your life. The best way to do so is in stages, rather than all-at-once. Start by going on **a 10-day or 30-day cleanse**, and also create **a daily routine**.

Here's what *I* did to apply all this wisdom and information, simply and effectively, in my day-to-day life. I started out by cutting out toxic personal care products, and cutting out **GMOs, Soy, milk, sugar, wheat, unhealthy fats, and processed foods** from my life (sugar was the hardest!). I then printed on an A4 sheet of paper the routine that I follow every day. I recommend you create something like this:

- I wake up at 6am. **I set the intention**: *"I am having an AMAZING day today!"*

- I drink a glass **water with aloe vera**, MSM powder, moringa olefeira, and add a few drops of Iodine, Marine Phytoplankton, and Colloidal Silver.

- I also take a shot of fresh **wheatgrass** juice.

- I use the **rebounder** for 2 minutes while I look at my **Visionboard** on my office wall and I do my 10 or so **affirmations** (*"Every Day In Every Way I Am Healthier & Stronger! Every Day In Every Way I Am Better & Better! I Love My Life! I Am Rich, I Am Loved, I Am Grateful! I Have Access To All The…"*)

- I do 100 **push-ups**, ten pull-ups, 200 **crunches**, and some basic **Yoga** stretches. The daily discipline and routine of *doing it* is more important than *how much* you do each day.

- I **walk** my dog in the forest… an opportunity to connect with nature and feel *grateful*.

- I **meditate** in the garden or in my home office for 20 minutes.

- Just before starting my meditation, I close my eyes and **visualize** PALE PINK around me and throughout me for unconditional love for myself, I breathe in MEDIUM GREEN in my Heart Chakra area (and blow out Red, Grey, Blue which represent anger, emotional confusion, and a mind pattern of isolation), I visualize ICE BLUE in my Thyroid Area *(to unblock my communication)*, I visualize the *Power Archetype* ⋀ (in red) in every cell of my body, and I visualize **My Perfect Life** as I have imagined it. I also do Stewart Swerdlow's *"T-bar balancing", "Golden Altar", "Child Within", "Ultimate Protection Technique", "Releasing To Oversoul",* and Chakra Spinning visualizations. These visualizations take just 3-4 minutes to complete. I then enjoy relaxing into my meditation, letting go of all thought, and bringing myself powerfully back *to the present moment.*

- My assistant prepares my **'Green Juice'** which helps me alkalize my body and provides my body with great nutrition. This typically consists of avocado (I have now removed it from the recipe, having developed a 'food sensitivity' to it), spinach, cucumber, and celery, apples to make it sweeter, and I also alternate with: fresh ginger, Udos Oil™; Beyond Greens™, Vitamineral™, Living Fuel™, or Doc Broc™; Maca, Ginseng, Spirulina, Chlorella, Kelp, sesame seeds, chia seeds, pumpkin seeds, apricot seeds, linseed, walnuts, Brazil nuts, almonds, wheatgrass powder, moringa olefeira, baobab, Turmeric, Pau d'Arco or Cats' Claw, Goji berries, blueberries, etc.

- I take daily a natural organic multivitamin, and Vitamin D3 and K2.

- I then work at my laptop. My subconscious mind is programmed thanks to positive subliminal messages flashing on my computer screen.

- I drink at least 2 litres of water a day.

- Around 4pm I **walk** my dog again, and I **meditate** again for 20 minutes.

- I do not eat past 7pm, and I go to bed thinking of **5 things I am grateful for**.

- I enjoy playing basketball, tennis, or squash once a week; I have a **sauna** once a week, and I have an **Epsom Salts bath** twice a month. Twice a year I see a chiropractor and do a thorough 10-day detox.

This type of routine helps you maintain excellent health and energy, rather than go on a "diet" or "fitness regime" for a short time and then revert to your old habits – which is what most people do. **Success comes down to your *mindset,* your *values,* and your *daily habits*.** It takes commitment and consistent work. It's not a one-off act or 'a diet' that will bring you success or good health. Make it a part of your daily life.

Here are a few more things you can do to skyrocket your vitality, health and energy:

Invest In High Quality Whole Foods And Nutritional Supplements

I recommend buying a Breville juicer, a Nutribullet blender, and a regular 1.5-liter blender, as well as some quality nutritional supplements such as the ones listed earlier in this book; the jars in the picture you see on the next page contain cacao, moringa oleifera, apricot seeds, sunflower and pumpkin seeds, pine nuts, goji berries, chia seeds, linseed, dried nettles and dandelion, pau d'arco, cats claw, dried wheatgrass, sesame seeds, brazil nuts, walnuts, hemp seeds, chlorella, spirulina, kelp, maca, baobab, schizandra, ginseng, turmeric, and bee pollen; I add a selection of these in my morning 'Green Juice' smoothie, as well as adding fresh ginger and berries.

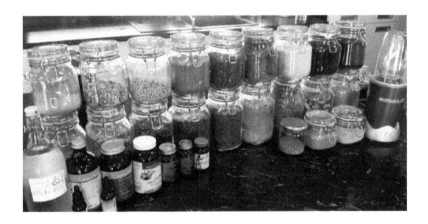

Grow Your Own Wheatgrass, Herbs, and Organic Vegetables

I also recommend growing your own wheatgrass (you'll need to get a small wheatgrass juicer) and your own organic vegetables. It's fun to do and you can get the kids involved too!

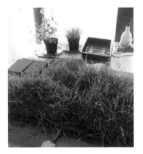

We source a lot of our vegetables from local farmers via our neighbourhood's Community Supported Agriculture program.

Get a House Water Filter and Natural Personal Care Products

It is important to switch to more natural brands of toiletries, makeup, and cleaning products; get a whole house water filter to protect your family from harmful fluoride, chlorine, and dozens more chemicals in the water supply!

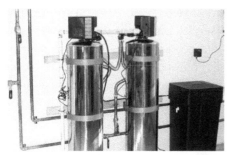 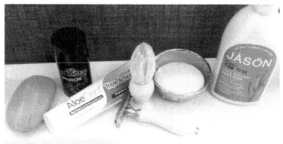

Meditate, Get a Rebounder, and Exercise!

Every day I take time to meditate, do some yoga, and use my rebounder, in a corner of my home office.

It doesn't matter initially whether you do this for 10 minutes a day or 30. *The important thing is to get into the habit!*

I also recommend creating a **visionboard** of your favourite aspirational pictures – images that illustrate your goals and the life you want to live. This way you can visualize your new exciting healthy, vibrant, and abundant life while you exercise!

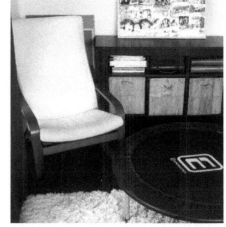

Do not feel overwhelmed if all this sounds like 'too much'. You don't need to do all this in one go. I integrated these changes gradually into my life. You can adopt and apply just one suggestion per month. For example, one month I invested in buying Q-link and Aulterra products to protect our house from harmful EMF. The next month I bought 5-6 whole foods and one multivitamin. The third month I bought natural personal care products for our bathroom. The fourth month I bought a rebounder. The fifth month I went on a meditation course, and I started doing yoga. The sixth month I bought a whole house water filter and went to see a chiropractor. The seventh month I started growing my own wheatgrass… This is starting to sound a lot like the song *The 12 Days of Christmas!*

FINAL THOUGHTS

Billions of pounds of cancer-causing pesticides, herbicides, and fungicides are sprayed on our crops every year. More than 10,000 chemical solvents and preservatives are used in food processing, and 13,200 chemicals are used in our cosmetics and soaps. 1,000 new chemicals are introduced each year in our environment. Our farm animals are fed millions of tons of antibiotics, anti-parasitic drugs, growth hormones, sex hormones, and anti-depressants. Our water supply is laced with dozens of drugs, chemicals, and deadly fluoride. Thousands of products are contaminated with deadly *aspartame*. Children are poisoned with mercury-filled vaccinations, and we let dentists fill our teeth with toxic mercury. Doctors destroy our immune system with X-rays, CT scans, and dangerous, toxic pharmaceutical drugs. And then we drink alcohol and consume sugar, junk food, and processed food. Is it really any surprise so many human beings are unwell, tired, diseased, and diagnosed with Cancer?

The Smartest People Are Taking Control of Their Health

Smart people are realizing that they need to take personal responsibility for their lifestyle choices. They are educating themselves about Health, instead of leaving it in the hands of the medical establishment. They are exercising daily, they are going to health food stores, eating LIVE foods, and taking nutritional supplements. They understand the price there is to pay if they *don't* do this is a mediocre life filled with pains, aches, Diabetes, Heart Disease, Arthritis, Multiple Sclerosis, or *worse*.

They are no longer willing to destroy their body, their health, their *life*, for foods that may taste good but that give them nothing. Their life is too precious. They value themselves too much.

You have a choice. **You can *use* this information to heal from Cancer naturally... and live an extraordinarily long and healthy life... or go on with your lives as before**. Either decision will carry its consequences. For what it's worth, I sincerely hope that you will put this invaluable information to good use, and I look forward to hearing how you have turned around your health challenges and taken back control of your life.

Get In Touch

We want to hear from you! Share your healing journey and your success story with us. Join our community, and get some support.

You may contact our team to book a personal consultation or some coaching at info@TheNewBiology.co.uk

You may join our mailing list to stay in touch at www.TheNewBiology.co.uk.

Download your complimentary Special Reports valued at over $300 at www.TheNewBiology.co.uk/bonus.

And finally, you can book yourself on a 7-day or 14-day detox retreat at www.TheNewBiology.co.uk/retreat.

I look forward to meeting you in person at one of our live events in due course. I wish you all the health and success in the world.

Ewan M. Cameron

About The Author

Ewan Cameron is a Vancouver-based journalist that has been exposing the disinformation tactics of the pharmaceutical industry for over a decade. A graduate of the Northern Alberta Institute of Technology, he completed his journalism studies in the early 2000's before joining a local newspaper, where he became disillusioned by his editor's refusal to publish health-related and pollution-related news stories. The reason soon became clear. These stories would upset their corporate clients on which the newspaper depended for advertising revenue. After setting up his own blog and publishing more than thirty health-related books under a pen name, Ewan was contacted by a whistleblower working at a U.S. pharmaceutical company. Some of the highly controversial 'leaked' material is contained in the pages of this book.

TESTIMONIALS

"You are amazing and what you're doing is such an extraordinary contribution to people. I am so excited that you're on a mission to spread the word to educate people about what's happening to the health of people worldwide, especially in the States and the UK. I'm a Chiropractor and everything you share to the public speaks the Truth about Life, Living, Happiness and Health. Thank you so much for what you are doing. Thank you for being there for me to find you so simply." – Dr. MaryAnne S.

"After reading your approach, I changed radically my behaviour. I feel better, I'm in good shape, my glycaemic level it's down from 240 to 140 and sometimes 128-130. Thank you for everything." – Dr. Niki I.

"I am a physician and what I read in your ebook makes a lot of sense." – Dr. Lazzarini

"Thanks Ewan for the gift of life!!! I wanted to say thanks for giving me my life back! I've been type 1 diabetic for 16 years now and on 68 units of insulin a day feeling virtually lifeless at the age of 29. I was sleeping 10 to 14 hour per day, still to awake feeling lifeless, weak and sick. My blood sugars were running 16 to 35, sometimes even off the meter. After reading over the material I finally realized and understood what was really going on in my body. I put the simple, down to earth adjustments into my lifestyle, mainly by changing my diet consuming nurturance, not food and eliminating poisonous foods from my diet and my life turned around in days. I now can have powerful, motivated days on 6 or 7 hours of sleep. And my sugars have come down to a range of 5 to 9. My insulin has also decreased 40%." – Matthew C., Canada

"I would like to thank you for sharing such valuable information. My sugar levels most of the time average 280's and sometimes even 300's. My glycohaemoglobin was 7.5 to 8.5 and the protein in my kidneys was extremely high. I felt terrible all the time. Then I found your ebook. Since I introduced all this lifestyle changing dietary habits in my life my glycohaemogoblin is now 5.4. The protein in my kidneys has remained at normal range keeping me from going on Dialysis. My sugar levels stay in a more normal range. My diabetic medication has decreased considerably until the point I think I will no longer use it. I am so grateful for your discovery of this information and for sharing it with the world." – Juan C. D.

"Ewan, your book is in my opinion a true candidate to the Nobel Prize. I had type-1 diabetes for 36 years, but not anymore. You make the impossible possible. Thanks for the cure!!!" – Sara W., Sweden

"I can't begin to express how much pleasure it gives me to send you my testimonial, as downloading your book & putting into action what I read, has literally changed my life! I was suffering from Fibromyalgia, Chronic Fatigue Syndrome, & all the awful baggage that goes with those two conditions. I also suffered from Type 2 Diabetes, Hypothyroidism, Hypertension, severe GERD, multiple environmental sensitivities, sinusitis, mood swings [because I felt so miserable], sleep deprivation because of constant pain & steady weight gain, even tho' I ate properly & prepared healthy food. You will notice that everything I mention in the above paragraph is in the past tense! After reading your book, I decided that I had nothing to lose. The changes that I began to experience were remarkable & began to take place within a few days of following my new regime. Now, I no longer take any prescription medications. My blood sugars stabilized & are now all in the low normal range & my blood pressure has also dropped & is in the 116/ 60 range. I am pain free for the first time in 15 years & now know what it is like to have quality sleep. I have energy I never dreamed possible. Indigestion & acid reflux are a thing of the past & I no longer have any sinus, eye or ear problems. The bonus is that I have lost 23 lbs. & know that I will continue to lose until my weight stabilizes to where it should be. I not only have amazing stamina, but also mental clarity & feel very positive & upbeat. Everyone I see tells me I look fantastic & that my skin is radiant. Every day I marvel at the positive changes that continue to take place & I am so thankful & happy. Thank you for the information that has allowed me to regain my health & to enjoy all that life has to offer. Because of the changes friends have witnessed in me, they have also decided to go the same route. I am excited to be able to help others to achieve good health. I can't say thank you enough. God bless." – Eleanor B.

"I want you to know that I am doing well. I had one lupus flare up in the summer, but it didn't last as long as it usually does. I look great, and more importantly I FEEL great. I thank you over and over for your book; I do feel blessed that you wrote it, that I found it, and that you continue to keep in touch! Thank you so much! You're MY angel! Stay healthy, keep doing what you're doing!!" – Sandi

"I came across your book and immediately "got" what it was about.... I've been on this new alkalizing diet for 2-1/2 weeks and have lost 9 pounds. Best of all, my Eczema is completely healed. Thank you for providing a MAJOR "link" to my next great life adventure." – Jacqueline

"Ewan, the preamble to your book was like a hand grenade thrown through the door. Your book has turned my whole life 180 degrees." – Bill A.

"I just wanted to drop you a quick email to let you know that your book was extremely helpful in getting my health back. I have been struggling with psoriasis for nearly a year and a half after I developed a bad case due to a period of stress-binge-eating after a traumatic car accident last year. The disorder developed and worsened at a very rapid rate to where it spread from shoulder to shoulder, from my chest up to just above my Adam's apple. It was so very uncomfortable, unsightly, and very scary. I purchased your book a few months ago and read it. It was your simple breakdown of the link between overacidity and chronic illnesses that gave me the lead I needed. In the past two months my itching is nearly gone; irritated, sore and itchy patches are shrinking, scars are healing. I just had to tell you, that your book was the real turning point in what was at times a hellish journey through illness. Thank you so much. Your advice has helped me to get on the path to health, sparing me from terrible discomfort. I hope to pass the word along to others as they deal with their own crises. I just wanted you to know it worked, and it's made a wonderful difference in my life." – Lee H.

"Thank you! I have detoxed. Wow! That just sure is live. It's like bubbling like coke. Amazing! I also lost two kg's in three days from just being on the liquids.

369

And I had NO pain [from my Multiple Sclerosis] on the days I was taking this mixture! No back spasms! Awesome, I felt like I was nineteen again, just wanted to do the things that I haven't had the strength or energy for. Thank you for telling the truth. God Bless and keep up the good work." – Antoinette R.

"I cannot tell you how much of a difference your book on Eczema has made already. I am no longer on any oral or topical medication as I was on doxycycline and olux (an antibiotic and a steroid foam). This is only after 1 week after beginning to apply your information. Thank you. I am already spreading the news of your breakthroughs." – Marilyn B.

"I was desperately looking for a cure for my psoriasis that I had 12 years, I visited a lot of doctors and spent a lot of money on creams and moisturizers, what was upsetting so much when doctors said to me that there is no cure for it. Then a few weeks ago I checked in internet the latest news about psoriasis, and thanks god I came across your e-book, and I bought it without a little hesitation. I followed the diet, and I feel so good, my psoriasis is all cleared, I couldn't believe it, it's a miracle! I wish I knew about it long time ago, so I could prevent all the trouble it has caused me last 12 years. Thank you so much, you've been great help." – Omar R.

"Nothing I tried before for my M.S. worked. In the last year despite all my efforts my health and in particular my walking deteriorated. Three days after taking [the nutritional supplement you suggest in your ebook] I already noticed an immense improvement. First this meant that at least I could comfortably walk to the bus stop, which is such a tiny step but a huge thing in comparison to before.

[After] roughly 7/8 weeks I noticed that I could easily walk 5 minutes and felt almost normal. Yesterday I walked for 15 minutes! Thanks so much." – Claudia

"Thank you. I love the book. I think my prayers for recovery from Multiple Sclerosis have been answered by your book, even after a couple of days. When I get up in the morning, there is no pain! I used to dread getting out of bed. My sister-in-law, who is visiting, is doing the same thing and she is having no pain either. WOW! Several people have told me I am speaking more clearly." – Dorrie

"The arthritis in my hands is GONE... I wake up in the a.m. and can easily and readily flex my fingers!! I think your PLAN FOR LIVING is totally amazing! and so simple!! Thank you once again for sharing this with me! Bless you!" – Sandi

"I am so thankful to you for all the research you are doing, and for being so generous by sharing it with us. Your book changed my life! I purchased your book the day after I was diagnosed with this horrible disease (Lupus). I was extremely depressed with my diagnosis, but was determined to beat the odds and actually get cured. I could not have done it without your help. I immediately started making the changes you suggested. After 6 weeks of following your advice, my sedimentation levels went down from 131 to 19 (normal is considered anything below 30.) Also my antibodies, which at the time of diagnosis were ALL positive, after the 6 weeks, were normal. My doctor called it "a miracle cure". I don't have enough words to thank you. I thank God for having led me to your website." – Maria C.J., New Jersey

"After 5 months of testing your theory, and its fantastic results, I must admit that it's completely right. I feel entirely different, and I would never, ever come back to my old way of feeding myself. Amazing! Not one sneeze since June (I used to get sinusitis, or bronchitis, at least once a month, nothing would work). No more gout symptoms, more stamina (including sex!), my hair does not fall like before, my lupus is no longer active, etc. The solution was so simple, and so efficient!" – JM

"I followed every point of your book, with no exception. The lupus spots on my skull are no longer red, but almost white. My dermatologist was surprised. He says he's never seen such a regression. I feel much younger than when I was 50! THANK YOU VERY MUCH, Ewan. I owe you a lot." – Jean-Michel C., Tahiti

"Thank you so much for the most wonderful and greatest book ever!" – Suraj B., Kathmandu, Nepal

"Thank you! God bless you for your efforts to awaken the people from the mass hypnosis that the medical society has affected and infected... so many. My father had Cancer and the alkalizing spirulina that I gave him put him in remission for 20 extra years." – Phyllis

371

"I read your book and did what you say. To be free of gout, "grateful" isn't strong enough." – Max

"My total cholesterol levels had gone up from 250mg/dl to well over 300. I was put on cholesterol-lowering drugs and beta blockers for my blood pressure. My total cholesterol levels have only gone up over the years to close to 400mg/dl. Things got worse though and I had a light heart attack. After having read your book, and using the supplements, my cholesterol levels have dropped by nearly 100 points and the other values improved dramatically in just two months." – Paul G., Spain

"I do not know if I want to laugh or cry, I am so thankful to you, how can I ever say thank you enough! You are a Godsend! Thank you, thank you a million times. May God bless you!" – Ria S.

"Almost a year to the day, the eczema is now GONE, my vitality is up & simply there is no looking back." – Chris

"The medical profession has been no help at all with my Multiple Sclerosis. I have only been following your programme for 2 weeks but have already noticed the benefits! Thank you for giving me hope. I feel so much better and other people are noticing the difference. It is working! No new lesions since my first MRI and very few symptoms." (Anonymous)

"I was diagnosed with Arthritis about 2 years ago. Because of these supplement I have gone from 9 pain pills a day to 2." – Anthony N.

"The arthritis pains in my joints, which have been very present over the last few years, have disappeared. Thank you. I will stick to the diet. And by the way, I have lost over 12 kilos." – Paul

"I bought your book. 85% of my psoriasis is now gone and I lost 72 lbs on your special diet plan. This is great information! Thank you!" – Carole G.

"You are an amazing man. Your book has really helped me and I am now well on my way to reversing my Diabetes. Bless all your endeavours and everything you touch." Hugh G.

"You are a great inspiration! We have both changed our diet drastically, and we no longer suffer from Lupus!" – Spyros B.

"Thank you very much! I have read your Health Book with a great, great, great.... interest and it has transformed me completely. Had I to be on NOBEL PRIZE COMMITTEE my pen would tick your name a thousand times!! You are now on my list of few THINKERS on this planet that I love most!" – Emmanuel A., Uganda.

"My wife has Multiple Sclerosis for 8 years and since buying your book and getting her on Glyconutrients she has for the first time in 7 years shown an MRI scan with reduced lesion in quantity and size." – Clinton van E., South Africa

"I was diagnosed with MS 6 years ago. I downloaded your book, and I am now walking with no problem, I know my body keeps repairing itself. I'd like to thank you with all my heart." – Cheryl

"I was diagnosed with Multiple Sclerosis in 1986. I have been taking the Glyconutrients for 15 months and most of my body that was taken away with the MS is slowly returning." – Santo

"I'm 30 years old and I've been a type I diabetic since I was 4. My mother was also diagnosed with Type I diabetes (along with her sister) when they were both about 16 years old. As I got older I had to inject more and more insulin. On some days I was taking upwards of 8 shots a DAY to try and control my sugars. Before I started this transformation a grand total of about 60+ units of insulin every single day! I was about 160 lbs. Then I read your book. I started doing it and lo and behold I started to feel great. I now take only 20 units of insulin in total! I FEEL PHENOMENAL!! I have never ever felt his good in my life! I have lost 20 lbs in 2 months!!! The benefits are tremendous. My energy is wonderful. My glycohaemoglobin went from 8.2 to 6.0!!! That's unreal! My doctors are so happy they said just keep doing whatever I'm doing. And they don't even know I've lost 20 lbs yet! I've never been so happy in my life. You are granting people long overdue miracles!" – Kristen

"I was having difficulty breathing and could not exercise, I had difficulty even walking upstairs, because of my Asthma. Since reading your book, my Asthma has steadily reduced and I now exercise quite vigorously for 20 minutes each day to the point of "getting a good sweat on" and I am starting to feel like my old self again. Also over the past few months I have drastically reduced my medication and am aiming to be totally off drugs over the next few months." – John

373

Milton Keynes UK
Ingram Content Group UK Ltd.
UKHW030653220324
439802UK00002B/42